Diane,
Thank you so much,
what a
great
class!
Be well,
JJ Wat

Tracking the Dragon

Dr. Janice Walton-Hadlock, DAOM

Tracking the Dragon
Dr. Janice Walton-Hadlock, DAOM, LAc
Illustrated by Ben Bateson

Published by Fastpencil, Cupertino, CA

First edition: 2010
©Janice Walton-Hadlock

Tracking the Dragon

Table of Contents

Originally, this book was written as a class text for students of Asian medicine who had already completed at least one year of study. Knowledge of the channel locations, acupoint locations, and basic terminology, including at least one system of "pattern" diagnosis, was assumed.

Since then, some beginning students and even readers with no background in Asian medicine have expressed gratitude for the explanations and demystifications in this book – but they have requested the inclusion of some basic, starter information.

Now, with the addition of point location/channel Qi maps at the back of the book and some acupuncture theory basics, and beginner can get up and running: feeling channel Qi by hand, using the findings to make diagnoses.

"Pattern diagnosis" refers to the Asian tradition of combining information from a patient's pulse, tongue, and other physical presentations, plus a patient's symptoms, into one of the official patterns. Various systems, or "schools" of pattern diagnosis abound; the systems include Eight parameters, Six Levels, Five Elements, and Zhang-Fu, to name just a few. Each system uses its own collection of patterns. Many practitioners use patterns from several schools.

Once a practitioner has settled on the official pattern that best describes the patient's condition, he then uses the appropriate acupuncture, moxa, massage, lasers, magnets, or herbal treatment that is recommended for *all* people with that pattern.

But whether the practitioner is using acupuncture needles, moxa, herbs, Tui Na, or Medical Qi Gong to treat the pattern, and whether the pattern is expressed in terms of "hot and cold," "Yin and Yang," "Wood Attacking Earth," or "Jue Yin level Fire," the *underlying* goal is always the same: restoration of channel Qi to its correct flow.

A very brief definition of channel Qi

As westerners, we first learn in high school physics that moving electrical currents create electromagnetic fields and electromagnetic waves. As a corollary, we learn the reverse is also possible: waves can create currents. The sequence in which we are taught these ideas influences our thoughts regarding matter and waves. We tend to look at tangibles, and consider their invisible, inherent wave properties to be side effects. This thinking is backwards.

To understand the ancient thinking behind Asian medicine, and to understand modern physics, we must reverse the preferred sequence of these ideas: we must think first, that waves can create currents; then, energy in currents can transform back into waves.

The ancient theories hold that, at the moment of initiation of the universe, what we now call the "Big Bang," all creation was purely vibratory, purely waves. Some waves condensed into matter. More exactly, the energy in waves transformed into the energy in currents. Or we might say, the energy in those waves condensed into energy formats that manifest as moving electrical units and other quantum bits. This charged movement constitutes currents. More simply, "waves can make currents."

This idea matches perfectly with our modern "string theory" of physics, which holds that all materially existing subatomic components (quantum particles) are made up of tightly coiled bits of vibrations. All matter is derived from vibrations, or waves. When matter dematerializes, it shifts back into a state of pure vibration.

As westerners, we tend to think that the chemistry in living systems creates any electrical currents that might be detected coursing over the surface of the cells, or streaming along the connective tissue. These currents, in turn, might be "giving off" waves. To understand Asian medicine, we must think more correctly: waves are forming the currents. The currents, in turn, create, sustain, and guide the cellular chemistry. The chemical behavior, in turn, creates further waves.

We cannot feel, by hand, the specific electromagnetic movement patterns (waves and electrical currents) that define and create each of the types of atoms. We cannot feel, by hand, the larger currents that flow in highly specific patterns over each cell's surface, directing the inner-cellular chemical processes. But in large organisms, we can feel, by hand, the highly specific routes of the relatively huge currents formed by the billions of iterations of extra-cellular currents, currents that flow near the external surface of the organism. We call these routes The Channels.

For the most part, when we speak of the channel Qi that is found in all living systems, the energy that allows living systems to *seemingly* defy entropy and remain stable in the face of environmental changes, we are speaking about the moving currents that direct all biological processes. But to better appreciate channel Qi, we must also think of it as the *waves* that create those currents *and* the currents. To even more accurately describe channel Qi, we can say that it is made up of currents *and* the waves of thoughts and emotion that create and drive the currents *and* the waves given off by the chemical structures that are derived from and which stabilize those currents.

And to be still more accurate, channel Qi is one more thing: channel Qi is not only waves and material currents derived from the waves, it is the energy absorbed or released in the *transition* from wave energy to matter (electrons), and back again.

The *locations* at which wave energy converts to matter – or the reverse, where matter converts back to wave energy – are known in ancient Chinese philosophy as pivot points. These are the *places* where energy pivots back and forth between vibrational energy and formed components of matter (electrons and other subatomic bits) at any given point in time.

According to ancient Asian physics, creation, in order to appear real, needed three parts: <u>wave</u> (known in Sanskrit as *Om,* or in Chinese as *Da* [Great] *Om,* also pronounced *Tao*), <u>matter</u> (*Anu,* often translated as "atom"), and the <u>location</u> (*Desa*) of the transition between wave and matter at any given point in time (*Kala*).

In Chinese theory, the vibrational, or wave, basis for a thing's existence, or you might say the *idea* of a thing's physical existence, is referred to as its "Heavenly," or Yang (closer to God, closer to the origin) aspect. The quantum bits that create the seemingly "real," or "material" version of that idea are referred to as that creation's "Earthly," or Yin (further from God, further from the origin) aspect. The Pivots, the sum of the *locations* at which, at any given instant in time, wave energy transitions into matter, or "pivots" back into pure vibration, is the third part of the system.

As an aside, "The Dragon joins Heaven and Earth" is a not uncommon expression in Chinese. The expression has many applications, including the idea that man's physical body resides somewhere between the skyey Empyrean and the soil of planet Earth. (This is sometimes rephrased as "Man stands between Heaven and Earth.)

Another common application interprets Heaven as man's soul, Earth as man's body, and the Dragon as the dynamic that, for the short span of a man's life, binds the two.

The application of the Heaven/Dragon/Earth metaphor to the three parts of channel Qi – electrical waves, electrons (and related "formed" matter of quantum physics), and the transitional Pivots that exist "between" them – is particularly apt – and may very likely be the metaphor's historical foundation.

Given this understanding, the sum of the pivot points in living systems, pivots that occur between the waves of "Heaven" and the chemical basis of "Earth," the sum of which is known as the flow of Channel Qi, can metaphorically be referred to as The Dragon.

I believe this may be the *original* understanding of the Heaven/Dragon/Earth expression.

If our eyes beheld truth, we would see that matter is constantly flashing in and out of existence at a nearly infinite number of locations, at the interface with the intangible surface that, in western science, has recently been named "the ether." Throughout the universe, the transition points between waves and matter, the individual pivots, are locationally determined by the same Consciousness that created Vibrations in the first place. The sum of the locations of the individual pivots over any specific period of *time* (anything from nanoseconds to eons) provides the basis for the seeming *movement* of all electrical currents during that time span. Given the popular use of the Chinese expression, "The Dragon joins Heaven and Earth," the name for this third aspect of creation – the *movement* in currents, the phenomenon that lies between wave and matter *over time* is the *movement* of the Dragon.

In large living systems, such as humans, this movement aspect of the Dragon can be felt, as it travels in its highly specific pathways, near the surface of the organism. What we call channel Qi are the areas in living systems where the movement aspect of current is in a feel-able, detectable format.

Again, in an orgainism, its *pure* vibrations (what a Westerner might call the Platonic Ideal) are referred to as Heaven. Its formed, seemingly "real" matter, ranging from electrons and subatomic particles to the chunky protons, is referred to as Earth. The seeming *movement* of the electron portion of the Earth aspect, created by transitions between wave and matter, or you might say "the flow of The (collective) Pivots," "the currents," or the Dragon, is the channel Qi. If the organism is large enough, its currents of channel Qi are so large that we can feel them.

The vibrations that bring forth the universe are *created* by Consciousness. the transitions from wave to matter and back again, and the movements of currents thus created, are *directed* by Consciousness.

The flow of a human's channel Qi is directed and influenced by a combination of Consciousness, the human's consciousness, the matter-based molecules in his body such as DNA, *and* his highly specific original vibrations, or fractal waves, the fractal waves that *define* each human being. These extremely subtle "defining" wave patterns, patterns unique to each individual, exist before conception, and continue to exist after death. These individual wave patterns, or vibrations, are all subsets of the Universal vibration, from which all formed parts (material existence) of the universe are derived.

Western science is just beginning to propose the relationship between vibrational, or wave, physics and humans. In *The Elegant Universe*, by Brian Greene, the author proposes: "humans are, in fact, 3-D holographic projections of two-dimensional [wave] data." In other words, the waves come first. Matter is an illusory derivative.

This is *not* a new concept. Twenty six hundred years ago, the philosophers of ancient India were writing and teaching these concepts in universities at Nalanda and Taxila. Traveling scholars from around the world were welcomed. Many famous Chinese scholars carried these ideas back to their homeland, where they contributed to the thriving philosophical debates of the Hundred Schools period of Chinese history, a period that preceded the violent, 221 BC "unification" of China.

Where is the channel Qi?

In living systems, currents of channel Qi bathe the surface of every cell. From the moment of conception, a specific pattern of electrical flow over the outside of the cell wall directs all cellular activity, including DNA expression. The specific pattern of this extracellular channel Qi flow is directed primarily by the wave-based Idea of the organism, and secondarily by the electromagnetic influence of the DNA molecule and other structures within the organism.

So long as the channel Qi of a cell is flowing over the surface of the cell in its correct pattern, that cell is alive. In any living cell, or any living system, it is the invisible wave energy and the wave's directing of the movement of the organism's channel Qi that allows the cell, or the living system, to exist in *seeming* defiance of entropy.

When the channel Qi *ceases* to be influenced by the Idea-wave patterns (Divine Consciousness), and merely flows mechanically, in the pattern defined by proximity to its cellular chemistry or the surrounding chemistry, the cell is dead. Its chemical structure may still *exist*, but the organism is dead, and its structure is subject to entropy.

As the cells of a multi-celled organism increase from their original single cell, the channel Qi patterns continue to flow in highly specific patterns over the cell walls, electromagnetically directing every process that occurs within the cells. As the growing cell cluster increases in size, alterations in the surface-to-volume ratio of the organism and other alterations due to changes in mass and shape cause derivative variations in the fractal flow patterns of the organism's channel Qi. These localized variations in the flow of channel Qi, in turn, trigger localized alterations in DNA expression. These alterations allow various cells to assume different roles.

In multi-celled organisms, in addition to the streams of current that run over the surface of each cell, the compoundings of the original fractal, or "Mother," pattern of channel Qi also flow over the exterior of the entire organism.

iv

Even when an organism vastly increases in size, iterations of the currents that direct individual cells continue to influence and maintain the currents that traverse the exterior of the organism. These exterior currents can become huge – in humans, these currents are large enough to be detected by hand. These currents that flow over the exterior of the organism (or, more accurately, just under the skin), serve to both reflect *and* direct the individual, cellular currents.

As stated before, in Asian medicine, we refer to these large, exterior (just under the skin) rivers of current as The Channels. The flow patterns of human channels are highly standardized: the mathematical formula (a non-linear equation) theoretically (according to modern physics' Chaos theory) derivable from the fractal that underlies the highly specific flow patterns seen in humans might even be considered a *definition* for the structural design of an embodied human.

In large organisms, the channel Qi flow patterns in the exterior channels influence the channel Qi flow patterns at the cellular level. The cellular channel Qi flow patterns help maintain the external channel Qi flow patterns. These mutual influences provide stability to the organism. An organism's body can be influenced by external events such as weather, food, physical impact, and so on, *via* changes in the large rivers of channel Qi that occur from exposure to these events. These changes are then transmitted to the smaller streams and rivulets of channel Qi, and then to the channel Qi that traverses each cell. These changes in cell-level channel Qi flow then exert a changed influence over cellular chemistries and structures.

At the same time, the large rivers of channel Qi are kept stable in *spite* of external influences, by virtue of the billions of cellular contributions of channel Qi wave signals: iterations that are held in place fairly well by virtue of the highly stable molecules of DNA and other cellular structures.

From jellyfish to great blue whales, this external-internal communication occurs between rivers of currents large and small, that is to say, the large currents of channel Qi in the close-to-the-surface channels and the small currents that bathe each cell.

The effect of these mutually resonant currents on cellular chemistry and functions *and* the effects of external influences on the currents *and* the stabilizing effect that cellular chemistry has on the channel Qi – all working together – are the basis for homeostasis.

Homeostasis is an organism's ability to *respond* to externals, while maintaining a high degree of structural and electrical constancy *despite* external fluctuations. We tend to think that homeostasis refers to the stability of the body's chemistry. In fact, homeostasis is the underlying-stability-amidst-change that occurs in the body's waves and currents and chemistry. Ultimately, the thing that does *not* change easily, the anchor that keeps the organism alive despite changes in the environs, is the underlying, unchanging wave *idea* behind the creation of the organism.

Errors in the flow of channel Qi

The underlying cause of all human health problems is a disruption, or glitch, in the flow of the channel Qi.

Errors in the rivers of channel Qi can be brought about by external influences such as injury, illness, extremes of weather, toxins, and so on. Errors in channel Qi can also be brought about by what Chinese medicine refers to as "internal influences": thought waves created by (self-generated) emotionalism (the Seven Pernicious, or negative, Emotions). Whatever the cause, errors in the rivers of channel Qi flow will immediately cause erroneous signals in the electrical instructions that flow to every cell in the body. These errors may result in wrong DNA expression and the subsequent malfunctions of cells and organs, and can even influence the mental state.

Treating the errors

The larger, coalesced, "external" streams and rivers of current lie close to the surface of the organism, and can therefore be easily manipulated using metal needles, magnets, lasers, Qi Gong (mental discipline of the currents), and so on.

All forms of Asian medicine are based, ultimately, on correcting glitches that develop in the flow of the large rivers of channel Qi. We use our methods of medicine to restore the large rivers of channel Qi flow to the "standard patterns" for humans: the patterns that are most perfectly aligned with the original wave patterns that define the Idea of "Human."

By restoring or maintaining the correct flow patterns of the largest rivers, the smaller bifurcated streams of channel Qi and the tiny, cellular streams of channel Qi are also restored to or maintained in the manner of current flow that reflects those specific waves that define us as healthy humans.

Resurrecting the art of working with channel Qi

During the most recent dark ages, which spanned the years from approximately 650 BC to 1750 AD, actual knowledge of a person's channel Qi flow was considered to be unknowable except to the great intuitive masters of medicine. These masters were able to discern the exact locations of any channel Qi disruptions. They could rectify these glitches by manipulating channel Qi at the exact point at which it was going astray. They had no need whatsoever of formulaic "patterns" to suggest treatments that *possibly* might be useful.[1]

As for the non-masters, during these dark times, even if a less-than-intuitive doctor *could* detect the movement of channel Qi, the comprehension and analytical skills required for assessment and correction of any disruptions were not available to most people. Hence the development of formulaic, cookbook style collections of one-size-fits-all treatments, based on the various schools of pattern diagnosis: everyone with a certain pattern should be treated the same way. The earliest of these patterns were codified in the Chinese medical classic, the *Nei Jing*.

The *Nei Jing*

The preeminent gospel of Chinese medicine is *Huang Ti Nei Jing (Golden Emperor's Classic of Medicine),* a tome comprised of two parts: *Su Wen* (Simple Questions) and *Ling Shu* (Divine Pivot).

---

[1] For more information on dark ages, higher ages, and the cyclical nature of human materialism, and spiritual and mechanical comprehension, please read *The Holy Science*, by Swami Sri Yukteswar Giri (1855-1936), published by Self-Realization Fellowship. In this succinct book, by translating directly from ancient Vedic texts, the author provides the dates and confirming historical manifestations for the current cycle of Dark and Golden Ages. He also explains the reasons for the errors in calculation that crept in near the beginning of the most recent dark age, yielding incorrect numbers, including those that say we are *still* in the most recent dark age.

More commonly referred to simply as "the *Nei Jing*," the long-revered classic was compiled during the dark ages (recent research suggests a compilation date of approximately 240 AD – approximately five hundred years after the unification of China). All subsequent traditional Chinese medical research has used the *Nei Jing* as its foundation material. When one refers to "the classics" of Chinese medicine, one is referring to the *Nei Jing*, unless other specific books are mentioned.

At the time the Nei Jing was compiled, much of the Chinese understanding of what we now call quantum theory and string theory, which is to say, the understanding of the physics of channel Qi, had already been lost.

The assemblers of the *Nei Jing* threw together all manner of profound spiritual aphorisms, residual concepts of the medicine of a higher age, the new, dark-ages pattern diagnostics, some budding medical superstitions, and misunderstandings inherent in a darkening era. They tied this mishmash together with sharp, thinly veiled criticisms of the long-dead, self-proclaimed "Golden" Emperor.

The first part of the Nei Jing is written in dialogue format, with the "Golden" Emperor who unified China in 221 BC asking questions, and the legendary medical sage Chi Bo answering.

If one understands the spiritual points being made in the *Nei Jing*, the book can be read as both a medical book, a spiritual guide, and a criticism of those who lack spiritual understanding, including the Emperor. In the *Nei Jing*, this Golden Emperor, who in real life had been a military despot who, for political reasons, had the scholars and philosophers buried alive in mass graves, is delightfully portrayed as an ignoramus, asking about, but unable to comprehend, the medical and spiritual knowledge of the wise doctor/philosopher who patiently answers his questions in phrases that simultaneously convey spiritual truisms with barbed criticisms of the Emperor.

However, for many centuries, the *Nei Jing* has been taken – by many of its readers – as a straightforward medical treatise: the spiritual aphorisms are completely ignored; the Emperor's dull-witted "contributions" to the dialogue are assumed to be intelligent and appropriate. Possibly because of the dialogue format, and unable to appreciate the odd bits of irony and even sarcasm, many scholars of the dark ages assumed that the book had been written by the Emperor himself. Even today, the book is often attributed to the Golden Emperor – a military dictator with no background in medicine.

Despite this somewhat common and enduring misapprehension, scholarly works, those of today and those dating back at least as far as the eleventh and twelfth century (works of philosopher/historians Cheng Hao and Zu Xi, respectively), provide firm evidence that the Nei Jing is a compilation assembled hundreds of years after the Emperor's death.

Today

We have long since emerged from the most recent dark age, the age in which the *Nei Jing* was compiled. Today, most would-be medical practitioners not only *can* feel channel Qi and any channel Qi disruptions, they have the intelligence to figure out how to *exactly* correct the specific disruptions in a person's channel Qi flow.

However, "official" recognition of the art of working directly with channel Qi has been squirming around uncomfortably for over a century. In an effort to appear "scientific," many modern individuals, and even the 20th century Chinese government, have dismissed the very idea of channel Qi, deeming it on par with the many other weird medical superstitions that developed during the most recent dark age.

Channel Qi is *not* one of the weird superstitions. It is the underlying basis of Asian medicine. Its use in medicine historically precedes the use of any and all of the pattern systems. The many diagnostic "patterns" of Asian medicine are simplifications created on behalf of people who could *not* feel channel Qi or understand the implications of incorrect channel Qi flow.

The various schools of pattern diagnoses were created during the dark ages. The patterns were an attempt to give generalized recipes and mnemonic devices to medical practitioners who would be "working in the dark."

The time has come to resurrect a science of medicine that uses easily accessible, feel-able currents to modify and correct the billions of cellular currents that go awry during poor health, sickness, and pain.

This book provides simple instructions that allow any student of Asian medicine to build upon the generalities of pattern diagnoses by adding the highly specific knowledge yielded by detecting the actual flow of channel Qi in a patient: by tracking the patient's dragon.

The practitioner of this medicine will be more successful if he *combines* his present-day, Asian medicine pattern theory training – which provides a wonderful vocabulary, and which remains indispensible if one is working with herbs – with the ancient, higher-age approach to medicine: directly detecting the flow of channel Qi, and performing treatments based on the idea of rectifying any errors in that flow.

As channel Qi glitches are repaired, the errors in the seemingly real, "physical," components of the body, components made up of condensed wave energy that resonates with the channel Qi wave energy, are also rectified.

The stunning, almost instantaneous, body-wide, physiological changes that can occur in response to *correctly* performed treatments of Asian medicine occur in response to rectifications of incorrectly flowing channel Qi. Oppositely, treatments that do *not* restore channel Qi to its correct flow do little, if any, good.

Merely adhering to generalities of pattern diagnosis gives a health practitioner a hit-or-miss chance at correcting aberrant flow of channel Qi. That's no longer good enough. The dark ages have ended. We can, once again, provide medical treatments that directly correct irregularities in channel Qi: corrections that then resonate with and correct the body's structure and chemistry.

In order to do this, we must be able to detect errors in the flow of channel Qi. Only by knowing exactly what the channel Qi is doing and where it is flowing, by tracking the dragon and thus detecting errors in its movement, is a health practitioner likely to obtain remarkable results with any degree of consistency.

A higher age has dawned. It is time, once again, to practice medicine based on the movement of energy: based on making straight the way for the Dragon that joins Heaven and Earth.

"It is by virtue of the twelve channels that human life exists, that disease arises, that human beings can be treated and illness cured. The twelve channels are where beginners start and masters end. To beginners, it seems easy; the masters know how difficult it is." [1]

Chapter one

Feeling Channel Qi

Feeling channel Qi is easy.

This book gives instruction in learning how to feel channel Qi, how to use that information to form a most accurate Asian Medicine diagnosis, and how to plan an appropriate treatment.

Feeling channel Qi in the hand

It can be extremely difficult to detect the flow of channel Qi in one's own body without simultaneously altering the flow as you go. Therefore, it is best to practice feeling the channel Qi of a friend or a fellow student.

It can be easiest, in the beginning, to feel channel Qi in the center of your palm, at acupoint P-8, by holding the center of the palm over a channel.

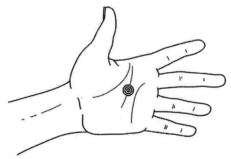

Fig. 1.1 The bulls-eye shows the location of P-8, pronounced "P-eight" or "Pericardium eight."

The palm should be held about one inch above the friend's skin. The hand should *not* touch the skin. The friend may remain fully clothed: clothing does not interfere with the perceptions of channel Qi. The energy emitted by channel Qi passes through clothing in the same way that radio waves pass through the wall of a house.

---

[1] *The Spiritual Pivot* [*Nei Jing*], chapter 17: translation taken from *A Manual of Acupuncture*, Peter Deadman and Mazin Al-Khafaji, 1998.

The "twelve channels" is a reference to the twelve, large, easily feel-able "primary" channels. Maps of these twelve channels are included at the back of this book.

Good channel locations on which to begin your practice are the lower leg portion of the Stomach channel, the arm portion of the Large Intestine channel, and the torso portion of the Ren channel. These sections of channel Qi don't crisscross with other channels, and your friend can be comfortable, lying supine.

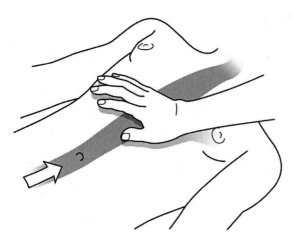

Fig. 1.2 The patient is lying down on a treatment table (or "couch," in England). The center of the practitioner's palm, acupoint P-8, is centered above the Ren channel. The hand is held about half an inch above the skin (or clothing, if any). The arrow shows the correct direction for channel Qi flow in the Ren channel. The hand may be stationary, or moving with or against the direction of channel Qi flow.

If the practice buddy has had any surgeries, severe injuries, or psychological issues that relate to the above-mentioned channels, either choose some different channels to practice on or choose a different friend. For example, a friend with a C-section scar may have moderately-to-severely reduced channel Qi flow in her entire Ren channel. It might be easier to work on her Large Intestine channel, instead – unless she also has a history of dislocated shoulder.

Step one: noticing the two directional sensations of channel Qi

Start by placing the palm of your hand over your friend's ST-36.[1]

Let your hand linger for a few moments over ST-36. Don't *do* anything with the energy in your hand. Be passive. Notice whether or not your hand notices any sense of a faint tingle, or even a faint movement, as if the *idea* of a gentle trickle of electrically charged air is moving against the palm of your hand.

---

[1] The drawing gives a general idea for locating acupoint ST-36. A person with no background in acupuncture point location may wish to go online to learn the *exact* locations of specific acupoints: simply search for ST-36 or Stomach 36. All acupoints mentioned in this book can also be found on the channel maps at the back of the book.

An excellent but expensive book on the subject, with beautiful, clearly detailed diagrams of channels and *exact* acupoint locations, is Peter Deadman's *A Manual of Acupuncture*, Eastland Press, Seattle.

If this is your first attempt at feeling channel Qi, you will probably feel nothing at all. That's fine. You are actually feeling something, but you have not yet learned to recognize the sensation as anything significant.

Next, let your hand move slowly *down* the Stomach channel, towards the ankle: "downstream" from ST-36.

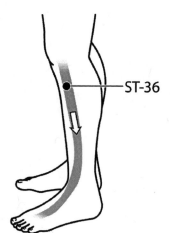

Fig. 1.3 The location of ST-36. The arrow shows the correct direction of the Stomach channel's Qi flow.

Relax your arm as you let the palm of your hand float down the path of the channel. Keep the palm of your hand about an inch or so away from the skin, hovering in the air, as you pass the center of your palm over the path of the channel.

Don't spend too long: only use three or four seconds, no more, going from the knee to the ankle.

Keeping the palm of the hand about an inch or less above the surface of the skin, bring the hand back *up* the Stomach channel at the same speed, moving "upstream," until you come to ST-36 again.

While you may not have noticed anything that you can refer to as "Qi flow," you may have noticed that your palm felt a difference between moving it downstream (with the flow of channel Qi) and moving it upstream (against the flow of channel Qi).

If you did not feel anything different between how your palm felt when moving downstream as compared to upstream, repeat the above exercise twenty or thirty times.

If, after doing this twenty or thirty more times, you still do not feel any difference in the sensation visited against your hand while moving your hand slowly upstream and downstream, an inch above the channel, you were probably making *the most common mistake*: you were trying to push some internal force of your own onto the patient. You cannot hope to feel the patient's channel Qi if you are trying to force your own thoughts, energy, or will onto the patient.

Feeling the air

If you can't feel anything different between moving your hand one direction along a channel's path compared to moving it the other direction, try this: hold your hand up in the air. Notice if you can detect, on your hand, the faint movement, if any, of the air in the room.

Notice this: while attempting to detect the movement of air with your hand, you never use your hand to "push" energy at the air. Instead, you wait quietly to notice any faint rustling that passes over the palm of your hand. This is the same type of perception used for feeling Qi: you let the outgoing energy in your hand become passive while you heighten your observational powers of the incoming energy.

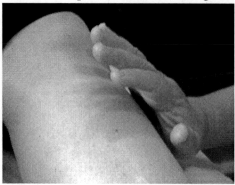

Fig. 1.4 Practitioner's P-8 being held over patient's left-side ST-36. (Patient's black pants are rolled up to her mid-knee.)

If you become convinced that there is no air movement whatsoever in the room, try blowing gently across the palm of your hand: let a faint stream of breath pass over the side of your palm, crossing from your thumb over to the little finger. Notice the sensation.

A student who can feel channel Qi right from the start does not need to spend any time blowing on his hand. The experiments with feeling air do *not* demonstrate what channel Qi feels like. The experiments with feeling air are only presented as a *tool for learning passivity*. This can be helpful for students who are accustomed to "feeling" the world around them by pushing on it.

Common errors

Pushing on a patient's channel Qi

In my years of teaching, I've noticed that some students with a strong background in physical therapy or massage therapy have a very difficult time feeling Qi, in the beginning. When I let them practice on me (while I amp up the applicable sections of channel Qi as much as possible, to make it highly "feel-able"), I sometimes notice an ugly sensation being perpetrated against my own channels by a few of these students. The genuine irritation to my own channels causes me to sometimes snap at them, "Stop that!" Sadly, in this situation, some students have been more proud of their ability to have "done something" energetic than they have been chastened by having done something *incorrect*.

I suspect that some students are so accustomed to pushing on patients instead of letting their hands passively "feel" the patient, that they can't help themselves: they force their own Qi onto patients instead of feeling the patients' channel Qi.

4

In a similar vein, those of my students who have been taught, incorrectly, that "medical Qi Gong" consists of tampering with a patient's channel Qi flow – as opposed to teaching the *patient* how to perform the Qi Gong exercises which might heal or restore the patient's own channel Qi –often have a very hard time feeling and respecting the patient's channel Qi flow. Instead, some of these students seem determined to *influence* the patient's channel Qi, rather than "merely" notice it.

If your past training lies in this direction, or if you learn from the world by pressing on it instead of letting it come to you, practice trying to make your hand's presence become invisible to your friend, as if you can feel him, but he can't feel you. This may help.

Drugs

When teaching classes for the general public in which I have taught how to feel channel Qi, I have noticed that *some* people who are taking antidepressant medications have had difficulty in feeling channel Qi. I have no idea if there is a relationship between the medication and the inability to feel channel Qi. I only mention the observation. For the most part, my general-public students, very often people with no experience in medicine, let alone acupuncture or bodywork, have had *no* problems quickly learning to feel channel Qi.

Using the fingertips

Another common impediment to learning is using the fingertips instead of the palm of the hand. It is *much* easier to recognize the *directional* feelings of channel Qi at the center of the palm of the hand. Of course, channel Qi can be felt with any part of the body, and once you get good at it, a patient's channel Qi can – and should – be felt from across the room, the moment the patient enters the treatment room. (Please be aware, to do so at any other, *non*-clinic, time may be a transgression of professional standards. It is just as foul to secretly spy on someone else's channel Qi flow, as it is to, for example, read other people's personal mail.)

But for beginners, I highly recommend using the palm of the hand, held above the surface of the skin, at a distance that ranges from a quarter of an inch to two inches.

Aside from these errors and exceptions, most students can start feeling the difference between "to" and "fro" channel Qi within about fifteen minutes. It may require several months to be able to feel channel Qi while holding your hand in one place, above a random acupoint. But learning to feel the difference between the sensations of moving downstream and upstream along the channel's path is the thing that is easy: it's also the thing that's of greater importance.

What am I trying to feel? Describing the "feeling" of channel Qi

My students have described in many ways the sensation that feels "different" when going upstream (*against* the flow of channel Qi), as compared with going downstream (*with* the flow).

Some of my favorites are as follows:

"When I go *upstream*, it's like rubbing velvet *against* the nap; downstream feels like rubbing velvet with the nap."

And from another student: "When I go *downstream*, it's like rubbing velvet *against* the nap; upstream feels like with the nap." (Note: this is the opposite of the first observation.)

"Downstream feels cool; upstream feels warm."

And the opposite from another student: "Downstream feels warm; upstream feels cool."

"Upstream feels more prickly; downstream is smoother."

And of course, "Downstream feels more prickly; upstream is smoother."

"Upstream feels weirder"

"Downstream feels weirder."

And so on. You get the idea: when attempting to describe, in words, a new, purely sensory experience, such as the sensation of channel Qi, metaphors differ, opposites abound. When a person, in striving to describe something inexplicable, describes it by comparing it to something else, the words don't necessarily help. This lack of cogent description doesn't really matter. All that really matters is that *you* learn to focus on the "something" that feels different depending on which way your hand moves. However *you* describe it is fine – just so long as you can tell a difference between upstream and downstream.

What channel Qi *really* feels like is the electromagnetic side effect of a moving electrical current.[1]

This moving current is the "Dragon" of Asian medicine, the moving dynamic that joins "heaven and earth." The channel Qi in all living systems is the sum of the places where electromagnetic waves and fields (the unseen energy of the vibratory realm: heaven) are directed, by consciousness (ideas, life force instructions), to transition back and forth, as needed, into currents of electrons (formed, tangible matter: earth).[2]

The current-like sensations given off at the more concentrated areas of the channels are palpable, even at a distance.[3]

For purposes of this text, the "distance" referred to is "approximately an inch away from the skin."

---

[1] I will not enter into the fray of current (so to speak) discussion as to whether or not the channel Qi is moving along a substrate that is fluid, fixed, or fascial (with fascia being the leading contender at present). Nor will I divert into the ongoing discussion as to what molecule, if any, carries the moving electron through the substrate. Popular ideas include nitrous oxide, oxygen, blood, "no carrier," and so on. Let us just say that flowing channel Qi has properties *similar* to those of an electrical current, including the propensity to follow the path of least resistance, and the ability to be encouraged by the presence of a voltage differential (as demonstrated by the effectiveness of using gold and silver acupuncture needles – or even stainless steel, or even the micro-differentials formed by even the tiniest physical manipulation of body tissues, such as acupressure or Tui Na).

[2] The currents created by the various waves are made up of electrons, photons, and other wave-derived subatomic particles. However, for the purpose of brevity and simplicity, the rest of this text will refer to *all* these current components simply as "electrons."

[3] The channel Qi of some patients who are taking high levels of anti-depressant, anti-anxiety, or anti-parkinson's medications may give off a weird, writhing, static sensation, instead of a somewhat straight line. Students have sometimes described this jumbled signal as being like snakes or like bugs crawling around just under the skin.

Sensations cannot be described in words – they can only be compared to other sensations. For example, one cannot describe the taste of an orange to a person who has never eaten an orange, so that the listener can say, "Oh. Now I know what an orange tastes like." For that matter, one person might say "Oranges are sweet" and the next person might say "Oranges are sour." Opposite descriptions, and both somewhat correct!

If three people tried to describe the taste of an orange, one person might say "bright and refreshing," another might try "acidic like a lemon, only sweeter," and a third might say, "slightly pulpy, but squirty with juice." But for a fact, despite their best descriptive efforts, the listener will have no idea whatsoever of what an orange tastes *like*.

Each student must experience for himself/herself what channel Qi feels "*like*." But in the end, it doesn't really matter what it feels "like." The important thing is to be able to feel it.

Very often, after about ten minutes of slowly moving his hand back and forth over the channel and noticing the difference between the upstream and downstream sensation, and then just holding the hand in one location while the Qi runs past his hand, the student blurts out, "I think I could feel this before, but I didn't know that it was something with a name!"

Yes. Channel Qi is very easy to feel.

On the other hand, students often have the opposite response: "I *think* I'm feeling something, I think, but I'm not *sure* it's channel Qi; I'm afraid I might just be imagining that I'm feeling something."

Building confidence

To help those students who are doubtful of their ability to feel channel Qi, I sometimes have students feel the channel Qi of a patient during "rounds" at the school's clinic. In "clinical rounds," the licensed instructor treats the patient, while up to five students observe at close range. In clinical rounds, we can ask the students to participate in a minimal manner: feeling the pulse and/or observing the tongue.

If, during rounds, I silently notice that a patient's channel Qi has an obvious blockage, I might make use of the situation in order to help students gain confidence in their channel-Qi detection skills. I don't tell the students that one of the channels is awry. I innocently name two of the channels, and ask the students to quickly run their hands upstream and downstream, over the paths of those two channels, just for practice. I also ask that, if they notice anything curious in the channels, they silently make of note of it in their charts.[1]

I may even casually remind the students to always maintain a professional, reassuring expression on their faces, and not linger too long while observing tongue, pulse, and channel Qi. My real motivation in asking them to keep a poker face is that I don't wish them to "give

---

[1] Teachers who are using this book as a text, who do this experiment, should be sure to remind their students to emit *no* outgoing energy from their hands. They must use utterly passive hands: observing, not seeking. Otherwise, an unthinking student might exert force on the patient's channel Qi, altering it. Once he's done this, it may take several minutes for the patient's channel Qi to revert back to its starting point – so the rest of the students will be feeling the effects of the pushy student instead of the patient's true situation.

anything away" to their fellow students. As I remind the students to make a quick note on their own student copies of the patient's chart about the condition of the channel Qi flow, the patient has no idea that I am requesting anything out of the ordinary.

Then, after inserting needles or other appropriate treatment for the patient, the students and I congregate in the discussion room. There, I ask the students to place their notes on the table. I ask the students to take turns going around the table, telling their classmates what they thought of the channel Qi, as supported by their notes.

And then, amazing to the students, they discover an unexpected, and highly comforting, *uniformity* of student observations! All the students will have felt the *exact* same "something curious" or "something wrong" at the exact same place. Even the students who, days earlier, had meekly protested, "I'm not sure; I don't think I can feel Qi; I don't know what I'm doing," have to admit – they felt "something is different" or "wrong" at the exact same location as their fellow students also felt that "something is different" or "wrong."

Sometimes I have to repeat this group experiment two or three times before the most self-doubting student is willing to admit that he or she is indeed feeling Qi – or is at least feeling the same thing that everyone else is.

The curious thing is that these students don't need to have been "following" the flow of Qi, necessarily (a skill described later in this chapter). They were just moving their hands up and down a channel, trying to notice if they could feel *anything*. And despite their doubts, they all felt the same thing, and could identify one specific area as "wrong."

While some students might never get the opportunity to experience the above "group" response, the very fact of this easily obtained uniformity in self-doubting students should serve to encourage every student to trust what he feels.

If you doubt your Qi-feeling ability, practice, practice, practice. For some people, as much as thirty minutes of practice is necessary.

If, after ten or fifteen minutes, you truly feel no difference at P-8 when moving your hand one direction along a channel, and then the opposite direction, don't worry about it. Try feeling channel Qi on a different person. Sleep on it. Sometimes we need a little sleep to process new sensations. The next day, try again. Practice a little every day, and very soon, you *will* be able to notice the difference between going with the flow and going against the flow.

Step two: associating the two different sensations with channel direction

Once you can feel a difference when you move your hand above the channel Qi, first one direction, and then the other direction, associate those feelings with what you already know about the "correct" direction of channel Qi flow.

For example, you already know that the direction of the Large Intestine channel flow goes from the wrist to the shoulder.[1] Therefore, the way that the channel Qi feels to you when you move your hand slowly over the path of the Large Intestine channel from the wrist to the shoulder, is going "with the flow." No matter what words you might use to *describe* the actual sensation, the wrist to shoulder direction is "going *with* the flow." We are assuming,

---

[1] If you are not familiar with the directions in which the channels are supposed to flow, look for the arrows on the channel maps at the back of this book.

of course, that your friend is healthy and has *no* history of significant injuries along the path of this channel.

Oppositely, the way that the channel Qi feels in the Large Intestine channel when you run your hand in the opposite direction, from the shoulder to the fingers, is how channel Qi feels when you are "going *against* the flow."

"With" the flow and "against" the flow will feel the same in all people. If you can teach yourself to identify a sensation as being "with" the flow, you will be able to recognize this same sensation in anyone when your hand is moving "with" his flowing channel Qi.

Step three: going with the flow

Once you have learned to recognize the sensation of channel Qi that is going "*with* the flow," practice letting your hand be carried along by this sensation. *Forget* about the sensations that occur when your hand moves *against* the flow. Those were just training devices.

When you let your hand move at the same speed and direction as the energy that is traveling "*with*" the flow, your hand will be moving in the same direction as the channel Qi.

By following the flow of current with your hand, and comparing the flow with the healthy, normal paths you learned in school or in this book, you will be able to tell if the channel Qi is flowing correctly or if it is flowing sideways, out of the channel's normal path, into another channel or into a divergent channel. You will be able to tell when a channel is running backwards, also called "running Rebelliously," which is to say, in the opposite direction of the pattern you learned in school.

Practicing passivity

Let your hand feel that it is being pulled along by the energy that is moving "with the flow." Or you might think of this as matching the movement of your hand with the movement of the energy that you can feel. But letting your hand be pulled by the energy is far easier, and more accurate.

If your ability to be a passive observer is good, you might even feel pleasure, like the sweet in-the-moment feeling of drifting in a canoe, as your hand is "carried along" by the channel Qi under your hand.

A dance example of "following energy"

A good "following" dancer is able to abandon any preconceived notions as to where the leading partner is going to go. By cultivating perfect relaxation with regard to *where* the movement is going, the "following" dancer is able to float around the dance floor, "carried" by the leading partner. In our busy lives, it can be pleasant to just follow, pleasant to *not* be in charge, for a moment or two, now and then.

In much the same way as the dancer, the dragon tracker, by perfect abandonment of any intention for where his hand might be led, other than to keep it parallel to the surface of the patient's skin, might begin to feel as if his hand could be being carried along by the patient's channel Qi.

Practice

Practice feeling channel Qi, back and forth, on several channels, on several healthy people. Then, practice letting your hand be carried along by the channel Qi flow on as many people as you can. The more you do this, the more you will feel comfortable with the idea that your hand can move "*with* the flow." Once you know how it feels when you're going with the flow, you can let your hand float along above the channel Qi anywhere on a patient's body. As you compare the direction of your hand's movement with what you know to be the correct pathways of channel Qi, you will be able to see your hand move in a "wrong direction" when a channel is flowing aberrantly.

Assessment

For example, if your hand is resting over a patient's Ren channel, and you feel your hand being carried up to Ren-13 and then being carried over to the Liver channel, you can be certain that something is amiss.

Or, if you are resting your hand over the patient's Du channel and your hand is carried a short way up the spine and then propelled up into the air, away from the body, the patient has a problem.

Again, no matter how you might *describe* the sensations of moving channel Qi, all that really matters is that you learn to 1) discern the direction in which the channel Qi is moving (going "with" the flow), and 2) learn to let yourself be carried by the flow of that channel Qi. After you can feel and follow the direction and route in which channel Qi is flowing, you can compare that direction and route with the correct pathways.[1] That comparison is the assessment.

More practice

If you aren't sure what is meant by "follow the Qi with your hand," put your hand close to your mouth. While blowing as gently and *slowly* as possible *across* the palm of your hand, move your hand at the same rate of speed as the breath. Breathe very *slowly*, and try to move your hand away from your mouth at the same speed as your breath. When your hand moves at the exact same speed and direction as your breath, you don't perceive the moving air of your breath. Let your hand get the full length of your arm away from your mouth as it moves at the same speed as the breath. Imagine that the energy in the breath is pushing your hand along.

Next, bring your hand close to the mouth again. Blow across your hand again, in the same way, but do not move your hand. You can again feel the movement of the air passing over your hand.

---

[1] If you've forgotten or never learned the directions for the flow of the channels, you can use the maps in this book or use any basic text that shows the location of the numbered acupoints. In most cases, the numbering sequence of the points shows the direction of the channel Qi flow. The overall direction of the channel Qi flow usually goes from the smaller-number point towards the larger-number point. For example, if the channel Qi is running from ST-36 to ST-45 (the numbers going from smaller to bigger), it's running the right direction in that segment. If it's running from ST-42 to ST-36 (numbers getting smaller), it's running the wrong way.

You have now experienced two styles of "feeling" the breath. You detected the speed of the breath by noticing the rate at which your hand is "moved along" by your breath *and* you experienced the sensation of having the breath move against your hand. In the first case, with the moving hand, you have felt both the direction and speed of the breath. In the second case, when you left your hand in one position and let the air move across it, you also felt the direction and speed.

Feeling channel Qi can also be accomplished either by allowing one's hand to be carried along by the flow channel Qi, or by holding the hand in one place and noticing the feeling of channel Qi moving across the hand.

I fear I'm making the learning seem far harder than it really is. Most of you won't need to blow on your hands.

The most important thing to remember is: "don't *think* about it." As soon as you start getting all logical on yourself, you can't be paying attention to your perceptions.

For example, consider the experience of listening to music: if you are busy *thinking* about what you are feeling, or *describing* to yourself how you feel when you listen to musician Jimi Hendrix, you will be missing the Jimi Hendrix *Experience*. Feeling channel Qi isn't *thinking* about sensations: it's having a direct experience of energy.

Thinking, or not

Of course, as soon as you *do* know how to feel channel Qi, you might *then* have to think about what you felt coming from your patient's channels. For example, if Qi was running the "wrong" way, or not running, you might need to ask yourself "Why?" Later chapters will help you answer this question. After you've felt the channel Qi, you will need to think about what the sensations might mean in terms of diagnosis and treatment. But while doing the actual feeling of channel Qi, don't be thinking about what the channel Qi is *supposed* to be doing.

Again, for most people learning to feel channel Qi, all they need to do is practice moving their hands back and forth over a few channels. When they do this long enough, *whether or not* they know what Qi "feels like," they do *eventually* feel a difference between the two directions. The difference is caused by running the hand either with, or against, the current of channel Qi. It doesn't matter what words the brain comes up with to "define" the experience. All that matters, in the beginning, is that you are able to notice that some gentle force is moving in the patient, and it feels different when your hand moves "with" it than when you move "against" it. After that, practice letting your hand be carried along by the sensation that moves "with" the channel Qi – and notice where the sensation leads you. It will lead you along the paths, right or wrong, that the channels are taking.

The width of the channels

Channel widths vary. For example, the Stomach channel is fairly thin, less than an inch wide, as it passes over ST-41. But in the vicinity of ST-36, the channel can be more than three inches wide, in an adult. When you are following the flow of Qi with your hands, you will notice that sometimes there is a narrow "line," only a quarter inch wide, or so, where the Qi feels strongest. This line, in many cases, will follow fairly closely the Traditional theoretical "line" created by the sequentially numbered acupoints. In some places where channel Qi runs in a very wide path instead of a narrow path, it can be harder to feel the movement of the channel Qi.

For example, on the relatively wide band of channel Qi in the portion of the Urinary Bladder channel that flows down the back, the channel is wider than the two parallel rows of acupoints that run down the back. The medial points follow the area of decreased electrical resistance along the medial border of the channel, and the lateral points define the area of decreased electrical resistance along the lateral border of the channel. The relative width of this channel spreads the channel Qi somewhat thinly over the back. This channel width can make the channel Qi harder to detect, in this area, than the flow in a narrower channel – for the beginner.

In general, when trying to ascertain "where" the Qi is going, just do your best. Until you feel confident, you can start off by tracking the imaginary "line" that connects the "dots" of the acupoints.

Case study #1

Restless leg at night

(The following case study took place in clinical rounds. The students were very new at feeling channel Qi. They had been instructed in feeling channel Qi the week before, for a period of fifteen minutes before starting rounds. I do not know if any students had done any practicing at home. I know that a *few* of the students had done no practicing at all. I only mention this so that the reader will understand how quickly, and with how little practice, the students had mastered the art of feeling channel Qi.)

Female, age 58, came into the clinic for increasing restless leg syndrome, at night, in her right leg. She was otherwise very healthy and fit.

Tongue and pulse diagnoses showed nothing remarkable. Although an intuitive pulse master might have been able to detect the source of her restless leg problem, there was *nothing* in the pulse reading to suggest a diagnosis. Her bearing was athletic and her demeanor cheerful.

While standing on the right side of the patient, while feeling her pulse, I noticed a channel Qi disruption. I hadn't used my hands to feel her channel Qi; I just became aware of a sensation of blockage in the lower right quadrant of my torso. (Feeling ambient channel Qi gets easier, the more you attune yourself to it.) I asked all the students to, one at a time, run their hands very quickly over her left *and* right stomach channels, from approximately ST-19 down to ST-36 – while making sure to not influence her channel Qi in any way.

I innocently asked the students then and there if they'd noticed anything, and where. They gleefully answered as if with one voice, "There!" They were all pointing at an area a few inches below her navel, on the right side. Quickly considering the most likely reason for the blockage, given the location, I asked the patient if she'd had her appendix taken out.

"Yes," she replied, "but that was *years* ago; I was a child."

I answered, "It feels to all of us as if something right here (I pointed) is preventing energy from getting into your leg. It's most likely the scar tissue from the appendectomy. May I take a look?"

12

She bared the abdomen in the suspect area. Right where we'd all felt the blockage, she had a moderately thin, quite long, indented scar running perpendicular to the Stomach channel. The students gave little gasps of excitement. They'd been able to pinpoint a Qi blockage!

I explained to the patient, "Scar tissue, like rubber, is non-conductive: electrical currents can't pass through. May I insert some acupuncture needles through the scar to see if you can get some energy moving along the surface of the metal needles, moving the energy *through* the scar tissue?"

I told her that I didn't usually like to needle scar tissue on a person who'd never had acupuncture before. Unlike some styles of acupuncture, needling scar tissue is often very painful. I gave her the quickest possible version of the flashback sensations and surgical memories she *might* re-experience when the needles penetrated the scar, and asked her if she was willing to let me try it.

She was game.

The main point of this case study is to demonstrate the uniformity of my student's experience. Be encouraged by this.

As an aside, to make this case study clinically relevant above and beyond the issue of feeling channel Qi, here's the conclusion: one week later, the patient returned to the clinic. Her restless leg syndrome was greatly reduced. Her symptoms had decreased the first night after the treatment, and continued to improve.

During the second treatment, I needled through the appendectomy scar again, placing the needles in slightly different locations from before, but still passing the needles through the keloid tissue at a right angle to the line of the scar. This second time, the sensations she experienced were more like the normal sensations associated with acupuncture.

Case study #2

Wrist treatment sends channel Qi to opposite foot

The following case study occurred in my private practice.

A female, age 60, retired semi-professional golfer, came in for wrist pain. She had sprained her right wrist a few weeks before, and now she was slicing all her drives off the tee. I palpated the right wrist. Several carpal bones were displaced. I did some very gentle, Yin-type, Tui Na (Chinese medical massage/manipulation), and the bones slid nicely back into place. I could have sent her home, knowing that the next surge of channel Qi through the Large Intestine channel, at 5:00 the next morning, would give the wrist the energy it needed to keep the bones in place. Instead, I decided to be on the safe side, and inserted a needle at *right*-side LI-4 to immediately increase the Qi flow through the wrist, thus strengthening the positioning of the restored carpal bones.

In just over two seconds (three seconds is about average for channel Qi to travel from LI-4 on one side of the body, to ST-45 on the opposite side of the body, following a needle insertion), she felt something in her toes on the *left* side. She asked me why the left side of her leg and her toes had tingled. I replied, "The side of the leg right here?" pointing out the path of the left Stomach channel on the lower leg. I continued, "And is it the second and third toes on the left side?"

She expressed surprise at my seeming prescience, but she agreed that I was exactly correct. I explained that the wrist needle was bringing up to speed the energy level in a current that flows up the arm to the face (Large Intestine channel), crosses over to the *other side* of the face, and then, on that other side, streams down the face, neck, torso and leg to the second and third toes (Stomach channel). She was pleased to know that her perceptions made sense according to Asian medical theory.

She asked why she'd felt the tingle during this treatment; in the past, she'd been needled at LI-4 and had not noticed anything subsequent in her opposite leg and foot.

I explained that her wrist injury had been causing significantly diminished energy flow in the Large Intestine channel. This, in turn, was causing significantly diminished energy flow in the Stomach channel on the opposite side.

She was a very healthy person. Ordinarily, there was enough channel Qi in her channels that she did not notice the difference when a slight increase pulsed through the system in response to a needle at LI-4. But because she had been walking around, for a few weeks, with a considerable insufficiency in those two channels (because of the wrist injury), she was able to feel the change when a full measure of channel Qi coursed, once again, through channels that had been depleted.

I gave her an example that one of my professors had given to me. "If a cup is full, and you put more tea into it, the extra will spill over the sides. You still have only one cup of tea. Your amount of tea has not changed. But if your cup is empty, and someone pours tea into it, you will have a changed amount of tea. You can tell that you have something more than before."

My patient was an athlete, and keenly aware of how her body felt. The sensations that she reported to me, and the sensations that many other patients have reported to me, have contributed to my appreciation for and personal knowledge of channels: channels do exist; they follow specific pathways.

More to the point, observant patients such as the one discussed above can sometimes feel channel Qi flowing in the locations described in the classic texts, even when they don't know to expect it.

This case study makes this point: the conformity of the sensations experienced by patients, together with the matching sensations that we can feel with our hands, serve as a confirmation that we are not "just imagining" the existence and sensations of channel Qi.

Self doubt

Probably the biggest impediment to using channel diagnostics is self-doubt. A novice may doubt that the sensations he is experiencing are the "real thing." But after overcoming the initial bout of thinking that feeling Qi is going to be very hard, most people can very easily feel channel Qi if it's running in the expected pattern. The real problems with self-doubt usually arise in cases where a patient's channel Qi is weak, missing altogether, running backwards, or attacking another channel.

I've worked with students and colleagues who do an excellent job of diagnosing channel Qi aberrations when the blockages are pretty straightforward. But these same practitioners, when confronted with something unexpected or unprecedented in their experience, suddenly don't trust what they're feeling.

Even colleagues who've been practicing this work for a few years will suddenly be hit by self-doubt when the signal behaves *very* strangely. They sometimes assume, in these cases, that they've lost the ability to feel channel Qi. In such cases, it's far more likely that the problem (the inability to feel the channel Qi at some particular location) is coming from something going on with the patient, not the practitioner. Still, self-doubt does crop up easily.

Some of the self-doubt may arise from the fact that we are dealing with something unseen *and* most of us grew up thinking that feeling energy was impossible. As long as we think that we're doing something that borders on the impossible, we are holding the door wide open for self-doubt.

Not so amazing, really

What we are doing when we feel channel Qi is not really that amazing. Many perfectly "normal" jobs require a similar level of sensory discretion.

For example, a musician, tuning his instrument, is listening for sound variations occurring at hundreds of vibrations per minute. If a violinist's A string is tuned to resonate at 443 beats per minute instead of the tuning fork's 440, he needs to be able to hear the irregular beat generated by the difference, and correct it.

It is said that Mozart once noticed more than one hundred notes and/or rhythmic variations in some bird's simple cry – a bird song in which I probably would have heard three notes and two rhythms.

Likewise, some visual artists can discern extremely fine gradations of color that most people cannot see. I've seen people who work in a house-paint store matching color swatches with an astounding speed and accuracy.

A tea taster can differentiate flavors that most palates don't know exist.

These skills are impressive, but we do not doubt that they exist. Because we have been raised to think these enhanced levels of job-related sensory perception are perfectly reasonable, we don't doubt that such attunement is possible.[1]

In our job, we work with channel Qi. After practicing acupuncture for even just a year or two, most of us can easily feel when an inserted needle goes from "connected to nothing" to "connected with something." When this happens, we say we've "Got the Qi." There's nothing really amazing about our ability to do this. This skill is only recognition of a sensation to which we've become attuned. There's nothing *amazing* about it.

---

[1] One of my favorite examples of "what is possible" occurred when a nine year-old girl stayed in the room while I treated her nineteen year-old sister. The younger girl had never heard of acupuncture, and had no expectations whatsoever. After the treatment, I asked the young girl if she'd enjoyed herself. "Oh yes!" She replied, "The best part was watching the blue-green light arcing between those [left and right side] needles down by her ankles."

She pointed to the needles at left- and right-side SP-6. I'd never seen that light, although I'd heard of it. I just smiled and said, "Yeah, that's really cool." I have to wonder, if I didn't already *know* that it's impossible to see that light, would I be able to see it, too? If students didn't start off with the knowledge that feeling channel Qi is nearly impossible, would they be able to feel it with more confidence?

And, leaping to a completely different subject, this anecdote also demonstrates why channel Qi is often referred to in the *Nei Jing* as "color."

When we are feeling channel Qi by hand, from an inch or so away from the skin, we are only noticing the exact same sort of energy that we can easily learn to recognize when the channel Qi pulls on a needle. We're just feeling it from a little farther away, without the medium of the needle.

Channel Qi is *not* a freakishly difficult thing to feel. In fact, when I run my hands over a patient and explain that I'm looking for an energetic glitch, I'm surprised at how often my patients say something along the lines of, "Well, I should hope so." These patients are *not* surprised that I can feel channel Qi. They *expect* it. I've had patients who've said to me, "When I was out of town, I went to an acupuncturist who couldn't even feel channel Qi! Can you believe it?"

We expect a violinist to know how to tune his violin, even though most of us do not have the sensory skills needed for such a job. Our patients have the right to expect us to know how to feel when we have "Got the Qi" or when channel Qi is flowing the wrong way, even if most people aren't used to noticing channel Qi.[1]

Looking ahead

Direct perception of the channels is often the most accurate and elegant method of forming an exact medical diagnosis and treatment plan. All of the "pattern" diagnoses of Asian medicine, ranging from Five Elements to Eight Parameters, are, at root, labels for pathologies that are set in motion, and maintained, via aberrant flow of channel Qi.

Channel Qi is the *leader* of the Blood, the leader, or driver, of all physical manifestation. Channel Qi is an electrical manifestation of waves set in motion, originally, by consciousness. These channels, in turn, generate physical manifestions (atoms and molecular structures) *and* the power to drive them into the correct behaviors. Channel Qi drives both the Yin (matter) and the Yang (energy) of our bodies, both the organs and their functions. All health issues that involve Yin, Yang, Qi, or Blood, or the Five phases of channel Qi can be most elegantly detected and treated by working directly with channel Qi for diagnosis and treatment.

In the realm of Asian medicine, the *exact* knowledge of where a patient's channels actually *are*, and the quality of the movement, held up against the knowledge of where and how they are *supposed* to be flowing, can often tell a health practitioner the *exact* nature of the patient's problem and, therefore, the exact treatment. Detecting the flow of channel Qi provides this exact knowledge. Almost anyone can learn to detect the flow patterns of channel Qi.

As the masters pointed out in the *Nei Jing*, "To beginners, it seems easy."

---

[1] Acupuncturists are not the only medical professionals that make use of the signals produced by channel Qi. Many chiropractors, naturopaths, osteopaths, craniosacral therapists, and even MDs take advantage of their ability to consciously or unconsciously feel the various signals and static created by incorrect channel Qi flow, and thus improve their diagnoses and treatment outcomes. What separates acupuncturists from these other professionals is that our medicine is *based* on the movement of channel Qi. If we fail to consciously work with these forces, we aren't actually practicing Asian medicine: we are guessing as to the underlying problem based on "pattern" generalities, and treating semi-blindly.

16

It *is* easy to detect the sensations of a patient's channel Qi and thereby derive an extremely accurate diagnosis and treatment plan.

As an aside, the hard part referred to in the *Nei Jing*, the part of channel work that masters "know is difficult," is a spiritual goal not directly related to the practice of doctoring others. This "difficult" part of channel work is the attainment of complete control of one's *own* consciousness, which then gives the ability to consciously regulate one's *own* channels – holding the channels, and therefore the body, in pathways of perfect health in spite of pathogens, climate, injury, or toxins. At the highest level, one can control one's own channels to the extent of consciously altering the body's energetics in order to enter the breathless state, in which one's energy and awareness can be consciously directed to leave and re-enter one's own body at will, and/or manifest other masteries of the physical realm. The masters recognize that this aspect of "knowing the channel Qi," which at the highest level involves complete surrender of ego, can be very difficult to master.

Again, the easy part is learning to detect the flow of channel Qi in patients, and using that knowledge to determine an elegant and effective medical treatment. Even a *beginning* student can arrive at a highly accurate diagnosis and effective treatment plan by noticing errors in a patient's channel-Qi flow pattern.

Sensing the flow of channel Qi requires only that one learns to recognize the distinct *physical* sensations emitted by the flow of channel Qi. Any person who is able to feel the sensation of gentle wind on his cheek, or who can tell the difference between the sensation of rubbing velvet one direction when compared to rubbing it the other way, should be able to quickly master the art of tracking the flow of channel Qi in a patient.

Then, if he knows the *correct* patterns of channel Qi flow, as described in the classics, he can quickly recognize if, and in what manner, the Qi flow in a patient is aberrant.

"By observing changes and movements, one can detect the secrets of nature in order to know the essential aspects of diagnosis, its yin and yang." [1]

Chapter two

Case study examples: Wood Attacking Earth

This chapter and the next will provide introductory case studies to show *how* knowledge of a patient's channels can be crucially helpful: *why* the exact location, vigor, or direction of channel aberrations can bring exactitude to a diagnosis and treatment plan.

The cases in this chapter feature Wood Attacking Earth: a very common diagnosis.

Before starting on the actual case studies, the following introduction points out a few problems that can arise from the "pattern" methods of diagnosis. The subsequent case studies then illustrate how these specific problems can be answered via channel diagnosis.

Introduction: A stab in the dark

Why are the patterns that we learn in school sometimes insufficient to provide a specific treatment plan? Why are they inherently ambiguous?

Consider the extremely common pattern of Wood Attacking Earth.

"Wood attacking Earth" means, literally, that channel Qi flow in the Gallbladder channel and/or the Liver channel (the two Wood channels) is so blocked or distorted that it is flowing into (attacking) the Stomach and/or Spleen channel (the two Earth channels).

---

[1] Su Wen, chapter 13-7, from *A Complete Translation of Nei-Jing and Nan-Jing translated by Henry C. Lu, PhD*; International College of Traditional Chinese Medicine of Vancouver, 2004; p. 114.

The word "movement" refers here to the movement of channel Qi – the actual movement of energy in the channels. The word "changes" refers here to the pulses.

As noted throughout this chapter of the Su Wen, moving channel Qi is Yang. Channel Qi is the real deal, the *source* of the body's energy. Like the sun, which is the *source* of all Earth's energy, and is therefore called Yang, the energy flowing in the channels is also a *source* of energy – also Yang.

In comparison, the pulse is Yin, like the moon. The moon merely *reflects* the energy of the sun: the pulse merely *reflects* what a person is doing, at any given moment, with his body's energy. The pulse has no true energy of its own. Thus the pulse, like the moon, is Yin – not the true, generative source, but merely a reflection. The pulses can change in the blink of an eye, in response to thoughts, activity levels, and mood.

But the main reason for including this quote is to encourage the self-doubting student. This quoted line from the *Su Wen* part of the *Nei Jing* confirms that "movement," the actual flow of Qi in the channels, *can* be assessed ("observed"). Learning to assess the flow of channel Qi is do-able, even simple.

From a purely *symptomatic* standpoint, Wood Attacking Earth means that something to do with Gallbladder channel- or Liver channel-related problems, ranging from suppressed or frustrated emotions all the way to viral hepatitis or gallstones, is causing trouble in Stomach channel- or Spleen channel-related systems, systems that range from regulation of appetite and metabolism to application of muscle strength.

If a practitioner of Asian medicine has decided that, based on tongue, pulse, and symptoms, a patient's problem is Wood Attacking Earth, he must then decide if he needs to eliminate the problem via sedating, strengthening, or "harmonizing" the Liver or Gallbladder channels, or by strengthening or "harmonizing" the Stomach or Spleen channels.[1] Or yet again, he might need to resolve the issue by strengthening the Heart, or even Pericardium channels – in hopes of thus calming the Liver channel. So many options for such a common diagnosis! Which is the "right" option? Is there such a thing as the "right" option?

Where's the logic?

In-school students of Asian medicine sometimes complain that, although many of their teachers clearly have a keen, intuitive sense of what is exactly wrong in their patients' various presentations of Wood Attacking Earth – sedating one patient or tonifying another – they often treat each patient a little differently, even when the patients supposedly have the same pattern, which is to say, the same diagnosis. The teachers do not always explain how or why they choose different treatments for people with the same patterns. Sometimes a teacher gives a beautiful explanation, but it usually only holds up for that one case, and does nothing to teach the student what to do when he confronts that same pattern in another patient.

These excellent doctors just seem to "know" which treatment approach to use in the various cases of Wood Attacking Earth. Sometimes they needle Liver points, or points along the Heart or Spleen channel, or points on all three channels, or something altogether different. The teacher might prescribe Xiao Yao Wan because the diagnosis is Wood Attacking Earth, or he might use Xiao Chai Hu Tang – for the same reason. However, if the teacher is pressed to explain his process of differentiation from one Wood-Attacking-Earth patient to the next, the teacher often falls back on, "It's a 'Wood Attacking Earth' treatment."

These teachers often have a hard time conveying their Insight Method to their students. The learning barrier may come from many sources, ranging from the traditional silence in matters of intuition, to Chinese political pressures for the medicine to be uniformly prescriptive (non-intuitive), and all the way to linguistic conflicts.

---

[1] "Harmonize" means, simply, "make the channels run in their correct paths, in the correct direction, and with the correct vigor." When the channels are running correctly, that is to say, the channels are running in the correct directions and in the correct locations, then and only then are their exquisitely balanced flow patterns "in harmony." When the channels are running correctly, then the *physiological* Yin and Yang aspects of the body are automatically balanced.

Excellent practitioners, now *and* back when I was in school, tend to justify their diagnostics to students by repeating, over and over, the name of the pattern.

They iterate, "It's Liver Attacking Spleen," or "It's Wood Attacking Earth," as if these repetitions will bring insight. Instead, they often bring education by rote: technical terms, without depth of understanding – and no way for the student to know why, in multiple cases that all manifested the same "pattern," different treatments were used for each case.

Again, the best doctors, who treat one patient with a wiry pulse and pale tongue very differently from how they treat the next patient with a wiry pulse and pale tongue, may try to *explain* their diagnoses and treatments in terms of refinements of symptoms, pulse, or tongue. But as every student knows, these *justifications* after the fact fail to explain how the student can learn to *anticipate* treatments in new situations.

Or oppositely, many teachers are unable to explain why some famous doctors treat every patient with the exact same treatment, regardless of diagnosis – and often get good results. (More about this later.)

Making it even harder to learn about diagnostic skills from this type of ineffective teaching, many students, and many long-term practitioners, aren't even confident in their pulse-diagnosis skills, let alone intuitive about diagnostics.

For these students and practitioners, even determining that Wood is Attacking Earth, based on pulse, may depend on an uncertain sense that the Liver pulse is "maybe wirier than it should be", or the tongue seems a bit "maybe more purple than it should be."

When the diagnoses of these would-be masters are shaky to begin with, their selection and application of an acupuncture treatment plan is very often a literal stab in the dark.

In comparison, consider the diagnostic approach in this chapter's case studies. Both cases feature Liver Qi stagnation and Earth deficiency: ostensibly, Wood Attacking Earth.

Case study #3

Liver Qi Attacking Spleen channel on the leg following Wind-Heat

Male, age 54. His symptoms, over the last five weeks, ever since having a brief bout of "stomach flu," have been lack of appetite, frequent and very loose stools, increasing lassitude, and depression. The Liver pulse was slightly wiry, and the Spleen pulse was slightly weak. The tongue had teeth marks, a slightly purple tone overall, and the tongue muscle itself seemed a bit tense, or "tight."

These findings suggested to me that I might do well to start my channel Qi investigation by looking for something amiss in his Liver channels.

Quickly running my hands over his Liver channels, keeping my hands about an inch above his clothing, I felt an area on his right lower leg, between LIV-5 and LIV-6, where Liver channel Qi stopped moving up the path of the Liver channel. Instead, Liver channel Qi was shunting medially over into the Spleen channel. There was almost no Liver channel Qi flowing in the leg portion of the Liver channel beyond this pathological "divergent" point where the Liver channel Qi flowed over into the Spleen channel.[1]

As an aside, there *was* some Qi in the Liver channel on the torso. The Ren channel serves as an auxiliary provider of channel Qi flow for all the channels. Even if the channels are blocked somewhere else along their path, they can pick up some amount of channel Qi from the Ren. In the case of the Liver channel, it picks up some channel Qi in the vicinity of Ren-3 and Ren-4. There are other auxiliary sources of channel Qi throughout the body as well. Therefore, evidence of channel Qi at the beginning and end parts of a channel does *not* mean that the length of the channel is unobstructed. To ascertain if the entire length of the channel is flowing, you must check the entire length of the channel.

I moved my hand quickly over his feet and ankles, checking the channel Qi flow in his Spleen channel for confirmation that his Spleen channel was being "attacked" by the Liver channel. The channel Qi from SP-1 through SP-6, and on up to the point where the Liver channel was dumping into the Spleen channel, was moving slowly. Because the Stomach channel Qi on the foot was running fine, and able to exit the Stomach channel and flow toward the Spleen channel at SP-3, the slowdown and weakness in the lower part of the Spleen channel was *not* coming from insufficiency of channel Qi flowing into the Spleen channel. This was not, primarily, a deficiency problem.

The Spleen channel *was* receiving a moderate supply of channel Qi from the Stomach channel, and yet the Spleen channel wasn't running very well between Sp-1 and Sp-6.
Consider:
1) The symptoms had started just after the patient had a Liver-attacking illness. (Although the patient had called it "stomach flu," the symptoms he described were a good fit for mild hepatitis.)

---

[1] A "pathological" or "unhealthy" divergence is one that occurs in response to some injury, illness, or emotion, as opposed to the healthy (classic) divergences, which occur instantly in response to the constant changes of physiological need.

Healthy divergent channels are segments of channel Qi that flow differently from the Primary-channel, and Du and Ren pathways that we learn in school. The flow patterns learned in school show the route of channel Qi when a person is awake, is physically relaxed, and is mentally in utter parasympathetic (relaxed, no fear) mode. In other neurological modes, such as sleep, sympathetic mode, or dissociation, or even when, in parasympathetic mode, specific physical activities require extra energy in a specific location, routings of channel Qi flow are significantly altered to accommodate the immediate physiological needs of that mode or that activity. These automatic, healthy alterations in channel Qi routing are called divergences. These healthy divergences are usually short-term, and occur in response to immediate needs for energy during the various neurological modes. They are also standardized: the healthy divergences are very similar from one person to the next.

Unhealthy divergences can also occur. Unhealthy, non-standard divergences can arise in response to injury, illness, or mental and emotional challenges. These divergences will be unique to the challenged person's physiology for the duration of the challenge. These divergences are pathological. They disrupt the healthy flow of normal, (Primary, Du, and Ren) channel flow patterns. So long as these pathological divergences are in place, the Qi no longer "goes through." When Qi cannot go through, "pain" (which means "less-than-optimal health condition") follows.

2) Exterior-Wind (pathogen-borne) illnesses that attack the Liver often impede the flow of Qi in the vicinity of LIV-5 or –6.

3) No foot or ankle injury, which might have caused a slow-down in channel Qi on the foot part of the Spleen channel, was apparent (using Tui Na to examine the foot and ankle).

And most important of all, the channel flow itself was providing hard cold proof of what was going on:

4) The Liver channel Qi was pouring into the Spleen channel part way up the lower leg.

Therefore, the most likely cause of the slowdown in the foot and ankle portion of the Spleen's channel Qi was the intrusive flow of Liver channel Qi into the Spleen channel – set in motion when the Liver channel Qi became stymied in the vicinity of LIV-6 during his recent illness. This would also account for the lack of channel Qi in the Liver channel from LIV-6 on up.

As suggested by his symptoms, and *proved* by the detection of divergent flow of Liver channel Qi into his Spleen channel, it was indeed a clear-cut case of Wood Attacking Earth.

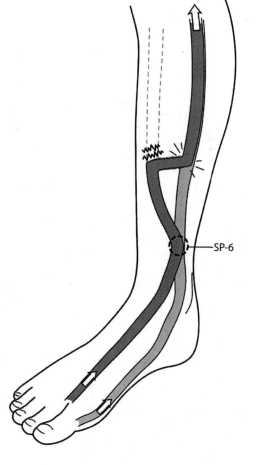

Fig. 2.1 The pale shading shows the Spleen channel. The darker shading shows the Liver channel. The zig-zag lines in the Liver channel show the site of the blockage. The dashed lines proximal to the blockage show what would have been the correct path of the Liver channel, a path that is now empty.

SP-6, where the Liver and Spleen channels meet, is shown merely to help the reader orient to the channels.

But in addition to knowing it was a case of Wood Attacking Earth, which I'd been able to guess from his symptoms and pulse, I now knew *where* the Wood was attacking from: just past LIV-5, on the left leg.

Since the Spleen channel had plenty of channel Qi flowing in it, albeit the wrong type, a beginning student may wonder why this patient was manifesting symptoms of "Spleen deficiency"(loss of appetite, loose stools, lassitude) as well as Liver channel stagnation and deficiency symptoms (depression, lassitude).

It is true that the Spleen channel had plenty of channel Qi. But it had the wrong *type* of channel Qi. Proximal to the point where the Liver channel Qi was flowing into the Spleen channel, the Spleen channel was loaded predominantly with Liver channel Qi, not with Spleen channel Qi.

Five kinds of channel Qi

Channel Qi is not "one size fits all." The currents that make up the channel Qi consist of five distinct types of currents – derived from five distinct types of vibratory phenomena. All five types of currents are present in every channel, but the *ratio* of the five types varies from one channel to another. These five types of currents are related to the theory of the Five Elements. [1]

---

[1] In the Yin, or materially discrete aspect of channel Qi energy, the units that make up the currents are electrons. These electrons move in one of five different movement patterns. The same forces that make up the currents, when considered in terms of the *vibrations* from which the electrons are derived (their Yang aspect), also occur in five different forms: different densities.

Although five types of vibrations, also known as Elements or Phases, exist, all the vibratory forms are derived from the first, most basic form of vibration: sound waves. The other types of vibrations (also known as Elements, or Phases) are four, successive condensations of the preceding type(s) of vibration. Sound waves, and the electrons created by them, constitute the first Element. In ancient Vedic lore, which greatly precedes Chinese Taoist philosophy, and from which Taoist philosophy was derived, this Element is known as Ether. The other four elements, Air, Fire, Water, and Earth, are compressions, or condensations, of Etheric vibrations.

If one's awareness is oriented towards the repulsion aspect of the sound wave (as opposed to the electromagnetically attractive aspect), the wave appears to generate electrons with a particular type of movement. Each of the other four types of vibrations, as well, if perceived from the repulsion aspect, creates vibration-related patterns of electron movement. In all, the five types of vibrations yield five types of electron movement.

The currents that flow through our bodies are made up of both vibratory motion and the electron-aspect of that vibration. Our perspective determines whether or not we perceive ourselves, and/or all matter, as pure vibration, pure matter, or something in between.

The manifestations of the first Element, sound waves, are formed by the vibratory waves emitted by pure thought. (By the way, thought waves are *not* the same things as the crude, electromagnetic *brain* waves generated by our neural activity.) The vibrations of this first Phase, or first Element, are referred to in some world scriptures as "The Word." For example, in the New Testament book of John, chapter 1, we read that, "In the beginning was the Word." In the Hebrew scriptures, Genesis1:1, this phase of creation is referred to as the "Spirit [consciousness, or thought] of God moving over the face of the waters [vibrations, or waves]."

24

Although, in Vedic lore, this element is named Ether, in Chinese medicine, this element might be called Wood. This Element is the most closely related to self-expression and the expression of consciousness. However, the Vedic understanding does *not* equate this Element with the Liver, eyes, and other correspondences that Asian medicine attributes to the Wood element.

While the ancient Vedic texts do associate each of the Elements with different sensory capabilities, directional movement, physiological functions, organs, and so on, the more ancient Vedic correspondences only *rarely* match up with the Chinese correspondences – the latter being only loosely based on Vedic science, and developed during the dark ages.

The reason for the lack of correspondence between the Vedic and the Chinese Five Element systems is historical: the Vedic elements are based on the actual physics involved in creating the illusion of changeable matter out of the indivisible and infinite. This physics was written up during a higher age. Although we know that this material was written down as long ago as 1600 BC, some historians consider the philosophy to have been codified much earlier, possibly as long ago as 6,000 BC.

Much later, the Chinese developed the Taoist precepts (the proposed dates for this range from 403 to 222 BC) and, probably around the same time, incorporated the idea of the Five Elements into medicine. Along with many other long-established Vedic principles, they adopted the name "Five Elements" or "Five Phases" from the Vedic system. However, they developed new, *metaphoric* meanings for these terms.

The Vedic understanding of the Five Elements held that the Elements are created in a linear fashion, with the sound wave being the basis for the formation of denser waves of feeling, known as Air, or feeling/awareness/Love. These waves of Air can condense further into waves of light, known as the Element of Fire. Vibrations of light can, in turn, condense further still, into the vibrations that form electrons with a more limited movement patterns that allow the electrons to clump together: the Element of Water. Finally, in the Fifth Element, which is to say, in the most dense, highly compacted format of sound vibration, electrons move in the particular, stodgy, manner that allows matter to appear solid. This element, in the Vedas, is referred to as Earth.

Oppositely, when *solid* matter ceases to exist and reverts back to wave form, its breakup releases, sequentially, vibrations of all the five types: all five forms are present in solids. Solids are not made up of one particular type of vibration: electrons in solids are made up of sound vibrations that have condensed through each of the other four phases until the ensuing vibrations, and the electrons produced thereby, are relatively constrained.

On the other hand, when the matter (electrons) formed by vibrations of pure sound (the Element of Ether) reverts back into wave form, only sound occurs – no feeling of movement, light, liquids, or solids, are released. In vibrations of the purely Ether type, the other four Elements are not present.

In other words, the Five Elements are sequential, not circular. The Five Elements are like nesting dolls. The outermost doll is Ether. The inner dolls are denser, tighter derivatives of the outer doll. These dolls must be created and stored sequentially: they do not describe a creative circle.

However, in the dark ages, the Chinese deemed all *five* of the elements to be metaphors for *physical* phenomena – hence the minimal number of parallels between the Vedic and the Chinese systems of "Five Elements."

When the Chinese decided that the Five Elements were circular, and referenced them to physical aspects of nature, the highly scientific correspondences described in the Vedas (relating each Element to an organ's dominant energy pattern, to a particular sensory function, to a direction such as upward or inward) no longer made any sense.

Based on studying both the Chinese and the Vedic, it appears that *some* of the ancient correspondences were retained by the Taoists, but shuffled around and redistributed amongst the elements in a way that *sort* of made sense from a very naturalistic point of view.

Most significantly, the latter-day Chinese, in trying to make sense of the Five Elements during a darkening age, did not understand that Five Elements, and the transitions between them, are constituents of a universe with a definite Beginning and End. The waves that create the various electron movements condense to bring about the progression from an unmanifested idea of a universe, all the way to the seeming world of matter. Then, when attraction-based perception alters the point of reference, the waves are able to uncompress: matter reverts back again into unmanifested idea.

Instead, incorrectly assuming that everything that was, *always* was, and always *would be*, and that the universe was inherently constant, albeit ever-changing, the faulty assumption was made that the Five Elements created each other in an unending *circle* (not a series of wave events of increasing density). For this reason, and many other reasons, the correspondences of the Vedic Five Elements and the correspondences of the Chinese Five Elements do not match up very tightly.

As an aside, one of the many reasons that the Illustrious Buddha incarnated at approximately 500 BC, one hundred and fifty years into the most recent dark age, was to bring his message of "Getting off the wheel, or circle," of matter-based consciousness. An avatar, he came to Earth when circular philosophy, despite its essential message of hopelessness, was becoming increasingly dominant. By telling his followers that they could "get off the wheel, or circle," inherent in matter-oriented living, he was reminding them to get in touch with the peaceful, non-material *waves* of energy that can carry a person back to the Origin (as opposed to the tension-sustaining electrical currents and matter). He was trying to remind us of the possibility of riding these waves to the infinite (not circumscribed), eternal (not circular), ever-new Joy, a joy unaffected by the physical cycles of higher and darker ages – or the fleeting cycles of nature.

The following is a brief comparison of the Vedic and Chinese correspondences to the Elements. The quasi-relationship between Ether (Vedic) and Wood (Chinese) has already been mentioned.

In the Vedas, the second Element is referred to as Air: in Chinese medicine, this phase is called Fire. In the Vedas, this element is composed of condensed sound waves that create the illusion of movement and the feeling of (awareness of) movement. The body's primary organ for processing the waves and electrons created by these waves is the heart and pericardium. In the Vedic system *and* in the Chinese system, the heart is the organ most closely associated with the second element, which is to say, the element that "follows" Ether/Wood.

Ether and Air, the first two types of vibrations and their corresponding electrical currents, play a crucial part in creating the human body via their performance in the currents of channel Qi. These two types of vibrations enter the body at conception and make up the vibrational energy constituent of the "straight and narrow" energy path in the spine that includes the spinal chakras. This particular manifestation of vibrational energy, anciently known as Zhong Qi, or "Upright" Qi, is the Qi that drives the Du and Ren channels, in particular. From the Du and Ren, this type of channel Qi is distributed throughout the primary channels, being condensed, as needed, into the denser forms of vibrations and electrons. The energy in this spinal (Zhong Qi) system enables a living system to *seem* to resist entropy, gravity, and the laws of thermodynamics. This energy cohesively shimmers away from the body at death.

Again, the waves and electrons of these first two Elements, though unmanifested as physical matter (matter in which electrons get paired up with other subatomic bits such as protons), nevertheless flow in the *channels* of living systems and constitute two of the five different kinds of channel Qi.

The next three phases, or elements, have waves that are much denser. The third Phase, or Element, is found at the etheric boundary where electrons (paired somewhere in the universe with matching protons) pop in and out of *nearly* perceptible (material) existence.

This Phase is associated with atoms in a gaseous state. In Vedic philosophy, this element is called Fire, and corresponds with locomotion (the dynamic movement of created particles at the etheric interface), color (the *electromagnetic* light waves and photons that are emitted during wave-current transformations), the eyes (which perceive the colors), upward, expansive movement (typical of fire and gases), and with assimilation (ideas becoming tangible).

Compare the above third-element Vedic correspondences with the Chinese Elements: in Chinese medicine, locomotion is associated with the Earth element, the eyes are associated with Wood, upward expansion is associated with Metal, and assimilation is associated with Earth. As noted earlier, the Vedic system is a description of the actual physics of the forces involved, and it does not match up with the Chinese system of cyclical nature metaphors. So, for the purposes of comparison, and in the absence of a clean match up, I'll say, only *somewhat* arbitrarily, based on the locomotion aspect, that the Vedic element of Fire is mildly related to the Chinese element of Earth.

I only expounded on these associations with the third Element as an example to illustrate my assertion that the correspondences for the elements in the two systems, Vedic and Chinese, do *not* match up very tightly.

The fourth phase has vibrations of even greater density, and electrons that are firmly associated with various other electrons, forming the atoms of liquids. The Vedic name for this phase is Water. Medically, this phase is associated with reproduction and the genitals. The Chinese element associated with reproduction is also called Water, but is considered to be a precursor of Wood, rather than a third derivative of Wood.

The fifth Phase, or Element, refers to the extreme denseness of vibrations that create the electron behaviors and currents that occur in solid matter. The Vedic name for this element is Earth. This element is medically associated with smells and elimination – the nose and the rectum. The Chinese name for this phase is Metal.

Again, everything that appears to have a solid, physical existence is using all five types of waves *and* the five types of currents that are generated by these waves.

For further reference, the five elements are referred to, in Sanskrit, as the *Pancha Tattwas* (Five Elements, or Five Electricities) or collectively as the *mahatattvas* (Great Electricities).

For gentle introductions to this subject, please see *God Talks With Arjuna; The Bhagavad Gita: Royal Science of God Realization*, by Paramahansa Yogananda, Self-Realization Fellowship, 1995, p. 867-875. Also consider *The Holy Science*, by Swami Sri Yukteswar (1855-1936), date of composition, unknown. For availability in the US, this title is now published by Self-Realization Fellowship. In the 1990 edition, see: p. 26-30.

For further information on the antiquity of Vedic philosophy and the regular, well-documented transmission of Vedic lore, including Buddhist teachings derived from the Vedas, to many Chinese scholars, *many* sites on the Internet are available.

As an interesting aside, string theory, once cutting edge, then discredited, then re-credited, requires five different *types* of strings (*types* of vibrations) to account for observed quantum behavior. The five phases of vibration/currents, historically referred to as the Five Elements, *may* turn out to be the five necessary differentiations of strings. Historically, this would mean that mankind is rediscovering the original meaning of the Five Elements – right around the same time that most educated humans are once again able to appreciate that matter is, in fact, an illusion. Considering that the higher understanding of the Five Elements was lost at about the same time that mankind was no longer able to understand the delusive nature of matter, this rediscovery adds further weight to the ancient argument that humanity's capacity for experiential knowledge (like all artifacts in the material universe) is cyclical in nature, and that a dark age of the mind truly did exist.

Finally, and more to the point, each of the various channels is supposed to be *predominantly* one type of current. For example, the Liver and Gallbladder channels, which are referred to as Wood channels, are supposed to be *predominantly* filled with Ether-type, sound wave-derived electron

For example, the type of current that should be *dominant* in Wood channels is derived from causal, or thought-based vibrations. This type of current is very different from the denser electromagnetic waves that *should* predominate in Earth channels.

So when the Wood-type blend of currents flows in the *Spleen* channel, an Earth channel, as it did in this case study, it's a problem.

The predominance of the wrong type of channel Qi in any channel's route can cause dysfunction of the cellular and organ functions that are directed by that channel. Therefore, in this case study, even though there was plenty of channel Qi flowing in the patient's Spleen channel after the Liver channel surged into the Spleen channel just past LIV-5, the channel Qi in the Spleen channel was predominantly the wrong kind. The Spleen channel had become loaded, predominantly, with Liver, or Wood, channel Qi.

Or, to put it most simply, Wood was attacking Earth.

Important note: from this point on, this text will refer to the currents of channel Qi as if they are made up solely of "generic" electrons. The reader will always bear in mind that wave energy and various forms of condensed electrical energy also exist in the channels. However, for purposes of brevity, together with the fact that nearly all of our treatments, except for comfort and counseling, address the *electrical* behaviors of the channel Qi, channel Qi will be described as if it was constituted from basic electrical forces, as studied in high school physics.

Treatment

I placed a needle into the Liver channel just past the location at which Liver channel Qi was shunting into the Spleen channel. Which is to say, the needle was inserted "downstream," or "proximal," or even "closer to the LIV-6 side of the divergence than the

---

currents, with a minimum of the denser, matter-bound electron currents. These Wood channels are associated with our ability to imagine, create, be artistic, and to express ourselves. The subtle and relatively unconstrained type of electron movement should dominate in Wood channels. These types of electrons have far more potential energy and are much less restrained than the other, denser currents. This is why the Wood channels are most likely to attack (flow into) other channels, if stymied. In comparison, in the stodgy Earth and Metal channels, thought waves have become condensed, to a large degree, into conglomerations of electrons. The dense, movement-restricted electrical currents that predominate in Earth and Metal channel Qi are rarely able to overpower the higher potential-energy forces that predominantly drive the currents of Wood energy. This is why, except in cases of *physical* injury or channel obstruction, we rarely see Earth channels successfully attacking Wood channels.

All of the channels have some representation from *each* of the five types of currents. Still, each channel is associated predominantly with *one* of the Five Elements. The body works best if the appropriate Element for that channel is *dominant* and if only small amounts of currents from the other four Elements are present, and present in the correct ratio, for that channel.

To truly understand channel theory, you must appreciate that the channels are made up of five kinds of channel Qi, and each channel should be predominantly one of the five types. And now, back to the case study.

LIV-5 side of the divergence." In other words, I placed the needle at a point in the Liver channel that *should* have had channel Qi in it, but which didn't.

I stimulated the needle. The needle functioned like a lightening rod, quickly attracting Liver channel Qi back into the correct path of the Liver channel. I soon felt the tug on the needle suggesting that Liver channel Qi had started flowing in its own pathway again.

At this point, I checked the Spleen channel Qi down by the foot. It was already picking up in tempo and vigor. I felt farther up the leg, making sure that the Liver channel Qi was now moving freely all the way to LIV-14. I even checked to make sure that I could feel channel Qi emerging at Lung-1; I wanted to be sure that Liver channel Qi was making it all the way through the chest and re-emerging by the clavicle, as it should.

The channel Qi was now "going through," as we say in Asian medicine. No other needles were called for.

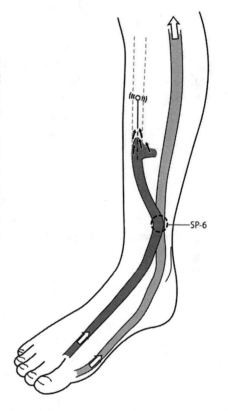

Fig. 2.2 A solid line topped by a vibrating circle represents the handle of the needle and a bit of the needle's shaft. A dashed line continuing down from the place where the solid line ends represents the under-the-skin part of the needle.
The needle insertion is just proximal to the blockage and perforates the blockage. With the needle in place, the blockage is no longer impervious to electrical flow – the needle provides a conductive path along which the channel Qi can flow. Liver channel Qi is thus able to flow in its correct path, perforating and breaking down the blockage.

Note the tiny arrows flowing towards the needle, showing the Liver channel Qi being actively attracted to the needle.

As the Liver channel Qi resumes flowing in its own bed, it ceases to attack the Spleen channel: the Spleen channel is once again filled with Spleen channel Qi.

Almost immediately, the patient felt better. He volunteered, "Something's changed." Several days later, in a follow-up phone call, he confirmed that he was feeling like his old self.

In terms of a western diagnosis, the area around LIV-5 and LIV-6 is often disrupted by pathogens that cause liver inflammation or, as we say in doctor-speak, hepatitis. The patient's "flu" symptoms, five weeks earlier, did match those of a mild form of Exterior-Wind (pathogen-based) illness moving Interior and Attacking Liver or, in this case, hepatitis.

In this patient, though the pathogen-induced portion of the illness was essentially over, Wood was continuing to attack Earth in the vicinity of LIV-5 and LIV-6 from mere habit. By directly treating the "attack site," the channel Qi flow was easily corrected – the patterns of the related health problems ceased.

Case Study #4

Wood Attacking Earth with emotional content

The following case study may seem more complex. However, it describes one of *the most common* patterns seen in our all-purpose acupuncture clinics in the United States. Although the principles may seem convoluted at first, just read through the case study for the overall sense of what is happening to the channel Qi flow. If you work regularly in a general-health clinic, within a few weeks of perusing this seemingly complex case study, you are certain to see a case in your clinic that will perfectly match the common scenario described below.

Liver Qi attacking Stomach channel in the torso

Female, age 52. The patient had experienced a mild "stomach flu" four weeks earlier.[1] She still had stomach discomfort, especially after eating, loss of appetite, frequent loose stools, acid indigestion, burping, depression and lassitude. She also had a wiry Liver pulse and weak Spleen pulse. Her tongue was pale, very slightly purple, and indented with teeth marks. Her diagnosis, based on pulse, tongue and symptoms, was Wood Attacking Earth, but quick scan of her channels using my hands showed a very different pattern than tht described in the preceding case study.

Channel Qi flow observations

The Liver channel Qi of her legs and torso was flowing correctly from her feet, up the legs, and even up so far as mid-torso, but it was not making it up to LIV-14, in the ribs. (Please refer to the map of the actual path of the Liver channel, at the back of the book.) Instead, a few inches inferior (closer to the feet) to LIV-14, the Liver channel Qi was flowing medially, into the Stomach channel. Stymied channel Qi will flow into whatever nearby pathway offers an opening with lower resistance. If the Liver channel is blocked, the Liver channel Qi (some of the most dynamic, powerfully driven channel Qi in the body) will flow into whatever nearby channel offers the least resistance. The powerful Wood-type channel Qi that predominates in the Liver channel can easily overwhelm the more modestly energized flow of channel Qi in a neighboring channel.

---

[1] I put the words "stomach flu" in quotes on behalf of the readers who know that "flu," technically, is short for "influenza," or "an infection settling in the lungs." However, the phrase "stomach flu" has become part of the vernacular. Patients often use the words "stomach flu" to refer to problems ranging from the rapid onset of food poisoning to the long-term gut discomfort of hepatitis, and even the butterflies in the stomach caused by emotional stress. In the above case studies, quote marks indicate that the *patient* referred to his own problem as "stomach flu," even though medical students know, technically, there is no such thing.

Her *Stomach* channel, which is supposed to flow downwards, towards the feet, was being flooded with upward flowing, head-bound, Liver channel Qi.

This surging of upward moving Qi was making palpable turbulence in the part of the Stomach channel that is superior (towards the head) from the point at which the Liver channel was dumping into it. In other words, because Liver channel Qi was flowing into the Stomach channel in the vicinity of ST-20, the Stomach channel Qi coming down from the head was not able to get past the attack location; below ST-20, very little Stomach channel Qi was present in the path of the Stomach channel. Very little Stomach channel Qi was flowing *down* through the torso, towards the feet.

Also, channel Qi in the chest portion of the Stomach channel that runs from ST-7 to ST-20 was moving in whorls – and its overall direction was *upwards*: towards the head! The channel Qi in the Stomach channel was being propelled upwards by the vigorous, headward-moving, Liver channel Qi. In the area below ST-20, the downward flowing Stomach channel Qi was deficient – hard to detect by hand.

Meanwhile, what about the Liver channel at LIV-14, and the Liver channel's path deep into the chest, emerging at LU-1?

Feeling for channel Qi at LU-1, there was no channel Qi to be felt: the Liver channel Qi was not getting through the chest and emerging at LU-1. Of course it wasn't – The Liver channel Qi was busy flowing sideways into the Stomach channel.

To summarize thus far: the Liver channel was attacking the Stomach channel at ST-20. The Stomach channel was therefore moving erratically in the area *superior* to ST-19, and was very weak (deficient) in the area inferior to ST-20. The Liver channel was *not* detectably flowing deeply into the chest and emerging at the surface again at LU-1. The Lung channel Qi flow was undetectable, deficient, at LU-1.

Now, we must consider the underlying cause of this very common pattern. Very often, the troublemaker, in these cases, is unrest, or tension, in the heart or pericardium.[1]

To understand this, a bit of preliminary information about the role of the heart and pericardium is in order.

The Fire element's influence on the channels in the chest

The electromagnetic fields of the heart and pericardium inform the Liver channel, as it flows nearby ("deep into the chest, beneath the Stomach channel") as to the manner (directions and amounts) in which Liver channel Qi should distribute itself upon exiting from the chest.

---

[1] The words heart and pericardium are *not* capitalized here, because they refer to the physical organs. When an organ name is capitalized, it refers to the Asian "organ system," a system that includes channels, physiological functions, and the organ itself. For example, a protozoa does not have physical organs of heart, kidney, and stomach, but it does have functions of Heart (internal cellular movement), Kidney (reproduction) and Stomach (digestion).

In general, when a word in this text is unexpectedly capitalized, the word is being used to represent an Asian medicine concept, rather than the usual English sense of the word.

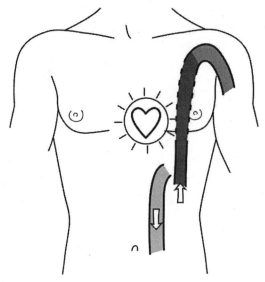

Fig. 2.3: A peaceful heart: the pericardium, represented by the circle around the heart, is open wide, relaxed, peaceful.

The Liver channel (indicated with the darkest shading) passes near to the heart when it flows deep into the chest. If the heart is at peace, the Liver channel Qi converts into Lung channel Qi (the medium shading) after passing by the heart.

The Stomach channel (the lightest shading) is shown traveling down the torso. The over-the-breast portion of the Stomach channel, which passes close to the surface of the skin, is not shown, thus allowing us to see the Liver channel, which travels more deeply inside (indicated by dashed lines), directly beneath the pectoral part of the Stomach channel.

If a person is calm, the electromagnetic fields of the heart and pericardium will project an "everything's OK" signal. When the Liver channel Qi passes deep through the chest in the presence of an "OK" signal, most of the Liver channel Qi flows back up to the surface of the skin at LU-1, and thence down the arms, following the Lung channel. Only a very small amount of Liver channel Qi diverts up to the vertex, and is distributed to various locations in the brain and to the eyes.

But if the heart is wary (in sympathetic, fight-or-flight mode), the heart and pericardium give off a different signal. This wary signal resonates with the channel Qi of the Liver channel in a way that causes much more of the Liver channel Qi to flow to the head. When a person is fearful, he diverts more Qi to the brain and eyes. And therefore, as the head gets more channel Qi than usual, the Lung channel gets less than usual.

Fig. 2.4 Mild emotional stress or fear: the pericardium is tightening up around the heart.

Notice that the Ren channel provides a "backup" supply of channel Qi to the Lung channel when more of Liver channel is being diverted to the vertex. The Ren channel Qi flows somewhat deeply (indicated by dashed lines) as it approaches the arm and flows into the Lung channel. Although you *will* be able to feel Lung channel Qi in the arm in this situation, you may *not* be able to feel any channel Qi in the near-clavicle points of LU-1 and LU-2, where the end of the Liver channel is supposed to transition into the beginning of the Lung channel – close to the surface of the skin.

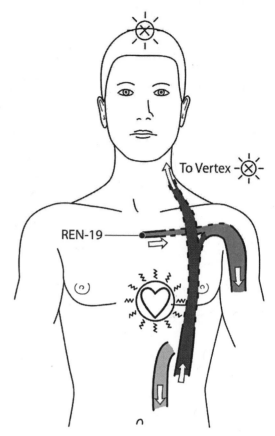

In yet another possible scenario, if the heart emotions have been *deeply* traumatized, the heart and pericardium may give such an altered electromagnetic signal that the Liver channel, or most of the Liver channel, will be unable to pass through the chest. In this case, when the Liver channel Qi is significantly blocked, or "stagnant," the Liver channel Qi will spill sideways, diverting into whatever nearby channel offers the least electrical resistance.

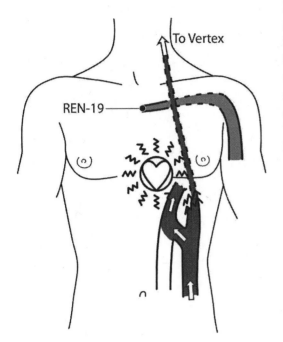

Fig. 2.5 A High degree of emotional stress or fear: the pericardium is tightened around the heart. The tightness may cause palpitations (awareness of the physical sensations of the heart-beat). The electro-magnetic signals from the heart signify "danger." The darker zigzag lines being given off by the heart are meant to illustrate a higher level of fear or anxiety than the milder zigzags in Fig. 2.4. The electro-magnetic field being given off by the heart creates a form of blockage, indicated by the double row of zigzag lines, obstructing the normal flow of Liver channel Qi. The degree of blockage depends on the degree to which the signal has been modified by stress of fear.

Note the various confusions that ensue in the Stomach channel: The darkest shading, signifying Liver channel Qi, is running sideways into the Stomach channel, and then flowing upwards via the path of the Stomach channel that runs *over* the pectoral area. This upward flowing Liver channel Qi in the Stomach channel can create an unsettled sensation in the stomach (burping, indigestion, acid reflux, and even the sensation of butterflies, or as it is called in Chinese, "Running Piglets.") At the same time, the lower part of the Stomach channel, below the point of attack, has been drawn with no shading in it, showing that it is nearly devoid of Stomach channel Qi. If the pectoral portion of the Stomach channel had been shown, it would be a jumble of Stomach channel Qi and Liver channel Qi, trying to flow both up (Liver) and down (Stomach) at the same time – with the Liver channel usually winning out.

Although the illustration suggests a neat "attack" point, the truth is messier. The decrease of Stomach channel Qi in the lower part of the Stomach channel will serve as a convenient "hollow" into which channel Qi can flow from other areas on the stymied Liver channel. After the initial attack creates diminished flow in portion of the Stomach channel inferior to the attack point, Liver channel Qi may well "spread out," attacking the Stomach channel from ST-19 or -20 all the way down the inferior end of the torso at ST-30. In the abdomen, the Liver channel and Stomach channel traverse much of the same turf. In the front torso of a healthy person, the Stomach channel flows closest to the surface of the skin, the Liver channel just below it, or "deeper."

Even if the heart is feeling peaceful, if Stomach or Spleen channel Qi is deficient somewhere, the Liver channel may well flow into the deficient areas – areas of lowered resistance.

If the heart is fearful or anxious, the "worried" route of Liver channel Qi will be triggered. Some portion of Liver channel Qi will flow to the vertex, but the main path, towards the Lung channel, will encounter a blockage: heart-generated high resistance. The Liver channel Qi will be unable to flow to the Lung channel. Instead, the stymied portion of the Liver channel Qi will flow into the path of least resistance or, as we say in Asian medicine, "Attack" whatever nearby channel happens to be the weakest.

To sum up, emotional tensions have an effect on signals generated by the heart or pericardium. These, in turn, influence Liver channel behavior at the point where the Liver channel passes near to the heart, deep in the chest.

A pathological "divergent" path

Getting back to the case study, I could feel with my hand that the patient's Liver channel Qi was flowing "sideways," into her Stomach channel, via a spontaneous, non-standardized, which is to say, pathological, divergent path. I started looking for the location at which the Liver channel was getting dammed up – the blockage that was causing the divergence.

Suspecting heart and pericardium, I let my hand move slowly up the patient's Ren channel. The Ren channel was barely moving, and stopped cold between Ren-14 and Ren-16. Channel Qi wasn't flowing at *all* through the heart/pericardium alarm points on the Ren channel.

Next, still curious about the heart and pericardium condition, I felt for the Qi flow in her wrists, in the Heart and Pericardium channel areas. The Pericardium channel's Qi flow was nearly non-existent. Because her Pericardium channel was very deficient, I wondered if the actual organ of the pericardium was being stressed (was deficient in Qi), and if so, why? Had there been physical damage to the pericardium tissues? Were there injuries along the Pericardium channel? I didn't know. Another possibility for this pericardium deficiency was that maybe the Liver channel wasn't providing enough channel Qi to the pericardium.

As an aside, the Liver channel, in addition to being influenced by the heart and pericardium, when it flows deeply into the chest, is also a major supplier of energy to the chest. In other words, the Liver channel itself helps provide vigor to the physical heart and pericardium. In this case, the Liver channel was no longer flowing deeply into the chest. I had to wonder if her Liver channel diversion was one reason for her pericardium channel Qi weakness.

In summary, we were looking at a somewhat complex, but fairly common situation: her Liver channel could not flow past the "I've been traumatized" signal in the chest emanating from the heart and pericardium. Then again, the pericardium channel might be deficient because the pericardium *organ* was receiving so little Liver channel support. Or, making it all the more interesting, the *deficiency* in the pericardium might now be the reason for the "trauma" signal being transmitted by the heart and pericardium – a signal that, in turn, was inhibiting the flow of Liver channel Qi through the chest! Which came first? Did it matter? Meanwhile, the Liver channel was shunting into her Stomach channel. Her channels were certainly not harmonized.

And what of the repercussions of these channel aberrations? Because the Liver channel Qi was dumping into the Stomach channel, the Stomach channel Qi was not able to flow the length of the body as it should, invigorating the legs and feeding the Spleen channel. This was inhibiting healthy digestion, and the energy that *derives* from healthy digestion (Earth, and particularly, Spleen energy).

Diagnosis

My thinking ran like this: most likely, when the patient's "stomach flu" caused the initial weakness in her Stomach channel, the pathogens and its toxins also caused a bit of extra work for her Liver. Her "stomach flu" may have even been a mild type of liver-attacking pathogen, a mild form of hepatitis. Or not.

Prior to her "stomach flu" episode, she'd had ongoing, low-grade emotional stress. This admitted stress had evidently not been strong enough to significantly impede the flow of healthy Liver channel Qi. But when the Liver channel Qi was weakened by the pathogen, the Liver channel Qi was no longer vigorous enough to get past her usual emotional (pericardial) block. Instead, it began flowing into the nearest channel that offered less resistance than the chronically somewhat-blocked path through the chest.

Because her stomach was mildly weakened by the bug, her Stomach channel Qi was temporarily less vigorous than usual. This weakness in the flow of her Stomach channel Qi created a condition in which it was easier for the Liver channel to flow in the path of the Stomach channel than it was for the Liver channel to get past the somewhat-impeding "I'm not *completely* OK" signal coming from the pericardium.

Even when weakened, Liver channel Qi, like all channel Qi, will follow the path of least electrical resistance. Under these conditions – a skittish pericardium and a weak Stomach channel – Liver channel Qi will find it easier to flow into the route of the Stomach channel than to flow in the "normal" Liver channel route that flows nearby the pericardium on its way to the clavicle, at LU-1.[1]

---

[1] The subject of electrical flow following the path of least resistance merits further discussion. But for now, in this quick footnote, it might be of interest merely to consider how modern scholars of Chinese medicine have given much deliberation to the translation of the ancient character that refers to what we, in English, call "acupuncture points." Many scholars feel that the word "hole," or "emptiness," best satisfies the meaning of the ancient, Chinese character.

But a better translation for the "acupoint" character might possibly be "hole: point of no resistance," or "point of less resistence."

As channel Qi flows through the body, it travels from one point of low resistance to the next. Research shows that, unlike, say, "trigger points," which are points of increased electrical resistance, the classic acupoints are points of decreased electrical resistance. That is to say, as channel Qi flows from one acupoint to the next along the course of the channel, it follows the path of least resistance. We might choose to say that channel Qi flows from one "hole" to the next, but if we speak in terms of "path of least resistance," it keeps the same meaning as "hole" and makes much more sense given our modern appreciation of electrical systems. With this translation, we can understand more easily why the channel systems can go awry: when pathologies occur, which is to say, when channels are blocked, creating resistance, and channel Qi then flows in an aberrant manner, the channel Qi still flows

With this new state of affairs – her Liver channel diverting into her Stomach channel – her digestion was thrown for a loop. The Liver Qi was upsetting the downwards flow of the Stomach's peristalsis – to say nothing of it filling the upper part of the Stomach channel with the wrong direction and type (wrong Element) of electron movement.

Then, with decreased energy because of impaired appetite and digestion, paired with a decrease in the amount of Liver channel Qi being delivered to her heart and pericardium, she didn't have the emotional, love-of-life energy needed to address her fairly mild, chronic emotional problems. She became depressed, with low appetite, and fatigue.

Now, based on channel movement (channel theory), her diagnosis was Wood attacking Earth with Fire deficiency. Was this channel diagnosis supported by her symptoms? Yes.

Lassitude and lack of appetite: these were very possibly caused by the lack of Stomach channel Qi and the ensuing Spleen channel Qi deficiency (Stomach channel Qi exits into, or "feeds" the Spleen channel). This looked like a case of "pain" (lassitude, loss of appetite), due to channel Qi not "going through."

Burping and indigestion: where the Liver channel was "attacking" the Stomach channel, it was causing the backwards and somewhat chaotic flow of Stomach channel Qi between St-7 and St-18. This chaotic Qi flow was preventing the normal flow of peristalsis: instead, the patient had burping and indigestion.

Depression: the diversion of the Liver channel Qi, which was taking a hairpin turn into the Stomach, meant that the Liver channel couldn't flow in the manner it flows best: rapidly and smoothly, with no resistance, from the feet to the clavicle, flowing easily past the heart. The ensuing slowing and lack of smoothness in the Liver channel as it careened into the Stomach channel was preventing the patient from feeling that creative, energetic zest for life that comes when the Liver channel runs rapidly, and smoothly, at the peak of its form.

Yes, the patient's symptoms could certainly be explained by this conglomeration of channel Qi confusions.

Inertia

Once channels start running in an aberrant manner, they might stay that way. If the altered, aberrant patterns are electrically *stable* enough, they can persevere indefinitely. A body at rest, or in motion, will tend to *stay* at rest, or in the same motion, until force is applied that alters its state.

On the other hand, if the signals from the heart and mind are correct and strong enough, they can correct any aberration.

In this patient, given her constant, though mild, levels of stress, her pathological channel divergences and ensuing weaknesses *might* have stayed that way indefinitely. Without treatment, or some sort of alteration in attitude, lifestyle, or shock, her Liver channel might easily have continued flowing into her Stomach channel indefinitely – even for the rest of her life.

---

according to the laws of physics: it still follows the path of least resistance: Like water, it flows to the nearest low spot, or "hole."

The patient hadn't developed the rare presence of mind and heart to recognize intuitively that her channels were running amok. Without a life-style change, brain wave change, some appalling, life-threatening, or otherwise intrusive event, or some form of medicinal shock such as acupuncture, magnet or laser therapy, or chemical medicine such as herbs, her channels could have continued like this for a long, long time.

In summary, her basic diagnosis was Wood Attacking Earth. More specifically, her Liver channel was being blocked at the heart or pericardium, causing the Liver channel to attack the Stomach channel, just a few inches below LIV-14. In addition, she could have been diagnosed with pericardium deficiency, Stomach and Spleen deficiency, and Liver deficiency.

In terms of root causes, it looked like one of those "which came first, the chicken or the egg" situations. So I stopped wondering about "initial cause." Whether the "flu" or some emotional crisis was the *start* of this jumbled state of affairs, *all* the incorrect channels – Liver, Pericardium, Stomach – had to be restored to health.

Where should I begin to treat the patient?

Treatment

The treatment would have to move Liver channel Qi past the pericardium. If successful, this restoration, or "harmonization," would restore energy to the pericardium, *and* bring an end to the Liver channel's divergence into the Stomach channel.

Before moving Liver channel Qi through the chest, I inserted a needles at right- and left-side LU-1 (Lung-1). I was soon going to get the Liver channel moving past her pericardium. When it did, I wanted the needles at LU-1 to act like lightening rods to make *most* of the Liver channel transition into the Lung channel – as it does in a relaxed, healthy person. If I didn't start by inserting needles at LU-1, there was the risk of *all* the newly released Liver channel Qi getting past the pericardium and flowing up the Liver channel's vertex pathway, to the head. This could potentially give her a powerful head-ache or make her feel edgy.

I tried stimulating the needles that I'd inserted at LU-1 but got no response in the needles. As noticed already, LU-1 was essentially a Qi-free zone. Still, with these needles in place, some of the Liver channel Qi might be attracted to them – once it was able to get past the obstructive signal, or "knot" in the chest.

I next inserted needles on the wrists, at HT-7 and P-6, to act as lightening rods to carry channel Qi into these channels when the Liver channel did start to flow through the chest. This would give an energetic boost to the heart and pericardium.

Then, I inserted the most re-directing point of the treatment, LIV-14. I immediately began rhythmically stimulating the pairings of LU-1 with LIV-14, first on the left side, then on the right, then left, then right. I stimulated each pair, thus encouraging the flow of channel Qi up through the chest from LIV-14 to LU-1. The needles at the clavicles soon picked up the faint trickle of energy that was now being forced, via the needles, to move past the pericardium. I checked for a sense of returning energy in the Pericardium channel and Heart channel points that I'd needled. A bit of Qi sensation now tugged back at me when I gently felt for channel Qi in the needles in the wrists.

38

To make a big surge in the Liver channel, now that the "Qi-directing" needles were in place and evidently working, I inserted needles at GB-41.

The Gallbladder channel runs from the head down to the feet. In a healthy, relaxed person, Gallbladder-41 is the point on the foot from which *much* of the Gallbladder channel Qi usually flows over into the Liver channel. Any remaining Gallbladder channel Qi flows down to the lateral toes where it either moves medially across the tips of the toes and into the Liver channel at LIV-1, or else grounds out, as needed. [1]

In this patient's case, the needles into GB-41 seemed to perk up the amount of channel Qi in the Liver channel. This increase in Liver channel Qi further activated the needles at LIV-14. With my hand running along the length of the patient's Liver channel, keeping my hand about an inch above the patient's clothing, I felt the channel Qi flow in the Liver channel. The amount of channel Qi in the Liver channel had increased noticeably. As, once again, I *very* gently moved the needles at LU-1 the tiniest bit, in an up and down direction, I began to feel a good increase in the "tug" on the needles. Channel Qi was flowing better now, from LIV-14 to LU-1.

I checked the wrists. The amount of channel Qi flow in the wrists had picked up further.

Most importantly, within a few moments, the Liver channel stopped flowing into the Stomach channel. At the same time that the Liver channel stopped flowing medially into the Stomach channel, the Qi flow into the LU-1 needles surged. The entire length of the Stomach channel also began flowing easily, and in the *correct* direction.

In summary, the treatment primarily involved restoring the flow of Liver channel Qi through the depths of the chest. This, in turn, ended the Liver channel's divergence into the Stomach channel. This cessation allowed the Stomach channel Qi to automatically resume its correct flow. At the same time, the pericardium and heart were invigorated because the Liver channel, the "liveliest" channel, the "channel of the blue-green dragon," was once again flowing past the heart and pericardium.

Almost immediately, the patient felt more relaxed. A few days later, a follow-up phone call found the patient feeling stronger. Her appetite had returned, her digestion was fine, and she was emotionally "smoothed out."

---

[1] Many acupuncturists needle LIV-3 to create a surge in the Liver channel. Some of my teachers prefer to use GB-41 when giving a nudge to the Liver channel: if the Liver channel is badly blocked, needling LIV-3 may just cause pain and increase the amount of Liver channel Qi that is being misdirected – while doing nothing to straighten out the Liver channel Qi. By using GB-41, we can increase channel Qi at the point where channel Qi becomes *available* to the Liver channel. The body can then decide how much channel Qi should go into the Liver channel, and how much should ground out in the toes. The body gets to decide how much it needs, rather than having a surge forced directly into the Liver channel at LIV-3. As one teacher who preferred GB-41 to LIV-3 said to me, "The Liver doesn't like to be pushed around."

Reviewing the above two case studies

Without using channel diagnosis

Using only symptoms and/or tongue and pulse, a diagnosis of "Wood attacking Earth" could justifiably been given to both these cases. The diagnosis would have been correct, so far as it went. In both cases, the Liver channel, known as "Wood," was attacking (flowing sideways into and disrupting) the Spleen channel or the Stomach channel, both of which are known as "Earth." Also, in both cases, the Liver Qi was stagnant – blocked up at some point along its channel, and therefore, shunting into some other channel.

But the diagnosis of Wood Attacking Earth or Liver Qi Stagnation does not tell the beginning practitioner what treatment to choose, or how to immediately *know* if he's successfully treated the condition. Consider the first case study in this chapter (case study #3) – where channel Qi was diverting from the Liver channel into the Spleen channel down on the lower leg. *If* the patient in case study #3, above, had received the treatment of case study #4, with needles inserted into the Heart and Pericardium channels at the wrists, and at LU-1, LIV-14, and GB-41, the Liver channel Qi might very well have continued attacking the Spleen channel on the leg. The patient's condition would *not* have improved.

Oppositely, if the patient in case study #4 had been needled between LIV-5 and LIV-6, which was the treatment from case study #3, the torso portion of the Liver channel would have continued diverting into the Stomach channel's path. Again, the patient's condition would probably *not* have improved.[1]

The "informed guess" treatment

In many cases, a beginning student, confronted with a condition that suggests either a pattern of Wood Attacking Earth or a pattern of Liver Qi Stagnation, performs a "treatment" by needling LIV-3 and LI-4 or some other "harmonizing" treatment. The more famous two- or three-point combos of acupoints, also known variously as "Four Gates," or, "When in doubt, Harmonize," sometimes work. They work because acupuncture stimulation at these strong "collecting" points is capable of sending a relatively large surge of current through the Yang Ming system (which includes the Stomach channel) and the Jue Yin system (which includes the Liver). (Some doctors prefer Lung or Spleen (Tai Yin) points, instead of Yang Ming, in combo with the Jue Yin for their basic harmonizing treatment. Either way, it works:

---

[1] Unlike the more general term "Wood Attacking Earth," the pattern known as "Liver Qi Stagnation" or even "Being Woody" is most often understood to mean the type of situation described in this chapter's second case study: an *emotional* blockage creating restriction in the area of the pericardium which, in turn, prevents the Liver Qi from passing through the chest easily. In these cases, the Liver Qi becomes somewhat "knotted," or "stagnant," in the torso as it wends its way into a less-than-ideal pathway.

When I was first studying Asian medicine, my fellow students and I, with an insouciance born of beginner's knowledge, often tossed about the term "Liver Qi Stagnation" for any Liver- or emotion-related problem. None of us really knew what the term meant: we certainly hadn't learned yet how to track down the underlying cause – the *real* diagnosis.

Now I ask my clinic students, before they start a patient's treatment, to explain to me *why*, as a *side effect*, the Liver Qi in the torso has become stagnant. A good diagnostician may implicate pericardium, heart, pathogen, scar tissue, or whatever is applicable, in explaining *why* the Liver Qi has become stymied.

the channel Qi is joggled loose from its incorrect path, and resumes flowing in the correct, or "harmonized" manner.)

The defibrillator method of acupuncture

This surge-based treatment works along the same principles of a heart defibrillator. A heart defibrillator does *not* reset the super-fast, steady-state, fibrillating heart to a predetermined slower pace: it shocks the heart into a completely random, highly charged state.[1] The hope of the person wielding the defibrillator is that, when the patient's heart falls back down into *some* steady state, the heart will *chance* into the particular steady state that is most healthy: seventy beats a minute instead of, say, seventy *times three*. Of course, sometimes, after applying the defibrillator, the heart shifts into a steady state that is still not optimal – maybe one hundred and forty, or two hundred and ten. If so, the defibrillator is applied again. Eventually, if defibrillated (destabilized) enough times, odds are good that the heart will chance into the more peaceful rate of approximately seventy beats per minute.

Until the heart settles down, by chance, into a *healthy*, which is to say, "slow" steady state, we can keep applying the defibrillator, destabilizing the system in the hopes that it will eventually settle back down into the system we want. It's not an *exacting* treatment, but it is a treatment, of sorts. Sometimes we get lucky, and it works.

An all-purpose Four Gates-type treatment for Wood Attacking Earth works in very much the same way as a defibrillator: by stimulating the strongest acupoints we've got for the channels that apparently aren't happy, which is to say, by creating a surge of energy that powers through the Wood and Earth systems, we cause them to surge, and possibly, jump out of their pathological flow patterns, just for a bit. After the initial shock, as the channel Qi settles back down, the odds are somewhat good that the channel Qi will resume flow in the *correct* pathways – no matter where they were prior to the jolt. After all, when in a state of physical and emotional health, the correct pathways do present the path of least resistance.

And yet, as many acupuncture students have learned, Four Gates only works sometimes. Four Gates is a "shake 'em up" treatment that doesn't necessarily get rid of an underlying glitch. It is an attempt to power-through a snafu in the hopes that "everything will be all right in the end if we startle the system violently enough."[2]

---

[1] The heart's electrical rhythms are usually in what is called a "steady state." A steady state electrical rate is a rate that can be maintained easily because the rate equals, or is a multiple of, some factor of the equation that defines the system. The electrical driver of an adult heart might be steady at, say, seventy cycles per minute, or at one hundred and forty (70 x 2) cycles per minute, or at two hundred and ten (70 x 3) cycles per minute, or at two hundred and eighty 70 x 4) cycles per minute, and so on.

[2] Interviews with people who have survived lightening strikes often elicit remarks such as "certain health problems were completely eradicated after the lightening strike." This is testimony to the ability of the body's channels to "drop back" into the most harmonized, "most relaxed" or "lowest" energy-requirement state following an "defibrillation-type" electrical shock.

Acupuncture needling, in some cases, provides a similar, but miniscule, shock. When the channels are harmonized (running correctly), they are running in the pattern that requires the least energy to sustain while, at the same time, providing energy in a manner that allows correct life-processes to occur most easily. When the channels are harmonized, correct living becomes nearly effortless. As a corollary, when one lives and thinks correctly, which is to say, in attunement with

If, instead of guesswork, we feel the flow of channel Qi in a patient, and then compare the *patient's* flow patterns with what we know to be the *correct* patterns, we don't have to guess, or use one-size-fits-most treatments. We can tell exactly what the problem is and where, and we know exactly what we need to do to fix it.[1]

---

natural law, the channels tend to remain harmonized. This latter point is strongly emphasized in the opening sections of the *Nei Jing*.

Then again, I recall reading a case study of a person who, shockingly, was hit by lightening *twice*. He was rendered instantly deaf by the first strike. Years later, his hearing was instantly restored by the second one. Another person who was hit by lightening reported that, following the shock, although he was a mail carrier in Minnesota, he was never again cold. After the lightening strike, he delivered mail, even during the depths of winter, never wearing more than his summer uniform of shorts and a short-sleeved shirt. Possibly, his body had been shocked in such a way that either he had a surplus of Yang (vibratory) energy for the rest of his life, or his ego-based delusion of sensitivity to temperature was destroyed by the blast. In any case, these are examples of *high* intensity electrical shake-ups. Acupuncture is far milder and less risky than a lightening strike, but an acupuncture guesswork treatment, such as Four Gates, nevertheless relies pretty much on the same principles.

[1] Although this book is written primarily for acupuncturists, the theory applies to herbology, as well. In the case of an herbalist, the discovery of unhealthy divergent channel Qi in both of these cases would have suggested that a *harmonizing* formula, such as Xiao Chai Hu Tang or Relaxed Wanderer, and not a tonifying formula, would best meet the case. We never tonify when a condition is excess.

A blockage is always what Asian medicine calls an "Excess" condition. The blockage is a form of Stagnation. Stagnation is always an "Excess" condition. A channel diverges into a second channel (Attacks) *because* of a Blood or Qi blockage in the first channel. Therefore, a divergence or Attack situation is always excessive.

The patients in these two cases had only *seeming* deficiency in their Earth channels (symptoms of lethargy, weakness, lack of appetite). This seeming deficiency was due to channel Qi diversions (Attacks) coming from their Wood channels. They did *not* have a true deficiency in the Earth channels. (For the benefit of the reader who is not familiar with Asian terms of Deficiency and Excess, causes of *true* deficiency in this case, if any, might have included poor nutrition or loss of blood.)

Therefore, an herbalist would avoid tonifying herbs, and focus instead on harmonizing (channel Qi-path rectifying) herbs for these two patients.

"There are a vast number of symptoms caused by unorthodox pathogens [also known as "Evil Wind"] that penetrate into meridians and then move forward into various parts of the body. If such symptoms are treated without reference to the root and fruits of meridians, pathogens will attack five viscera and six bowels." [1]

Chapter three

Case Study Examples: Exterior Evil-Wind

A stab in the strep

Next, let's briefly consider a case study from another set of conditions: Exterior Wind, or, pathogen-based illness.

When a person is first sick with a pathogenic illness (symptoms are still on the exterior), or just *before* he becomes overtly sick, assessment of his channel Qi flow will already reveal that his channel Qi has become disrupted at some location that is crucial to either the immune system or mental clarity or both. Some of the common locations that manifest disruption during attack from a pathogen are Du-14, UB-11 and -40, LI-4 and -11, LU-7, LIV-5 and -6, and Yin Tang.

Curiously, in any given flu season, when a specific germ is making the rounds, all the people who have the same bug tend to have the same locations of disruption in their channel Qi. It almost seems as if a particular pathogen's nature causes the destabilization of a particular location on a channel. It's possible that a sick body's alterations in channel flow correspond to electrical fields inherent in the structure and function of the pathogens. [2]

---

[1] *Ling Shu*, chapter 5-1, from *A Complete Translation of the Yellow Emperor's Classics of Internal Medicine and the Difficult Classic (Nei-Jing and Nan-Jing)*, Henry C. Lu, PhD, International College of Traditional Chinese Medicine of Vancouver, 2004,

[2] As western researchers in the field of pathogen proliferation are aware, many pathogens can lie low in the human body, replicating slowly but not causing detectable illness, until they amass a certain quantity. When the quantity is sufficient, the pathogens suddenly start wreaking havoc: replicating in a different, more blatant, manner. The body, finally aware of the invader, then starts fighting back. Western researchers have no idea what the signal is that the pathogens send to each other signifying that they now have enough members on board to begin the aggressive phase of their invasion.

But western researchers do know that a *possibly* concomitant factor can be neurotransmitter levels. Researchers have seen that the decrease in norepinephrine that occurs with stress or mood changes *sometimes* precedes the sudden proliferation. For example, in cases of some "dormant" pathogens residing in the body, such as the chickenpox virus (Herpes Zoster) that hides in the spine after the initial outbreak of chickenpox, and which later causes shingles, it has been proposed that the dormant pathogens may "wake up" in response to specific chemical changes in the body, such as an

As an aside, from the perspective of pure biology, one measure of a truly effective pathogen might be its ability to turn off its host's immune system, while still allowing the host to stay alive and provide a site for replication of the pathogen. Therefore, most human pathogens, in order to be successful, must have a method by which they can destabilize the human immune system to some degree, without actually killing the host.

One important factor in keeping the immune system optimized is correct "mental posture," an aspect of what one might call "will power." If a pathogen can diminish mental clarity, or otherwise alter the mind's ability to use focused will, so much the better – from the perspective of the pathogen. This is why, in sick people, we often see that Du 14, UB 10, or Yin Tang has been destabilized. Many highly successful pathogens destabilize the immune system *and* inhibit mental function.

We can hypothesize that the electromagnetic waves inherent in the structure and electrical function of the pathogen serve to *counter* some crucial electrical flow in the human host. Very possibly the human's channel Qi is altered when the pathogens have slowly, stealthily generated sufficient units of the pathogen. Then, the *sum* of the electromagnetic fields of the many pathogens units is large enough to contradict or alter, and thus destabilize, the electromagnetic field in some crucial channel Qi flow pattern in the human host. In other words, when enough of the microorganisms have been created within a human that the sum of the electromagnetic fields of the pathogen is large enough to influence the human channel Qi flow pattern, some pathogen-specific, crucial spot in the human's channel system ceases to flow correctly. When this occurs, the ensuing changes in the human's channels, organs, and

---

observed decrease in norepinephrine levels. Then again, perhaps the actual trigger is something else, and lowered norepinephrine levels preceding outbreaks of illness are circumstantial. For example, many people are familiar with the ability to stave off the flu until the stress level drops. When a long-awaited vacation finally begins, or the Big Project at work is finally over, so that the channel Qi shifts back into parasympathetic mode from sympathetic mode, the latent flu manifests.

For most pathogens, which multiply slowly until some critical "attack" mass is reached, the actual trigger that tells them when to go forth and multiply aggressively is not yet known to those western researchers who study the surge phenomenon. At present, western researchers are looking for some pathogen-produced *chemical* that allows the pathogens to "communicate with each other" that the critical mass has been attained.

The changes we can detect in pathogen-induced channel flow irregularities suggest a completely different, non-chemical mechanism: the alterations that occur in human channel Qi flow due to resonance with the electromagnetic properties of the pathogen may provide the "attack signal." A stealthy increase in the number of pathogenic warriors causes an increase in "amperage" in the pathogen's signal. Then, possibly, when there is enough "amperage" in the electrical signal deriving from the pathogen that the host's channel Qi pathways are slightly altered, the subsequent, channel-based changes in the *person's* chemical and organ function create the situation that signals "Go!" to the pathogen. Or even more directly, it's possible that the actual alteration in electromagnetic signals generated by the person's altered channel Qi may initiate the "replicate more quickly" segments of the pathogen's genetic material. At any rate, a change in pathogenic function based on electrical forces (channel Qi of the pathogen and the host) would be far simpler than the postulated chemical event proposed by western researchers. And truth tends to follow the simpler path.

44

overall chemistry may serve as the signals that instruct the pathogen to "tear of his mask" and get down to the vigorous business of replicating as fast as he can.[1]

The various types of pathogens each have somewhat different electromagnetic fields, and therefore, the destabilizing patterns vary from one bug to another. Assessment of channel Qi in people with early stage "Evil-Wind" (pathogen-based illness) shows that some pathogens destabilize the channel Qi flow at the back of the neck, near Du-14 and UB-11. Others disrupt the channel Qi flow at LI-4, LU-7, or in the Luo channel that connects LU-7 to LI-4. Still other common sites that, if disrupted, will turn down the immune system's ability to give peak performance are UB-40, LI-11, and Yin Tang. Following disruption at these points, some type of body function will be compromised. The compromise may be in immune function, mental function, or some other body function, or a combination.

Following the poor function of whichever system has been compromised, the pathogen is able to thrive quickly. The body does then respond (hopefully), but its optimum response has become inhibited by the alterations in channel Qi flow. The channel alterations, plus the less-than-elegant response that the altered body is then able to perform, together with the body's responses to both the presence of the pathogen and any toxic by-products of the pathogen, is what we call illness "symptoms." The time at which channel destabilization occurs is the point at which symptoms start to appear. This is the point when, based on symptoms, tongue, pulse, and other patterns, we can determine that the illness is starting to generate symptoms of either wind-cold or wind-heat.[2]

---

[1] Of course, the type of pathogen that is able to lie dormant for long periods of time (weeks or years) must have an electrically invisible resting phase in which his channel Qi pattern is in relative harmony with his host's until such time as the host is destabilized by some other event. Oppositely, the type of pathogen that kills within twenty-four hours or so need not bother with destabilizing the host's immune system. A hyper-virulent pathogen simply starts munching on his host, throwing off toxins, and boom: the host dies quickly. From a purely biological perspective, these pathogens are not necessarily the most "successful" in the long term: they kill off their own food supply. The pathogens that cause plague, for example, have very little activity in the decades that follow one of their feeding binges.

The "two-week viruses," on the other hand, such as measles, chicken pox, and other "common" illnesses, are able to find a home in nearly every human. Because they rarely kill their host, they are able to travel more, infect more people, and allow their hosts to replicate – providing new generations of hosts. These are the pathogens that tend to have a mechanism for destabilizing, somewhat, the host's immune system. These are also the pathogens that "weed out" the weakest hosts, helping the host species naturally "select" for the stronger immune systems. In terms of pure biology, both the pathogen and the host species benefit from this type of relationship.

[2] In Asian medicine terminology, if a "wind-borne" (or invisibly transmitted, at any rate) pathogen does not generate symptoms, it is as if the pathogen did not exist – it certainly is not a problem. The invisible pathogen is only *Evil* Wind if it is making a person sick. If a pathogen is minding its own business, being a part of nature, and not causing problems in a human, it is *not* being "Evil." It is just being itself. As for the word "Wind," this word applies even if the pathogen is food-borne, blood-borne, mosquito-borne, or whatever. "Wind-borne Evil," in the Asian medicine sense, refers to any *transmittable pathogen* that is *too small to see*, which is making the patient sick.

"Evil," in this case, means "not good for the highest manifestation of human health." For example, in Asian medicine, seasonal "Wind-derived" pathogens are considered to "arise" during that season, as if the pathogens aren't present during the rest of the year. The philosophy here is that these pathogens only become *problematic* during those seasons. (Continued on next page.)

If a person's body is robustly healthy, or if he already has immune history for a particular pathogen so that his immune system is primed and ready to produce the exact, corresponding antibodies for the pathogen, the person may never develop symptoms. His body will fight the invaders without the person even knowing that he is doing anything. On the other hand, in people that develop obvious symptoms from a pathogen, those symptoms tell us that the person's body – and his channel Qi system – have been, to some extent, altered, via the pathogen.

If we can determine the point(s) along the channel at which the channel Qi has been destabilized by the presence of the pathogen, we automatically know the most effective treatment. The best treatment will be one that restores the normal flow of channel Qi at the destabilized point(s).

This all relates back to the idea of the importance of feeling channel Qi for diagnostic purposes. If a health practitioner can find the spot that's been turned off by the bug, he can also turn it back on, instantly, with a bit of judicious needling.

For example, if the patient's channel Qi has obviously been disrupted at Du-14, then Du-14 is a location at which correct Qi flow must be restored. If the disruption has occurred at LI-4, a common spot for pathogen-based disruption, one must restore channel Qi flow at LI-4.

In school, I was taught a collection of points to "use for Exterior Evil Wind." This collection included the acupoints LI-4 and Du-14, to name just a few. Looking for some sort of cause and effect logic, I leaped to the assumption that needling LI-4 and the others always pumped up the immune system, and this immune system surge then provided the artillery to destroy the pathogens.

I have since learned that treating LI-4 only *restores* vigor to the immune system if channel Qi has been disrupted at LI-4. If a patient is dealing with a pathogen whose *modus operandi* involves destabilizing UB-40 *and* the patient's channel Qi is moving perfectly freely at LI-4, needling LI-4 might *not* provide any benefit. Or there might be a slight, temporary benefit: needling LI-4 *may* shift the body closer to sympathetic mode (white cell producing mode), briefly. There *may* also be potential benefit of body-wide defibrillating any over-all channel confusion by strong needling at any of those popular acupoints where

---

This actually makes a lot of sense. Oppositely, in western medicine, pathogens are always pathogens, whether or not they are causing any harm at the given moment.

This western philosophy has led to our current culture of over-sterilization and the subsequent growth of super-bugs. We even propagate pathogens in labs, and investigate their qualities with or *without* hosts. The pathogen, even if not making someone sick, is considered problematic. This is similar to the western (historical) idea that many species of animals, from mice and crows to wolves and bears, are pests and therefore should be unquestioningly destroyed whether or not the individual animal is actively threatening a human or the human's livelihood. Historically, an organism, large or small, that might *ever* present a threat to *any* human was considered inherently "evil" to many westerners.

But in historical, classical Asian medicine, if a pathogen is not actually affecting a person, it is not "evil." The pathogen only becomes identifiable as an Evil-Wind (a transmittable, pathogenic problem) after it has inhabited a person and affected that person's channel Qi – when that person has responded by "*coming down*" with it: has begun to show symptoms.

46

channel Qi runs vigorously – such as LI-4. But needling acupoints is *most* helpful when those selected acupoints are the site of pathogen-induced channel Qi confusion or blockage.

The "use for Exterior Evil Wind" collection that I learned might better have been referred to as "acupoints *frequently* disrupted by pathogens." In other words, those points are merely the "usual suspects." They aren't necessarily the *correct* ones in any given patient. They may also help, in a clumsy, generalized fashion, but this is not the ideal.

When channel Qi flow is restored in the areas that had been altered by the pathogen, all the human's systems that had become turned off or misguided, including the immune system, are *instantly* able to perform correctly, once again. A person with pathogenic illness can feel *much* better within a very short time, if the destabilized area in his body is restored to correct form via channel-restoring needling or channel-specific herbs.

We might even conjecture that, if a particular pattern of pathogenic Qi creates an electromagnetic field that is counter to the human's field, it makes sense that, oppositely, by restoring the human's field, we are resuming an electromagnetic pattern that runs counter to that of the pathogen: when the human's channel Qi flow is restored to proper alignment, the pathogen is electromagnetically stymied.

More elegantly than any antibiotic, a surge of human channel Qi that is in opposition to, which is to say, negates, the channel Qi pattern in the pathogen should, theoretically, be able to stop replication of, or even destroy, any of the pathogens that are in full-bore (exposed) replication mode.

An acupuncturist or herbalist will find that he gets extremely quick results at stopping the pathogen in its tracks by restoring the channel Qi flow in the destabilized area.

Of course, the patient may still have to deal with sequelae from his infection: the toxins and phlegm generated by both the pathogen proper and the battle with the pathogen. But it does seem, based on experiences with treatments that restore disrupted channel Qi flow, that the pathogens can very often be stopped cold by the resumption of the patient's correct channel Qi flow.

Case study #5

External wind attacking the Ren channel

In my own practice, an illustrative manifestation of this channel Qi disruption phenomenon occurred in fall of 2008.

Male, age 47. The patient was in fairly robust health. He came to see me because he'd been having such severe chest pains that he thought he'd had a heart attack. He'd been to the hospital and given a complete heart work up, but the hospital found nothing except a mild fever. They sent him home, after telling him that he "just" had some kind of sinus flu.

While I was checking his tongue and pulses, he mentioned something that he thought was humorous. Three students at the small, private high school where he teaches had gone to the hospital over the weekend, thinking they were having heart attacks. Of course, they all got full heart work-ups, and were all sent home after being told that they had a low fever and probably nothing more than a flu bug – "some sinus thing." It had occurred to him that his own "heart attack" had played out the exact same way.

I was deeply curious. It can be reasonable for a middle-aged man to have chest pains from a lung infection, and *then* think that he might be having a heart attack.

But this was the first time I'd ever heard of a cluster of healthy *teenagers*, who weren't using drugs, with presumably good hearts and no overt symptoms of influenza, all going to the hospital because they thought they were having heart attacks. And *three* students, in a school of only three hundred? This sounded more like the same infectious pathogen that, without causing actual heart damage, was causing heart-attack type pain (which is to say, blockage) in its victims' chests.

We learn in our Asian medical theory classes that the source of pain in humans is "Failure to go through" (often translated as "No go through").

If they were having chest pain, something was causing blockage in the area of the heart or a heart-related channel. Might the heart blockage be related, somehow, to their flu symptoms?

First, I checked my patient's pulses. His heart and pericardium pulses were small, but within normal limits. His lung pulse was floating, suggesting that his body was fighting something. In school, we are taught that a floating pulse indicates that the Wei Qi, also known as the Protective Qi, has been activated – the body has begun to recognize that it is under attack.[1]

---

[1] A common English translation of Wei Qi is "defensive Qi." This is an incorrect translation, as it conjures up an image of bulwarks, artillery, and warfare. Wei Qi means "Protective Qi." Wei Qi refers to the safe feeling a person gets when he's being held lovingly, snugly, in the arms of his mother, a loved one, or Divine Mother. When the body is being attacked from the outside, the protective energy can swaddle the body, confirming the *physical* existence of loving support from within and without. Wei Qi thus helps to *define* the body and *define* the correct paths of the channel Qi – thus restoring the correct channel Qi even in the face of the pathogen's alterations to the channel Qi. In light of the destabilizing energetics of pathogens, the Wei Qi's loving support for remembering one's self-definition plays a large stabilizing role. To the extent that he is able to summon up his Wei Qi, his sense that he is whole, safe, and protected, a human can defiantly resume his true channel Qi flow pattern even in the face of attempted alteration-by-pathogen.

In Asian classics, the loving-mother goddess, Kuan Yin, serves as a personification of Wei Qi. In Sanskrit writings, the protective energy is often exemplified by Divine Mother: the loving, creative aspect of the Om (Sacred Breath, or "The Word") vibration. Om, in Sanskrit, became *Spiritus Sanctus*, in Latin, which means, literally, Sacred Breath. (In English, hundreds of years ago, *Spiritus Sanctus* was translated into the somewhat spooky "Holy *Ghost*." We still cling to this weird translation.)

In any language, the idea of a loving, protective energy is quite different from the artillery and bulwark images conjured up by the modern English translation of Wei Qi into "defensive Qi."

I have asked *many* of my respected Chinese teachers about this. They all agreed that Wei Qi is a loving, protective energy, and not a form of battle-oriented, germ-killing Qi. Wei Qi is neither defensive nor attacking. It is love made tangible. It helps us to recall our true nature, which includes the harmonized patterns of our channel Qi flow – as opposed to the *false* nature being created in our channels via the channel Qi of the pathogen.

Pathogens are referred to in Chinese medicine as Wind-borne Evils. The word "Evil" in this case can be understood to mean "that which distorts Truth." Pathogens are "Evil" because they distort our true nature. Wei Qi is tangible energy arising from Love and Truth. The loving support of Wei Qi helps us remember the Truth of who we are, and how our channel Qi is supposed to run, and reinstates it.

48

The floating Lung pulse matched up with the "only a sinus flu" findings of the western doctor.

I decided to quickly run my hand over the patient's Heart channels, and the Heart alarm areas of his Urinary Bladder and Ren channels. I wondered if I might find a spot in his channel Qi that, if turned off, could logically account for his chest pain symptoms. I suspected that it would *not* be the usual suspects: *not* LI-4, Du-14, or UB-11.

The channel Qi flow in his Heart and Pericardium channels was weak, but running, and running in the correct direction. I was planning to check his back Shu points, UB-14 and UB-15 in particular, but first, I felt his Ren channel.

Fig. 3.1 The *healthy* Ren: a close-up view of a section of the Ren channel, showing just two of the many side branches: branches emerging from Ren-15 and Ren-17. These side branches supply the pericardium and heart.

To understand the findings of this case study, one must appreciate the role of the Ren channel in distributing channel Qi throughout the torso and neck, via side branchings, as needed.

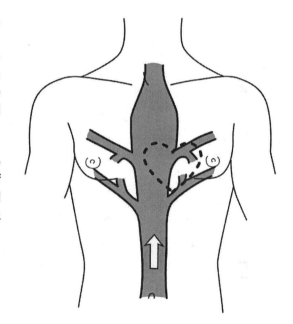

Bingo.

The Ren channel Qi was utterly stymied from Ren-14 to Ren-24. The Ren channel energy felt as if it were dissolving as it approached the xyphoid process; it was dispersing laterally, towards the sides of the torso. By the time it approached the sternum proper, there was no channel Qi to be felt along the path of the Ren.

Of course, many lung infections can *cause* problems in the chest that then *result* in problems in the vicinity of Ren-17. But my patient didn't have obvious lung symptoms – yet. And neither did any of the high school students who had thought they were having heart attacks.

I was fascinated. I'd never run across any pathogen whose immune-system turn-off mechanism worked by blocking the Ren and upper Kidney channels at the inferior end of the sternum, so that the Ren and Kidney channel Qi got shunted somewhere into the interior of the torso.

No wonder all these pathogen-infected people had felt as if they were having a heart attack. They were all hosting a pathogen whose "shut-down" method included blocking the flow of channel Qi at the inferior end of the sternum, thus drastically cutting off energy supply to the pericardium, heart, and lungs.

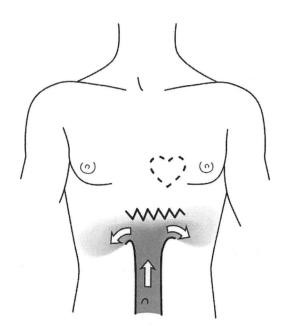

Fig. 3.2 In this case study, note the absence of Ren channel Qi flowing over the sternum, due to the blockage. The side branches that should carry channel Qi to the heart and pericardium, in such a case, are not able to flow.

The heart has been drawn smaller than usual, to represent the lack of channel Qi getting to the heart and the subsequent pain in the heart, from channel Qi "not getting through."

Getting my mind back on my patient, I needled his Ren-17 with a 2.0 cun needle, threading it down towards Ren-14. I inserted another 2 cun needle at Ren-15, also threading it towards Ren-14. I was using the needles to pull Ren channel Qi in the area of Ren-14 upward, towards Ren-17, forcing it to flow past the problem area. As soon as I did this, Ren channel Qi began to flow from Ren-14 up to Ren-24. The patient felt his chest relax. His low grade, ongoing "heart attack pain" subsided. The Heart and Pericardium channels became more vigorous. After the treatment, I instructed him to gently rub his sternum several times a day, in an upward direction, from Ren 12 to Ren 17. He recovered apace.

The next week, at school, I was teaching clinical rounds. My first patient was a male, age 42, who seemed very fit. He was starting to describe his symptoms, beginning by saying, "My doctor says it's just a sinus flu, but…" I stopped him gently, by asking him to please be quiet for just a moment, as I wanted to check something. I reached over and felt the channel Qi in his chest. It petered out just before Ren-15. I asked him if he'd been to the hospital because he thought he'd been having a heart attack.

"How did you know?" he exclaimed.

The startled look on his face registered surprised approval for the "mysteries of Asian medicine." The five beginning acupuncture students in the rounds class seemed equally, or even more, surprised.

I explained to the patient and students that I wasn't using Divine insight: I'd already seen this heart-pain/flu pattern in this year's flu season. I also took the opportunity to share a tip that had been taught to me by my teachers: always pay close attention to the first flu cases that come in each fall; very often, many of the later flu cases in that fall and winter will be of the same nature. If, early in the season, the health care provider can figure out the particular channel-disruption trick of whatever is making the rounds for this year, the provider will be able to diagnose subsequent flu patients most quickly and effectively, and even teach his un-sick patients some appropriate, *preventive* self-massage.

But the main point is this: feeling a floating pulse does not tell us whether the external evil (pathogen) is wind-cold or wind-heat. Even with an articulate patient who is just starting to have symptoms that enable the health practitioner to confirm either wind-cold or wind-heat, we must still guess at the best form of treatment if we are treating an unfamiliar pathogen using only tongue and pulse diagnosis. We compile as many symptoms as possible to determine if we are dealing with a pathogen whose *modus operandi* involves destabilizing the back of the neck, the forehead, the branch of the Large Intestine channel that crosses over to Du-14 (causing achy shoulders), and so on, so as to distinguish whether or not we are looking at a Yang Ming disorder, a Bladder channel attack, and so on. We try to come up with the best treatment plan based on the part of the body that is showing the *most* symptoms at that moment: not *pure* guesswork, but not an exact plan of attack either.

And very often, by the time we see a sick patient, his symptoms have become spread over many organs. At this point, we often ignore the pathogen's initial presentation altogether, and devise a treatment to relieve symptoms, and "Release the Exterior (Get rid of the pathogen that came from outside myself)."

If, instead of guessing, we can detect the exact location where the pathogen has deranged the channel Qi system, and restore Qi flow to that area, the patient's own body will quickly be able to fully recognize, and battle, the presence of the Evil visitor. The channel Qi restoration may even neutralize the unwanted guest.

Then, *after* the channel Qi flow has been restored, we may also perform treatments that dissolve the phlegm or address the other side effects that built up during the time of the illness.[1]

---

[1] Not every Evil-Wind case is this simple.

A neighbor, age 58, dropped over to my house asking for help with his flu. Normally very healthy and vigorous, for several days he'd been running a fever of 101.6 (F) every afternoon, for six hours. He had no appetite. His mind was cloudy. He felt terribly weak in the arms. He had an unproductive cough. He had severe insomnia – he was only able to sleep between the hours of five and eight in the morning.

The blockage in his Ren channel was easy to feel. He felt a shocking amount of uncharacteristic pain when I needled Ren-19, -18, -17, -16, and -15, but the channel Qi finally started flowing through his Ren channel. The next day he came by again – his condition was unimproved. I noticed a blockage at UB-13, and needled the blocked sections of that channel and got the UB channel flowing nicely. The next day, he came over, as requested, and reported that his symptoms were unchanged. That day, the leg portion of his Liver channel was noticeably blocked. Also, the Ren channels and UB channels were somewhat blocked, again. There seemed to be no channel Qi whatsoever in his Large Intestine channel.

Every day, I treated a different blockage, and nothing I did seemed to last. I also used all the appropriate traditional herb formulas, and even performed a tuning fork treatment. Finally, after seventeen days during which my treatments seemed to do no good at all, it was apparent that his bacterial pneumonia was winning the battle. Much as he distrusted western medicine, he yielded to advice and started taking antibiotics. Within twenty-four hours, he felt much better: the cough and fever, his primary Wind-Heat symptoms, were both gone.

All the channel theory and herbs at my disposal hadn't been enough to conquer his infection.

Some pathogens are stronger than our medicine. Pathogens that cause Ebola and plague, and even the mundane ones that cause bacterial pneumonia might be said to have a stronger "will to live" than we humans. The dynamics of their channel Qi may be stronger or more stable than ours.

Within a week of starting antibiotics, this patient was eating better. However, he was still very weak and could barely raise his arms over his head. He still had severe tachycardia, an irregularly irregular heartbeat, palpitations, random attacks of low blood pressure and orthostatic hypotension (low blood pressure when changing to standing from a seated position), extreme weakness, and his ferociously pounding and highly irregular heart rate were still keeping him from sleeping. After two weeks of this, he'd lost another ten pounds. These continuing symptoms, I was to learn, were a condition called "sepsis."

Sepsis can occur following a pathogenic illness when the body cannot handle the debris from dead cells quickly enough. The heme released by dead cells, if not processed rapidly enough, converts to a toxic form. A buildup of this toxic variant of heme can lead to poor regulation of the autonomic nervous system, with symptoms that include racing heart, highly irregular heart beat, low blood pressure, confusion, build up of fluid in the lungs, and death.

Had I insisted adamantly, earlier in his illness, that he take antibiotics for his bacterial pneumonia, and had he complied, he most likely would not have developed sepsis. Happily, the sepsis did not develop to the stage of fluid build up in the lungs or brain. But he now had a chronic heart condition and chronic low pressure that made it nearly impossible for him to work, exercise, or stay focused. He spent many hours every day simply resting in bed, hoping for the day when his heart would calm down and his strength would return. He also worked actively at calming his heart: he did his yogic breathing, calming visualizations, and affirmations. However, his body seemed to be stuck in a new pattern. As for his channel Qi, it was almost non-existent in his arms. It was blocked at various spots in the Ren, UB, and Liver channels, and very weak everywhere else. It was too chaotic to use, diagnostically.

I felt I had failed him. I referred him to the most brilliant professor at the acupuncture college where I teach: Dr. Jeffery Pang, MD (China), LAc. Dr. Pang prescribed Tian Wang Bu Xin Dan, a formula that replenishes Heart and Pericardium Yin. The herbal pills worked within ten minutes! All the heart symptoms ceased. With the cessation of the erratic pounding, his mental clarity returned. He could even fall into a deep, untroubled sleep…for four hours. As soon as the dose wore off, every four hours, all his symptoms were exactly as before. For nearly a week, he managed his symptoms by taking pills every four hours. But this herb formula can be mildly habituating – a person can become somewhat resistant to the formula. Five days after he started this formula, his coverage became noticeably decreased. He needed to increase his dose of tablets by nearly 50% in order to get the same hours of coverage. The herbs were only masking symptoms, not treating them.

This case study concludes in the last chapter, when you will have enough information about channel theory and the different neural modes to understand exactly what was going on in his body.

Summary of the introductory case studies in chapters two and three

All emotional problems, organ problems, and all other symptoms of imperfect health manifest in the channels. Conditions of deficiency or excess, interior or exterior, Qi, Blood, Yin or Yang, all manifest in the channels.

In some cases, such as malnutrition and physical injury, the external, causative nature of the problem comes first, and the damage to the channels then follows. In other cases, particularly in problems that have pathogenic or mental/emotional components, the channel disruption comes first, and is the cause of the subsequent physical problems.

By correcting the flow of channel Qi at the exact point where it has gone astray, health can very often be exactingly, rapidly restored.

Of course, the most elegant method for instantly restoring the course of channels to their correct pathways is for the patient to think correct thoughts: thoughts that are in line with, or in tune with, one's true nature. Thoughts generate highly specific electromagnetic waves. These waves influence, for better or worse, the movements of the channels.

Because most humans are not yet able to control and focus their thoughts in such a way as to maintain correct flow of channel Qi in the face of all challenges, doctors of every culture practice the art of medicine.

In Asian medicine, detecting and correcting the actual flow of channel Qi is one of the most logical and elegant ways to practice this art.

"Color and pulse are valued by Gods, and they were taught by the teachers of former times." [1]

Chapter four

Channels: the diagnostic tools of the masters

Questions that arise

With regard to detecting a patient's channel Qi and using this to form a diagnosis, the two questions that most often arise are: 1) Isn't pulse diagnosis the most perfect form of Asian medicine diagnostics? and 2) If channel diagnosis is such a powerful tool, why isn't it mentioned in the classics? This chapter will address both of these questions.

Is pulse diagnosis the apex of diagnostic skills?

Knowledge of the flow aberrations in a patient's channel Qi can yield objective, "hard" diagnoses as to the exact underlying nature and energetic location of the patient's problems. Diagnosing based on the actual flow of channel Qi is highly objective and does not require the use of intuition. Almost anyone can quickly learn to do it.

---

[1] Su Wen, chapter 13-5, *A Complete Translation of the Yellow Emperor's Classics of Internal Medicine and the Difficult Classic (Nei-Jing and Nan-Jing)*, Henry C. Lu, PhD, International College of Traditional Chinese Medicine of Vancouver, 2004, p. 114.

These skills were taught in olden times! And they are no longer taught. Why not? Refer back to the first chapter of the Nei-Jing...where it is written that people used to have deeper understanding, but now [in 221 BC] they do not – so of course, the more sophisticated techniques of diagnosis were no longer being taught.

As for my sense that the word "color" in this part of the *Nei-Jing* refers to the light-wave related energy of channel Qi, I wrote to Wallace Li, L. Ac, DAOM, professor of Chinese medical classics. I asked if the word "color" in this section of the Nei-Jing might be referring to light, as in, the light waves that are involved in the generation of channel Qi. He replied, "When the Taoism/TCM classics use the word "color," it implies Qi and color (Qi Se) [aka vibratory energy and color], unless they address the "Qi" part specifically and separately. Your perception is the same as mine."

As a further suggestion that the ancient term, "color," refers to an energy source, we learn in the *Nei-Jing* that "Color is Yang." In particular, Color is Yang when compared to the relative Yin of the pulse and other, merely physiological, sources of diagnostic information. This further supports the idea that "Color," in this usage, refers to the energy derived from and associated with light. Although, in modern times, the word "complexion" is sometimes used to translate the Chinese character "color" into English, thus suggesting that the original author was writing about facial tone variations, this translation does not fit with other references to "Color" in the *Nei Jing*, such as Color being like the sun, or Color being associated with movement and dynamics, or "Closer to the Truth (or Sun)" (which is to say, Yang), when compared to the pulse.

Comparatively, the other forms of Asian medicine diagnosis are, for most medical practitioners, highly subjective: open to interpretation and error.

For example, merely learning the objective, word-based descriptions for tongue and pulse diagnosis does *not* give one the ability to ascertain and interpret the appearance of the tongue or sensations of the pulse with enough certainty to form an exact diagnosis. Most students must spend years, at a minimum, learning how to feel the pulses. Even after years of study, many acupuncturists never really master the art of forming an exact diagnosis based on pulse.

Tongue appearances can be equally inexact and somewhat subjective.[1]

Diagnoses that do not lead to an exact treatment plan

Even if one is able to derive a likely "pattern" diagnosis from the pulse, the exact treatment plan, based on that diagnosis, remains a matter of choosing from the collection of treatments that are known to be most effective, in general, for that type of pattern.

For example, even if a diagnosis of External Wind-Heat attacking the Bladder channel (pathogenic illness causing fever and aches between the shoulder blades) has been made using tongue and pulse, the doctor must then guess whether the most elegant treatment will begin with the Large Intestine channel, the Bladder channel, the Lung channel, or some other primary channel – or all of them.

Many acupuncturists "err on the side of safety" and treat several. But even then, there are some pathogens whose mode of attack involves other channels, even the Du channel and/or the Ren.

Without knowing which channel is at the root of the problem, let alone the exact location on that channel that has become altered by the presence of the pathogen, many acupuncturists or herbalists do not *know* which of the many "Wind-Heat" treatments to select. Guesswork, for many, remains a major factor in selecting a treatment plan.

The role of intuition

When it comes to tongue and pulse diagnosis, why are the best doctors, the masters of this medicine, able to recognize subtleties that remain hidden to most practitioners and students? How are the master doctors able to determine an exactly appropriate treatment plan for each individual?

The masters use *intuition* or, as it is translated from the classics in Ted Kaptchuk's *Web That Has No Weaver*, "Penetrating Divine Illumination." Intuition may be used *in addition* to the more objective observations of the tongue's appearance, the pulse's kinetics,

---

[1] One of my most brilliant teachers, Jeffery Pang, MD (China), LAc – and a profoundly successful practitioner – was wont to say, "If either the tongue or pulse or both clearly doesn't match up with the symptoms, mentally throw away what doesn't match. *Forget* about it."

Jake Paul Fratkin, a respected authority in TCM, author of *Chinese Herbal Patent Medicines*, and editor/organizer of Wu & Fischer's *Practical Therapeutics of Traditional Chinese Medicine*, says, "While all the textbook information is accurate concerning coats, colors, shapes, etc., I feel that the tongue offers no helpful information 85% of the time." From "Treating Complex Multilayered Cases;" *Acupuncture Today*, 11:4, April 2010, p.22.

and the other body language clues. Even though an intuitive diagnostic master might insist that he is using classic definitions of face, body language, tongue, pulse, or smell to arrive at his brilliant and exact diagnosis, be assured that the master is performing these classic diagnostics while *also* applying his highly developed intuition.

The "mechanics" of that intuition varies from one master to the next. One may have an intuitively developed ability to "see" areas of darker and lighter energy in the patient. Another may "hear" an intuitive voice whispering to him as he touches the pulse. Indeed, some translations of the classics instruct the doctor to "listen" to the pulse, not "touch" it. Or the medical master may be able to kinesthetically feel, within himself, temporary alterations in his own body-electric due to proximity to the patient's aberrant electromagnetic fields.

These subtle, seemingly *non*-objective methods of "seeing," "hearing," and "feeling" are all based on a heightened ability to perceive subtle shifts in a patient's channels and other electromagnetic forces: these perceptions rely on the sixth sense: the "energetic sense;" intuition.

Defining intuition

"Intuition" does not mean the same thing as "hunch" or "gut-level feeling."

Very often, unrecognized personal biases or subconscious memories push a person to have a strong hunch based on a "gut feeling." However, these feelings are merely opinions. They are just as likely to be wrong as to be right.

Intuition, on the other hand, is based on precise information that is fielded by the heart. Electromagnetic aspects of the heart and pericardium work like a receiving/transmitting radio. The heart and pericardium are able to "receive," or resonate with, electromagnetic fields – including the fields being generated by a patient. A person who is able to accurately attune his heart's radio to the patient's "station" can feel the resultant shifts in his own heart and pericardium. This information may be instantly assessed using the *buddhi* (heart-attuned, wisdom) portion of the mind as opposed to the opinions that flourish in the *manas* (sensory and ego-based) portion of the mind.

In the field of medicine, very often, the heart attunement will give a vastly different, even an opposite, diagnosis from that which springs into the doctor's mind or "gut." [1]

----

[1] Years ago, when I was a student at acupuncture college, it took me an embarrassingly long time before I noticed that my fellow students and I repeatedly had diagnostic "hunches" that corresponded to whatever syndrome or illness pattern we'd been studying in class the previous week. For example, on a given week, many of us might insist that most of our patients were clear cut cases of Phlegm Misting the Heart. The week before, most of our patients were, beyond a doubt, showing Heart Fire causing Bladder heat. We could be passionately convinced of the certain truth of our "hunches." We would argue our cases with the clinic teachers, unable to understand why the teacher didn't always respect what we referred to as "intuition."

This "You See What You Are Looking For" syndrome is *not* driven by intuition. It is driven by a combination of subtle, ego-based desire and personal experiences that combine with ego-based sensory interpretation and emotional events. A syndrome almost as common, but far harder to recognize, is the human tendency to project one's own mental and emotional baggage onto the patient. In either case, we students often defended these glaringly incorrect diagnoses by claiming that they were based on our "intuition." (Continued on next page.)

For example, a highly intuitive doctor may *think* to himself something along the lines of, "Everything I've learned is telling me that the patient's problem, acne, is Damp-Heat. I know exactly how to treat it – *but* a small, still voice within me is calmly saying, over and over, 'She doesn't even know she's pregnant, but she has a dangerous fallopian pregnancy.' *That's* what I have to treat, immediately." That small, still voice, a voice that may fly in the face of the "facts" or the "feelings," is intuition.[1]

Intuition is the actual basis for a medical master's seemingly miraculous diagnostic skills. His process is based, at least to some degree, on the sixth sense. His superior diagnostic skills are *objectively* inexplicable: not teachable through books, lectures, or examples.

A medical master often performs his intuitive assessment during the quiet time during which his fingers rest on the patient's pulse, or he may be listening to his intuition while gazing at the patient's tongue. The medical master may *say* that his diagnosis is based on tongue or pulse. He may *not even realize* the extent to which he is using his intuition. A few excellent doctors will even admit that they "just know" what the patient needs but, since the knowing comes to them *while* they go through the motions of checking tongue and pulse, they insist that their knowledge comes *from* tongue and pulse.

Rest assured, the great masters of Asian medicine, and for that matter, the great masters of *every* school of medicine, are using far more than mere textbook information. The great Asian medicine masters, for example, are using more than word-based descriptions of pulse or tongue patterns while arriving at their conclusions. A *great* doctor's diagnosis is based on his ability to access his intuition – a skill obtained through practicing humility and regularly sitting in silent meditation: "observing himself," as it says in the *Nei Jing*.

On the other hand, by feeling the movement of channel Qi, a sensory, *non*-intuitive evaluation, we can get much of the same information. Even if you can't yet access Penetrating, Divine Illumination, you *can* easily learn to feel the movement of channel Qi. The diagnostic process is a bit slower, but it gives much the same information.

History of the texts: from the exactness of knowing to the approximation of the written word

If intuition and sensory knowledge of the channels are so important, why weren't these skill sets written up in the great medical classic, the *Huang Ti Nei Jing*?

They were.

As another non-medical but common example of ego being misinterpreted as intuition, consider the affairs of the heart. Many failed relationships started off with a "gut level" attraction that proclaimed "Soul mate, forever!" But when the fires cooled down, the attraction turns out to have had nothing to do with intuition and wisdom, and everything to do with ego and desire.

[1] This was an actual case, observed in clinical theater, when I was in school. The doctor said she needed to go to the hospital immediately. The patient insisted that there was no way she could be pregnant. The doctor refused to touch her, repeating his instruction that she go to the hospital. She left in a huff. We heard from her several days later. The doctor's conviction had worried her. She'd gone to the hospital. The doctors were dubious, but an ultrasound revealed the ectopic pregnancy. We students were enthralled. When we asked the doctor how he'd known, he didn't reply, at first. Then, after thinking a bit, he said, "Pulse and tongue."

Ch'i Po (the medical authority in the *Nei Jing*) even says, "There should be *no doubt* or confusion as to the application of the meaning of complexion [A better translation would have been "color": the movement of channel Qi] and pulse... all good (medical) practices were revived from the spiritual men who had attained Tao, the right way of life." [Italics mine][1]

And in the same chapter, he says, "The utmost in the art of healing can be achieved when there is unity."

Only by possessing intuitive knowledge of Truth can one make medical diagnoses that are "free from doubt." "Unity" refers to the oneness with the universe that can be experienced, at will, by those who have attuned themselves to Tao, or The Way.[2]

In the same chapter of the *Nei Jing*, book five, the point is made that using direct perception of the channels was "taught by the teachers of former times."

And as for the importance of knowing exactly what the channels are doing, whether discerned intuitively or using sensory perception, the *Nei Jing* states clearly, "It is by virtue of the channels...diseases can be treated and cured."

I used to demand of my teachers, "Why aren't the classics, and the *Nei Jing* in particular, more explicit on these subjects of intuition and feeling channel Qi? Why does our modern, "classics-based" medical training focus primarily on pulse and tongue diagnosis instead of meditation, intuition, and learning to detect the actual flow of channel Qi?" Why weren't these things in our books?

It turns out, generalized sensations of pulse and appearance of tongue *can* be described in a book, and tested on a quiz. Intuition cannot.

Also, historically, feeling the flow of invisible forces such as channel Qi may well have been an art that came across as increasingly mystical over time, even to the point of arousing suspicion of dark forces at work. Finally, it is highly likely that information about detecting channels was held back from the Emperor and his henchmen when the *Nei Jing* opus was being compiled.

The way of the masters: the transition to pulse and tongue diagnostics

The ancient masters of Asian medicine did not slowly develop their medical knowledge by trial and error. They did not try various treatments and then assess whether or not their patients seemed to benefit, thus accumulating a collection of data regarding "what works and what doesn't."

In very ancient times, certain people were recognized as master doctors because they were able to intuitively behold, and fix, the energetic problems that created illness in their

---

[1] *The Yellow Emperor's Classic of Internal Medicine*, translated by Ilza Veith, 2002, University of California Press, Berkeley. *Su Wen*, Book 2, chapter 13. Following one of the modern conventions, the word color was translated in Veith's text as "complexion."

[2] The Tao, often translated as "The Way," is known in other cultures as the Om, the Amen, Amin, the Word, and other words and phrases that refer to the knowable, vibratory foundation of the universe. Stilling the ego-based mind and using heart-feeling to *follow* these vibrations back to their origin leads one to attunement with all creation and, eventually, its source. Thus, it is "The Way."

patients. By *intuiting* their patients' problems, they could then perform or suggest the antidote.

In recorded, *written* history, when these intuitive masters either chose to, or in some cases were commanded to (possibly under the threat of death), *explain* their methodology in terms that could be written up for posterity – a posterity that, in those darkening ages, would no doubt include many *non*-intuitive students – the masters of medicine came up with descriptions of easily noted physiological traits that *often*, but not always, accompanied some specific types of energetic problems.

For example, an intuitive medical master might be able to notice, from across the room, an audible, palpable, or clairvoyantly visible blockage, or knotting, of energy in a patient's Liver channel. It would be obvious how this blockage was directly causing the patient's symptoms.

The master would *not* be able to explain to a non-intuitive student or colleague *how* he could hear, feel, or see this Liver channel stagnation. Looking for some way to convey a bit of word-based or written information about such cases to his fellow doctors and the students of posterity, the master would have to fall back on other, more tangible symptoms in the patient's body.

For example, the master would know from his past experience that, in *some* cases, the blocked Liver channel energy in a patient *might* be reflected in the patient's pulse, presenting a tense, rebounding (wiry) pulse.

Of course, the master also knows that some patients with knotted, tense Liver channel problems or pain do *not* have a wiry pulse. *And* he knows that some people have a wiry pulse now and then even though they have no Liver channel problems whatsoever. For that matter, he knows that some perfectly healthy people *always* have a wiry pulse.

Still, although the wiry pulse may or may *not* be indicative of a stagnation problem in the Liver channel, a master of intuitive medicine might fall back on this somewhat helpful wisdom: sometimes, a wiry pulse *might* be related to Liver channel Qi stagnation. While trying to instruct a less-than-intuitive student of the dark ages, or trying to put his wisdom into writing in response to royal command, the master might suggest, "If the pulse is wiry, you *might* want to treat the patient for Liver channel stagnation."

These attempts at explaining intuitively perceived channel disarray in terms of *likely* objective tongue and pulse behaviors are the types of instructions that have been carried down to us in the oldest classics. The subsequent "classic" works on the same subjects are sincere, but they nevertheless, by cultural decree, require that any new information must fit with all precedents.[1]

---

[1] Some subsequent scholarly works of Asian medicine remind me of the theorists in Galileo's day. Even when the invention of the telescope gave astronomers more hard data about planetary movement, traditional theory kept the Earth at the center of the universe. Attempts to pair new facts with traditional, earth-centric theory resulted in hideously complex hypotheses of planetary trajectories, in which heavenly bodies underwent leaps, backsteps, and temporary disappearing acts. The simplest solution, of course, was to throw away centuries worth of "classic," but incorrect, theory, and create a new, simple, sun-centric solar system theory that worked beautifully with the new data. This simplified approach also allowed for more accurate predictions of celestial behavior. The revolutionary theory was hailed by scientists of the day. Nevertheless, in response to Galileo's

But despite what the earliest masters wrote down for posterity, they knew that, across the human spectrum, the wiry pulse is only a *probable side effect* of the Liver channel problem. In other words, it's not the wiry pulse, per se, that *proves* a condition of Liver channel-Qi stagnation. The thing that *proves* Liver channel-Qi stagnation is accurate perception of the actual knots (contortions of channel Qi flow) in the Liver channel Qi.

If a would-be doctor cannot detect what the Liver channel is *actually* doing, a pulse diagnosis may be helpful – but then again, maybe not.

The basic diagnostic methods of Asian medicine that are taught in the classic texts, pulse, tongue, face, and so on, can sometimes be extremely helpful. They are, after all, the masters' notations of objective, definable, *fairly* common side effects, also called "patterns," of underlying problems. Taking notice of these side effects, if any, *might* be helpful in getting to the root of a patient's problem. But these diagnostic methods, unless accompanied by intuition, do not yield direct *perception* of the problem (the incorrect flow of channel Qi) – and, therefore, might well be incorrect.[1]

The mere tactile manifestations of the pulse only show what the patient is *willing* to show. If pulse reading results in brilliant accuracy, it is the doctor's use of intuition, rather than his physical pulse taking skills, that is revealing the subtler illness patterns in the patient.

---

promotion of the new theory, the Catholic church demanded obedience to the traditional view, and put Galileo under lifetime house arrest.

[1] When I was a student, I was determined that a pulse, if read accurately enough, would always yield a Truthful Diagnosis about a patient's condition. I was fortunate enough to have teachers who were able to demonstrate for me, over a period of a few minutes, how they could alter their own pulses to manifest conditions of wiry, slippery, deep, weak, and so on. My teachers did *not* do this to show off that they could alter their own pulses: this teaching was done to drive home the fact that pulses do not necessarily indicate the Truth about a patient's condition.

Eventually, my teachers helped me to understand that a vigorous patient who does not trust the doctor may bring his pulse so deep beneath the skin that, while in the doctor's office, his pulse appears "deep and weak." Or patients with a meditation practice that encourages withdrawing the energy from the physical body sometimes purposely enter into this "deep" state while the doctor is feeling the pulse. Whether from a desire to show how "still and calm" they can be or from a desire to "get out of the way while the doctor works," the results will be the same: a mentally altered pulse. Usually, this type of "stilling the mind" creates a pulse that exhibits a false slowness and extreme depth, and a temporary inhibition of any pulse characteristics that might have shown the pains or problems from which the patient suffers when he isn't in his "deep" state.

My teachers took care to point out other, more obvious forms of "altered pulse": the patient who has been running hard to get to his appointment on time, the patient who is taking pulse-altering medications or herbal treatments, and so on. I finally had to admit that the sensations given off by the pulse do not "tell the Truth."

Every patient has an inherent ability to subconsciously or consciously alter his pulse so that it reveals only those qualities he is willing to reveal – and he can *hide* those qualities that he does *not* want to reveal.

The Nei Jing states: "Using pulses, the doctor cannot make an error"

Then again, pulses can be highly accurate at providing information regarding *changes*: a doctor can compare a patient's pulse before, during, and after stimulation (even momentary stimulation via acupressure) at various acupoints. He can compare the before, during, and after pulses in response to placing herbs or patent medicines on a patient's hand or abdomen. The pulse changes that occur almost immediately, in response to these stimuli, can provide a *highly* accurate representation of how the person's body is *responding* to these specific treatments or treatment suggestions – at the moment.

It is in *this* sense, the sense that "relative *changes* in the pulse during and after treatment show how the patient is responding," that the *Nei Jing* claims a person "cannot *make* an error" [in treatment] if he uses the pulses [*to test the treatment*].

Mere tactile perceptions of the pulses do not provide an absolute measure of a person's health status. The pulses do not show a particular Truth. But the short-term changes in a pulse can very accurately show how a person responds – at least in the short term – to the doctor's treatment. Also, if a patient's pulse has been felt in the past, and the present pulse reading presents a perceptible change, this *change* may yield valuable clues.

In other words, the tactile sensations of the pulse, as described in the classics, do *not* necessarily give us a way to know the True Condition of a patient. The *relative* changes in a given person's pulse, changes that occur in response to illness or treatment, may be diagnostically helpful. The *relative* changes in a person's pulse that occur while the doctor experiments with various treatment plans may show whether or not the doctor is making a correct treatment – or an error.

Flawed diagnoses

If a would-be doctor is unable to intuitively know the cause of a patient's problems – which is to say, the exact channel flow aberrations that are occurring in the patient – the doctor must fall back on sensory diagnostic cues: looking, smelling, feeling, listening. But undeveloped and/or faulty senses can provide faulty information. Next, the information thus obtained is processed by inference – reasoning based on limited experience. Medical diagnoses built on faulty data, processed with inaccurate inferences, may be inherently flawed.

For those practitioners of Asian medicine who do not yet have a highly developed intuitive sense, the classic "teachable" diagnostic techniques of face coloration, body language, tongue, pulse, and smell might be the only techniques they have to fall back on in the beginning. But those techniques give only a *fairly* good idea of where to look for the problem, and a middling good chance of selecting an appropriate treatment.[1]

---

[1] Even so, pulse reading, observation of the complexion, listening to the tone of the voice, and the other forms of diagnoses can be important, powerful tools. Even though they might not yield precise diagnostic information, all students should practice listening to the pulses and noticing the other qualities in a patient's presentation.

For example, a patient came to my office because of mild "stomach" pain. Her symptoms suggested *possible*, early-stage appendicitis – an excess condition – but her weak pulse suggested a deficient condition. Contradicting the pulse, the shocking, hideous, patch of velvety, pure-black tongue coat at the back of her tongue, highly uncharacteristic for her, confirmed that something was *dangerously* wrong, even necrotic, in her intestines. Based on her tongue, I did not treat her, but

Even when combined with symptom "patterns," such as Eight Parameter patterns or Five Element patterns, those diagnostic "patterns" are just helpful, hopeful suggestions as to what the actual, underlying channel disorder *might* be. These so-called diagnostic methods are indirect. By themselves (without intuition), they may or may *not* lead to a correct diagnosis or treatment plan.

A run-in with my own intuition

Shortly after becoming licensed, a calm voice contradicted my thoughts as I was about to start treating a patient. The voice said, "Check his ankle." I silently rebuked the voice, pointing out that the situation was obviously Liver Wind causing tremor in the hand. My diagnosis was supported by a slightly wiry pulse. The other pulses felt about right, and the tongue was unremarkable.

The voice repeated calmly, "Check his ankle." I silently replied, with more resistance, "I don't want to waste his time. He obviously has Liver Wind in his hand." Again, calmly, "Check his ankle." I silently shot back, with some resentment, "I know what I learned in school! This is Liver Wind!"

This time, the voice came from a deeper, more ancient feeling deep in my heart. It merely said, "You know I'm always right."

I was stunned motionless. I thought about this statement: "You know I'm always right." Much as I resented it, I felt the truth of it. I paused, checking if any negative or fearful sensations had accompanied the inner voice. There was nothing fearful in my heart – only a peaceful stillness.

Immediately humbled and sheepish, feeling like I'd just been slapped by my guardian angel, or maybe my patient's guardian angel, I set down the needles that I'd been preparing to insert in his Liver channel and his hand. I felt his ankle. His anklebones were glaringly displaced.

I tried to assess the quality of the channel Qi flowing through his foot. No channel Qi was getting past the bone displacements. No channel Qi was flowing down into his foot from the Stomach or Gallbladder channel. Channel Qi even seemed to be flowing backwards in his Stomach channel, from the ankle upward.

I used no needles on this patient. For about twenty minutes I used gentle, Yin-type Tui Na to support his anklebones so they could reposition themselves, if *they* wanted to. After the bones suddenly jerked themselves back into place, Qi instantly began flowing normally into the patient's foot and legs. His intermittent tremor ceased, never to return.

Had I only used needles on his Liver channel, a slight increase in channel Qi might have temporarily moved through his foot during the treatment. But after removing those needles, the significantly displaced bones in his ankles would most likely have quickly resumed their blockage of the channel Qi in his foot and leg.

The ankle displacements from his childhood injury were probably being held in place by fear. It was the *fear* that needed to be treated, even more than the ankle displacements.

In retrospect, I understood that the slow, gentle, very supportive Yin Tui Na assuaged the fear in a way that mere needles never could have done. Logically, based on tongue and

---

immediately sent her to the hospital, where tests confirmed that she had a raging infection and a ready-to-burst appendix. Tongue was the crucial key for correct diagnosis, in this case.

Tongue is not *always* helpful, but it *can* sometimes be very valuable.

pulse, I could not possibly have known to perform this style of treatment. I doubt that any mere hunch could have overridden my arrogant confidence that wanted to use needles for Liver Wind. But the channel Qi aberration told the truth, even if I needed the corrective voice of my intuition telling me to pay attention to what the channel Qi was doing.

Our "hunches" and our "book learning" often lead us into error. Worse, the more certain we are of ourselves, the more easily we can slide into error, blinded by ego. True intuition is not so brash, so confident. It calmly tells us what *is* – with no sense of urgency to make itself heard. Whether we listen to it or not, whether we act on it or not, it will remain humble and modest. Intuition is easy to ignore. It is very polite – it rarely speaks unless spoken to.

Meditation and diagnostics

As noted in the *Su Wen*, "*By observing myself I know about others and their diseases are revealed to me...*"[1]

In other words, by calm, regular meditation and introspection ("observing myself"), a master develops the ability to still his distracting waves of ego consciousness and pay attention to his sixth sense. Using attunement with his sixth, or intuitive, sense, he can "feel," "see," "hear," or otherwise "understand" those processes that have run amok in the patient. In some cases, the intuition skips over the diagnosis altogether, and merely tells the doctor the appropriate treatment. Very often, it is by intuitively knowing what the *treatment* needs to be that the master can put into words the diagnosis.

For example, in the above example of displaced anklebones, I realized *after* the treatment that the diagnosis must have been Blood Stagnation – an unhealed, physically tangible injury – mentally held in place and rendered numb by willful Pericardium Qi blockage – a mental response to profound, dissociation-triggering *fear*. The patient's tremor was a fear-based symptom. Fear, not Wind, had been the underlying, or root, problem.

Channel diagnostics

Be of good cheer! Almost everyone can quickly learn to feel channel Qi.

Feeling the flow of the channels yields direct sensory information about the very forces that determine a person's health. Therefore, feeling the movement of the channels is of direct, not indirect, value. It yields information that does not need to be interpreted via obscure theory. Sensing the actual movement of the channels yields actual *knowledge* of a patient's channel Qi locations, directions, and strengths.

Ultimately, all health problems, all illness "patterns," derive from incorrect flow of channel Qi. This truth is expressed in the oft-repeated mantra, "Go through, no pain; no go through, pain."[2]

---

[1] *The Yellow Emperor's Classic of Internal Medicine*, translated by Ilza Veith, 2002, University of California Press, Berkeley, p.124.

[2] It took me years to understand what was meant by this phrase. While I was in school, I used to badger one excellent practitioner/teacher in particular, Sharon Feng, MD (China), LAc, as to how acupuncture *really* worked. I demanded regularly why a certain needle would correct a certain condition. For example, I *keenly* wanted to know how, exactly, a needle inserted at Ren-4 might stimulate ovarian function. Sharon answered me every time with "Tong Zhi Bu Tong; Bu Tong Zhi

Diagnosing the flow of channel Qi, the very essence of Asian medicine, can be *guessed* at by feeling the pulses, looking at the tongue, considering the patient's symptoms in light of the Eight Parameters, the Five Elements, or any other method of diagnosis.

Then again, the direct method of feeling the *actual* movement of channel Qi is easy to do and requires no guesswork. The diagnostic method of detecting the actual flow of channel Qi can yield a highly accurate diagnosis and suggest a confirmable treatment plan.

The most elegant method of diagnosis, aside from intuitive, heart-resonant awareness, is direct perception of the channels.

This method of diagnosis is not discussed in the versions of the Asian medical classics that have been handed down to us. We can only conjecture as to the reasons for this omission.[1]

Tong." When, in my increasing frustration, I regularly demanded a more technical answer, she patiently translated it for me, "Go through, no pain; No go through, pain."

She must have thought I had no memory skills whatsoever because, for several years, we went through this drill at least once a week. It became pure routine.

Many years after I'd graduated, while treating a patient in my private practice, I suddenly realized that the patient's problem was arising from an incorrect, diverted pattern of channel Qi flow in an area distal to the problem area. As soon as my acupuncture treatment corrected his diverted flow of channel Qi, the channel Qi began to flow correctly – it coursed all the way up his leg to the problem area in the torso. The person's pains and tensions in this area immediately released: the patient felt warmth and healing energy coursing through the problem spot.

At the same moment that the patient began to respond, I suddenly realized what had happened: the Qi was now "Going Through." Now, there was "No pain."

I suddenly realized that "Go through" means "the channels flow in their correct pathways." The word "Pain" means "anything that is detrimental for a human." I've finally come to understand that the word "Pain," in this context, can mean aberrant conditions ranging from influenza, cancer, indigestion, insomnia, self-pity or anger, all the way to gallstones. These are all included under the heading of "Pain."

As I realized this, I first wondered why my teacher hadn't explained this to me. Then, in a humiliating flash of belated insight, I realized that she *had*. She had told me, day after day, week after week, "Go through, no pain; No go through, pain." She had told me exactly, concisely, the essence of Asian medicine. But because I was not yet able to feel channels and work with channels, I wasn't able to understand her.

Eventually, I came up with the following English "expanded translation version" of what she meant: "If the channels are all flowing in their correct patterns, a person's health is correct. If the channels are not flowing correctly, the person's health is being negatively affected": Tong Zhi Bu Tong; Bu Tong, Zhi Tong. Now, twenty years later, Dr. Sharon Feng is still very patient with me when I come to her with questions.

[1] In the last few decades, a few practitioners have been trying to bring channel theory and diagnosis back into play. Dr. Ju-Yi Wang, a highly respected professor and practitioner of Chinese medicine, and for many years the editor of the Chinese journal *Chinese Medicine*, has written an excellent book in English (not available in Chinese) on the subject: *Applied Channel Theory in Chinese Medicine: Wang Ju-Yi's Lectures on Channel Therapeutics*, by Wang Ju-Yi and Jason Robertson, Eastland Press, Seattle, 2008.

Dr. Wang recommends that students look for problems in channel Qi flow by feeling for the small bumps of fluids that accumulate when channel Qi is flowing too slowly over a long period of

Leaving the dark ages behind

In modern times, invisible forces are no longer considered magical. For example, cell phones receive invisible signals from practically invisible satellites and medical diagnostics are done with the invisible forces inside of magnetic resonance machines. For the most part, a doctor is no longer suspected of being unscientific or in league with the devil when he works with "invisible" forces such as electric static, electrical currents, electromagnetic fields – and someday soon, channel Qi.[1]

Nor is it, in this century, in many countries, unduly immodest to pursue detection of channel Qi in close proximity to (within a few inches of) a patient's body. Such proximity would have been considered immoral only a century ago.[2]

---

time. By limiting his channel diagnostics to obviously palpable bumps, which he calls nodules, rather than feeling the Qi directly, he avoids the inevitable discussions about working with invisible, electrical forces. These nodules develop along the paths of channels that have been running poorly for a significant period of time – like silt building up in the bed of a slow moving stream.

However, I have watched him work. Sometimes he demonstrates that he is feeling for bumps. Other times, he seems to be assessing the channel Qi flow without touching the patient's body – but if asked, he insists he is feeling for nodules. Dr. Wang kept many of his ideas on channel theory under the radar during the decades when, in China, the very *idea* of channels was sweepingly dismissed as dangerous superstition. After the turn of the millennium, the political climate in China changed enough that "belief" in channels was no longer politically dangerous. Dr. Wang told me during a lunch (via translator Jason Robertson), "Now, in China, you can no longer get in trouble for insisting on the existence of channels – but on the other hand, no one in the medical realm will be interested in hearing about them or discussing them."

Nevertheless, because of his extraordinary success in treating unusually difficult cases, and in spite of his eventual "coming out" regarding his use of widely and *officially* scorned channel theory, he has become a National Treasure.

[1] Students who were born in these "modern" times may not realize just how mysterious and "work-of-the-devil" the invisible forces used to seem, even in the early twentieth century, even after witch burning had ceased to be fashionable in most countries.

One of my favorite stories by American humorist James Thurber recounts how, after his grandmother's house was put on the power grid in the early part of the 20th century:

"Grandma was always "horribly suspicious that electricity was dripping invisibly out all over the house. It leaked, she contended, out of empty sockets if the wall switch had been left on. She would go around screwing in a bulb, and if it lighted up, she would hastily and fearfully turn off the wall switch. She was satisfied then that she had stopped not only a costly but a dangerous leakage. Nobody could ever clear this up for her." (From *The Thurber Carnival*, James Thurber, Kingsport Press, 1945, "The Car We Had to Push," p.186.)

Happily, in these modern days of radio, TV, and cyber communication, we no longer are guilty of witchcraft when we make use of – or are able to detect – "invisible" forms of energy. In much of the world, doctors can safely admit, once again, that the flow of channel Qi is real, and is easy to feel.

[2] We've all heard how, during one of history's "modesty" crazes, doctors were not allowed to feel the pulses of high-born women in China. Instead, the doctor had to sit a respectful distance from the patient and feel her pulses via a piece of silk thread that had been tied around her wrist. I cannot verify the truth of this persistent story. (Continued on next page.)

66

It has *always* been possible to detect by hand the flow of a patient's invisible channel Qi. However, for at least two millennia, we can be fairly certain that such detection, requiring both proximity and the acknowledgement of invisible forces, would not have been culturally acceptable to the general public.

We cannot know if this method of diagnosis was explicitly described in the original *Nei Jing* and then discarded when it became suspect, or if it were merely alluded to, and dropped when it became incomprehensible. It is even possible that the ancient medical masters, having been commanded to write up their knowledge for the benefit of the self-proclaimed emperor, intentionally left out their most important technique: detecting the flow of channel Qi.[1]

But today, in the twenty-first century, diagnosis via direct perception of channel Qi is once *again* explicable and morally free from suspicion.[2]

In conclusion

Working diagnostically with channel Qi flow is not new. It was used in ancient times: "Beginners think it is easy."

I am more certain of the authority of the following case study demonstrating twentieth century medical modesty: a woman had received a jagged cut on the buttocks that needed to be stitched up, and soon. The "mortifying" injury had occurred on one of three unmarried, elderly sisters. The sisters lived together in genteel antebellum style in America's south in the early twentieth century. Their high point of each week was an evening of cards with the elderly town doctor – the only doctor in their small village. Of course, if the doctor were to put in stitches in "such a place," the sister in question would never be able to face him again. Their quartets of cards would be impossible. The solution? A maid fetched the doctor and led him into the silent parlor of the Victorian-style mansion. In the parlor, only the patient was present – the other two sisters were hiding upstairs. The patient was anonymously swathed in sheets except for the site of injury. The patient made no sound, spoke not a word, throughout the ordeal of being stitched up. The same conditions prevailed when the doctor returned to remove the stitches, one week later. At the card game the following week, all three sisters were sitting on soft cushions. Thus, modesty had been preserved, and life resumed as usual.

These two examples, the pulse-via-thread and the anonymity required of stitches to the fanny, are given here merely to make the point that the need for false modesty in the patient-doctor interface has greatly lessened in recent times, in many nations.

[1] Given the "Golden" Emperor's fondness for having scholars buried alive and other heinous acts of political expediency *and* his fearful obsession with aging and death – and his early demise – it may well be that the best doctors of the day knew about the Emperor's lurking health problems and kept silent on any subjects that might have provided medical assistance to the tyrant – particularly the subject of diagnosing via channel Qi flow.

[2] I may be premature in stating that working with invisible energy is no longer suspect; I've had patients who, prior to making their first acupuncture appointment, have sought council with their pastors to determine whether or not acupuncture was "safe for Christians." Happily, in all the cases that have come to my attention, the Christian pastors have affirmed that acupuncture is, indeed, safe for Christians. As one pastor put it, "All healing comes from God."

In my mere twenty years of practice, I've seen acceptance of energetic (invisible) medicine growing steadily.

The knowledge of channel Qi flow in sickness and health is not only absolutely consistent with principles of Asian medicine, it is the underlying basis for the development of the diagnostic "patterns" of Asian medicine. The "patterns" are merely systematic ways of assembling information so that one can make an educated *guess* at what the channels are doing. The patterns can be extremely helpful – or not. But knowing what a patient's channels are actually doing gives a practitioner a much better chance of diagnosing the *exact* story.

Diagnostics via channel Qi flow might not have been used overtly, publicly, for more than two millennia. Now, though some might say, "Once again," we live in an era where electricity, electromagnetic waves, magnetism, and other forms of "invisible" energy are socially acceptable forces. Knowable channels, "by virtue of which all human life is possible" are, once again, forces that we can use – and we can once again admit that we are using them.

Perfect intuition will always be the best method of diagnosis. But second best is direct perception of channel Qi flow. This highly accurate, *easily taught* method for determining a medical diagnosis is once again socially acceptable.

Let us rejoice in the morning of a higher age. The ancient masters rejoice with us.

"Change of colors corresponds to pulses of the four seasons, which is valued by gods because it is in tune with the divine being and which enables us to flee from death and stay close to life." [1]

Chapter five

The healthy paths of the channels: part I

Parasympathetic mode

Introduction: The four healthy modes

These next four chapters will describe the healthy paths of the channels: the four main categories of *correct*, healthy channel Qi routes. These four routings of channel Qi occur in 1) parasympathetic mode, 2) sympathetic mode, 3) sleep, and 4) dissociation.

The parasympathetic routes are, more or less, the primary channel paths that we learn in school. The other three routings for channel Qi occur in response to daily activities, as a person shifts from parasympathetic mode to sympathetic mode, or sleep mode, and once in a great while, into dissociation mode.

This first-of-four chapter includes introductory details about the four main modes and then will focus primarily on the parasympathetic mode pathways.

---

[1] *Su Wen*, chapter 13-9, from *A Complete Translation of the Yellow Emperor's Classics of Internal Medicine and the Difficult Classic*, by Henry C. Lu, PhD, published by the International College of Traditional Chinese Medicine, Vancouver, BC, Canada, 2004.

The "four seasons," in this case, are the four neural modes. The first mode, full blown parasympathetic, occurs in deep meditation, joy, or contentment, when we are, as it says in the above quote, "in tune with the Divine Being." The sympathetic mode, sometimes called "fight or flight," enables us, as the quote says next, "to flee from death." Dissociated mode, which is a last-ditch attempt by the body to stay alive in the face of mortal wounds, lets us "stay close to life." The fourth season, sleep, is not mentioned in this stanza of the *Su Wen*. Very likely, it was included in the original, but fell by the wayside when someone either misplaced the original or felt that sleep was not a medical condition and so decided to leave it out.

This selection from the *Su Wen* might best be translated into modern English as "The changes in channel Qi (electrical and wave energy in the channels, aka color, or light-wave energy) correspond to the four neural modes. These four modes consist of parasympathetic (at peace), sympathetic (fearful), dissociative (dealing with mortal injury), and sleep. These modes, in turn, cause changes in heart rate and organ functions, and are *reflected*, somewhat, in the pulses."

Introductory details about the four modes

1) Parasympathetic

Back in the 1960s, I was taught in high school to think of parasympathetic as the "mindless, cud-chewing" mode. Now, we consider parasympathetic mode to be far more complex: animal behaviorists consider parasympathetic mode the mode that dominates during contentment or during "seeking" behaviors such as eating, reading, flirting, singing, following up on curiosity, ambling about. Pretty much any activity that does *not* involve fear can occur while a person is in parasympathetic mode.

The parasympathetic routes of channel Qi are the routes of the twelve primary channels, routes that we learn in school. These routings are considered an ideal, and manifest in a person who is relaxed, at peace, joyful, and utterly without fear.

The closer one's channel Qi flow patterns resemble the parasympathetic, or "ideal" routes, the healthier that person is.

Of course, in reality, it might be safe to say that almost no one has channel flow patterns that correspond *exactly* to those ideals. Certainly, a patient with health problems does *not* have channel Qi flow that conforms exactly to the ideal routes.

2) Sympathetic

Another major mode is sympathetic mode.[1] Sympathetic mode is sometimes referred to as "fight or flight" or, more correctly, "fret, fight, flight, or freeze."

In this mode, channel Qi does not flow in the same patterns as it does when one is content or joyful. In sympathetic mode, channel Qi is redirected ("diverges" is the verb usually used in acupuncture texts) primarily to the heart, adrenal glands, and the sides of the brain (the precuneus, or "ego assessment" areas), and to specific, adrenaline-driven motor functions. The channel Qi from digestion-serving channels is diverted away from digestion, and applied to the adrenaline-based needs of the moment.

3) Sleep

During sleep, also, the channels do *not* flow in the parasympathetic pattern. Sleep is a condition that, physiologically, electrically, neurally, is considerably different from parasympathetic mode. The channel Qi divergences that occur during sleep drive the *subsequent* physiological changes that occur during sleep. These changes allow for diminished consciousness, reduced digestive function, and muscle inhibition.

---

[1] Some students confuse sympathetic and parasympathetic, possibly because the word "sympathy" suggests peace and calm. The neural mode nomenclature has *nothing* to do with our modern meaning for the word "sympathy." This nomenclature was applied, in the 1780s, to those nerves that became *activated* in response to stress. (The "stress" was Galvani's electrical shock, applied to frogs.) At the time, all *other* nerves were assumed, incorrectly, to run automatically, without triggers. This *activation* in response to stress was considered "sympathetic" which, back in the day, meant "responsive." Over time, we began to apply this "sympathetic" nomenclature to all the adrenaline-based systems: systems that *respond* to fear.

4) Dissociation`

During dissociation, the channel Qi flows *very* differently than during parasympathetic mode – including running backwards, in some channels, and back and forth in others.

Briefly, dissociation is a normal, correct response to a near-mortal injury, extreme loss of blood, or excessive slicing or puncturing of the skin. This mode, the least frequent (hopefully) of the four main modes, nevertheless provides the most exquisite understanding of the extreme variability of normal, correct channel Qi flow patterns.

Generalities about the three *non*-parasympathetic routes

The channel Qi routes that are not part of the parasympathetic system are referred to in the *Nei Jing* as "divergent" routes, which is to say, they diverge from the ideal (parasympathetic) Primary paths of channel Qi.

In the classic literature, information about the various channel divergences is currently scattered across several chapters. Some information appears in the divergence section, in which a sampling of the many divergent channel possibilities is described. Descriptions of other common divergent paths are found, incorrectly, in the descriptions of the primary channel routes, mixed in with the descriptions of the primary channels. The inclusion of possible divergences in with the basic description of a given channel's primary routing can give the reader the incorrect idea that the channel Qi *always* flows in *all* of the possible routes that are mentioned for any given channel. A quick assessment of the channel Qi, by hand, will be enough to show the curious student the errors of these inclusions.

Given the great antiquity of the *Nei Jing*, it is not surprising that a few bits have gotten jumbled or displaced. However, by actually feeling the channel Qi routes of patients, in sickness and in health, you will be able to learn where the paths actually go in each of the four modes and what constitutes a healthy divergent (*non*-parasympathetic) path.

Parasympathetic mode

The channel Qi flow patterns that we learn in school are an ideal. They represent the Qi flow patterns that occur in a person of perfect health who is 1) awake and 2) in full-bore parasympathetic mode. Parasympathetic mode is the neural mode that dominates when we are without fear, which is to say, "close to the Divine," and possibly engaged in "seeking" behaviors.

A note to those seeking licensure: do not remember the following information when you are taking the licensing board exams. For the exams, recite all point locations and channel properties exactly as they are taught in the official books. The material in this book is NOT referenced in the board exams.

From one channel to another

The twelve primary channels are not twelve distinct segments of current. The channels are *one* continuous, looping stream of electricity. We say, for the sake of convenience, that the flow of the primary channels "begins" at LU-1, at the beginning of the

Lung channel. At the very end of the "last" primary channel, the Liver channel, the channel Qi flows back into the beginning of the "first" channel.

In a healthy person who is awake and relaxed (in parasympathetic mode), the channels *flow* in the same sequence that you were *taught* these channels, in school.

The first channel you studied, the Lung channel, flows into the second channel you studied, the Large Intestine channel. The Large Intestine channel flows into the third, or Stomach, channel. The Stomach channel flows into the Spleen channel, and so on. We are *taught* the channels in this sequence, all the books on Asian medicine *present* them in this sequence, because the channel Qi *flows* in this sequence. Or, to be more correct, they flow in this sequence up to seventy percent of the time, *at most*, in a perfectly healthy person.[1]

Prove it to yourself

If you've taken these pathways on pure trust, up until now, the time has come for you to prove to yourself that these flow patterns do exist. Track the paths of all the primary channels.

If you have some extra time, you can even feel for the channel Qi flow at the Luo (extra connecting) channels, as well. Discover for yourself the tangible routes of the Exit/Entry connections.

You now *know* how to *feel* the flow of channel Qi: you can prove to yourself whether or not the classical teachings regarding the primary channels and the four modes are actually correct. Start with parasympathetic mode. Confirm to your own satisfaction that the paths of the channels, as taught in the texts, actually do conform to the channel Qi flow in a relaxed, healthy human: a person in parasympathetic mode.

Start with a patient who is contentedly relaxed, which is to say, in parasympathetic mode. See if his channels flow in approximately the same locations and directions that you learned in school.

Often, an easy place to feel one of the highly specific "bends" in the flow of channel Qi is the mid-torso part of the Stomach channel after the channel Qi has passed over the breast. I was thrilled the first time I felt it: my hand was pulled closer to the midline as it flowed from ST-18 over to ST-20. Just like the pictures in the books!

To help you understand some of what you will feel, the following discussion takes you on a channel-by-channel trip through the channel transitions of parasympathetic mode.

If you have not yet learned the paths of the channels, you can refer to the "actual" channel maps (as opposed to the modern "traditional" maps) in the appendix, at the back of the book.

Details of channel transitions

Approaching the end of the Lung channel, near the wrist, a small amount of the Lung channel Qi flows into the Large Intestine channel, from LU-7 to LI-4. The rest of the Lung channel Qi spreads out into various paths: some flows over the palm and up the palmar surface of the index finger, some makes its way down to the tip of the thumb via the palmar surface and the sides of the thumb.

---

[1] This statement was made by Dr. Ju-Yi Wang, world authority on channel theory, in a doctoral program lecture in 2007. Even a healthy person sleeps about 30% of his day. During sleep, the channel Qi flows very differently, hence, the "70%" statement.

After getting all the way to the tip of the index finger, some of this Lung channel Qi flows back up the dorsal side and the "closer to the thumb side," or "medial side" of the index finger.[1] Whenever the thumb makes fleeting contact with the index finger, the Lung channel Qi that makes it to the tip of the thumb will also flow into the medial side of the index finger. Otherwise, channel Qi in the thumb can be discharged as static onto any surface that is touched.[2]

Any excess channel Qi, channel Qi that is not needed by the body, will be discharged out the tips of the fingers or toes into whatever surfaces touch the fingers.

The proportion of the channel's Qi that flows from LU-7 into the luo vessel, shunting directly to LI-4, *relative* to the amount that flows over the thenar prominence of the palm, or out to the finger tips, varies from moment to moment, depending on the amount of channel Qi that is being needed for use in the fingertips *or* on what neural mode the person happens to be in at the moment.

A similar variability in channel routing occurs in *all* the channels that terminate in the digits: some channel Qi is routed directly from the channel's Exit point into the Entry point on the next channel, some gets routed to the fingers or toes and thence into the next channel, with any excess being discharged as static.

The more a person is leaning towards parasympathetic, the greater amount that goes to the tips of the fingers and toes. (Consider how the hands and toes grow sweetly warm when a person becomes deeply relaxed.) Oppositely, the more a person is leaning towards sympathetic mode, the greater the amount that goes directly into the Entry point of the next channel – unless the fingers or toes are being called upon to perform some specific task, in which case they may receive a larger share of channel Qi for the moment.[3]

Yin Tang, the meeting place

After the Lung channel Qi has flowed into the Large Intestine channel, the Large Intestine channel flows up the arm to Yin Tang.

Yin Tang is the meeting point of all three arm-Yang channels (Large Intestine, Small Intestine, and Triple Burner). Although all the channel Qi in the body is actually one, continuous stream, all the arm-Yang channels are said to end at Yin Tang, and the three leg-Yang channels (Stomach, Urinary Bladder, and Gallbladder) are said to begin at Yin Tang.

The flow of channel Qi is one continuous stream, even though the ratio of the five *types* of channel Qi is different in the various channels. Still, for the sake of convenience and

---

[1] The awkward phrasing, "thumb-side" of the index finger, is used here because, in posing the hands for the "standard medical posture," the hands face opposite ways in Asian and western medicine. Therefore, Asian and western terminologies assume opposite meanings for the directional word "medial," when applied to the hands.

[2] The famous hand posture, or "mudra," in which the tip of the thumb rests against the tip of the index finger is a position that stimulates more Lung channel Qi to transition to Large Intestine channel Qi via parasympathetic mode, as opposed to having more Lung channel Qi transition via the Luo channel, on the wrist – which is a sympathetic mode pattern.

[3] Maps of all the channel paths can be found at the back of the book. This chapter contains only a selected few of the actual channel paths – those few that are significantly different from the paths that are currently taught in school as "traditional" channels.

nomenclature, we speak of the channels as if they stop and start. And Yin Tang, "the meeting place," is the spot at which the arm-Yang channel nomenclature ends and the leg-Yang channel nomenclature begins.

As Large Intestine channel Qi flows into Yin Tang, its Yang Ming characteristics route it into a path that we call the Stomach channel.

While this Yin Tang business may seem like an insignificant detail for now, Yin Tang will appear over and over in discussions of the different neural modes.

The Stomach channel path

Stomach channel Qi flows down from Yin Tang, the point between the eyebrows, and spreads over the face.

As the Stomach channel Qi flows down to the cheek bones, it spreads wide, spanning the distance from ST-3 to ST-7. The Stomach channel Qi of the face is still somewhat "wide" as it spreads between ST-4 and ST-5, and then narrows as it collects at ST-6. The Stomach channel stays somewhat narrow as it makes its way down the front of the neck, along the sternocleidomastoids.

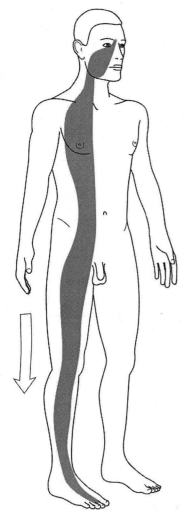

Fig. 5.1 Actual main path of the Stomach channel. The smaller, connecting paths and internal paths are not shown.

As the Stomach channel pours down the chest, it widens out as it crosses over the breast. It narrows a bit as it moves closer to the Ren channel. Then, when it crosses over to the hip, it widens again.

On the lower leg, at ST-36, the channel is quite wide. The "location" of ST-36 activity is sometimes said to be up to three inches across. Needling almost anywhere into the vicinity of this "Sea of Qi" (aka ST-36) will elicit a channel Qi response. The channel becomes very narrow and strong when the channel Qi flows over ST-42.

As an aside, the flow of the Stomach channel over the face does *not* follow a skinny line that connects-the-dots of the Stomach channel points. Whoever decided on the modern numbering system for the Stomach channel acupoints numbered them in such a manner that the channel seems to zig-zag back and forth. For example, ST-1 is at the eyes and ST-6 is at the back of the jaw. But ST-8 is up on the forehead. And ST-9 is

74

down on the neck.[1]

A quick detection of the Stomach channel Qi will show that this channel does *not* jump back and forth, from the chin to the forehead, and back to the neck.

From ST-42, the Stomach channel Qi bifurcates. Some of the channel Qi flows over to SP-3, making a graceful arc across the top of the foot. The rest of the Stomach channel Qi flows out the tips of the second and third toes. From here, any excess channel Qi can either ground out into the earth (or shoes and socks) or flow medially over the tips of the toes until it flows into the Spleen channel at SP-1.

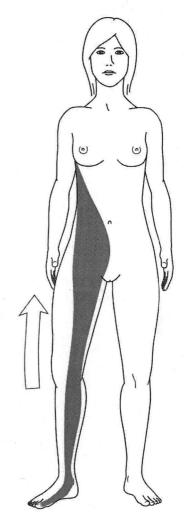

Fig. 5.2   The actual path of the Spleen channel.

Transitioning into the Spleen channel from the Stomach channel

When a person is, to a high degree, in sympathetic (fight, flight, or freeze) mode, nearly all the Stomach channel Qi flows directly into SP-3 instead of flowing out to the toes.

Only when a person is in parasympathetic mode or in sleep mode does a significant amount, a detectable-by-hand amount, of Stomach channel Qi flow all the way out to the tips of the toes, before flowing medially, along the tips of the toes, into the Spleen channel, in the vicinity of SP-1.

The spleen channel flows up the legs and much of the torso. In those areas where the Spleen and Liver

---

[1] Compare the actual path of the Stomach channel with the "traditional" map of the Stomach channel, in the back of this book. In the "traditional" drawings, the Stomach channel Qi caroms back and forth, and up and down, as it traverses the face, as if the channel Qi travels in all directions at all times. This is not the case: the branch of the Stomach channel that supposedly travels from the chin to the neck is not active in parasympathetic mode.

channel pass through the same zone, the Spleen channel passes under (closer to the muscle, farther from the skin) the Liver channel. (In the historical texts, this is usually referred to as "The Liver channel crosses *over* the Spleen channel.") Just below the armpit, as the Spleen channel passes by the heart and pericardium, the channel Qi changes names, and becomes known as the Heart channel.

Going past the heart

As an aside, the ever-changing electr-magnetic signals emitted by the heart and pericardium, signals that alter in response to every thought, regulate the transitions in channel Qi flow as all of the three leg Yin channels (Spleen, Kidney, and Liver) traverse the torso and head into the arms. The signals from the heart tell the channels how much channel Qi can transition from the leg Yin channels into the next channel along the primary route (an arm Yin channel, in every case), and how much channel Qi should go elsewhere, as needed at the moment.

For example, when a person is in pure parasympathetic mode, almost all of the Spleen channel Qi flows into the Heart channel, almost all of the Kidney channel Qi flows into the Pericardium channel, and almost all of the Liver channel Qi flows into the Lung channel.

However, if the heart's electromagnetic signals broadcast stress or fear, each of these channels will divert some portion of channel Qi towards the physical heart and the head, "shortchanging" the arm Yin channels. The Liver channel, in particular, will send a significant amount of channel Qi to the top of the head (the vertex), in response to stress. The amount of channel Qi sent to the heart and head is directly related to the amount of stress being broadcast by the heart.

Heart to Small Intestine

At the wrist and/or fingers, depending on mode and mood, respectively, the Heart channel Qi transitions into the Small Intestine channel Qi, which then flows up the arm.

As Small Intestine channel Qi approaches the shoulder, it widens, becoming broad enough to encompass both SI-9 and SI-10. Then, staying wide and shallow, it flows over the shoulder blade SI points. The path narrows again as the channel approaches the neck. The back and shoulder blade parts of the Small Intestine channel and the Urinary Bladder channel overlap a bit. In these cases – as is evident by the location of the shoulder blades themselves (bones that are formed by the currents in the Small Intestine channel) – the Small Intestine channel is closer to the skin. The Urinary Bladder channel, which helps grow and regulate the muscles that run down the back, runs deeper, going "under" the Small Intestine channel in these areas.

The Small Intestine channel flows up the neck and under the ear. It passes from the ear up to the eyebrow, where it flows under the Gallbladder channel during its approach to Yin Tang.

Urinary Bladder channel

From Yin Tang, the ever-flowing channel Qi flows up over the head and is referred to as Urinary Bladder channel Qi.

The Urinary Bladder channel flows down the left and right sides of the spine, in a stream several inches wide. The "inner" and "outer" rows of UB back-acupoints are *not* two separate streams of channel Qi. The inner and outer acupoints merely delineate the two strongest areas of flow in the fairly wide channel.

The Urinary Bladder channel is wide enough to span the distance from the Du channel to the Gallbladder channel. Take a moment to feel the Urinary Bladder

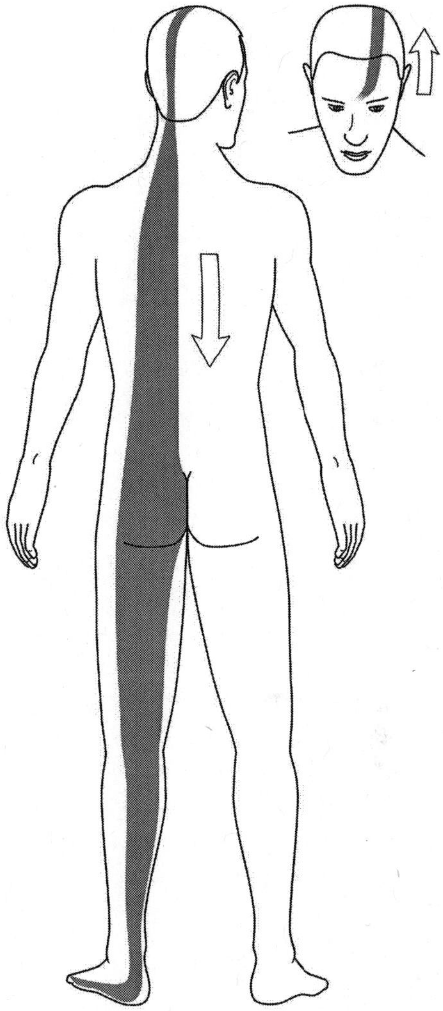

Fig. 5.3 The actual path of the Urinary Bladder channel.

The Bladder channel Qi flows into Kidney channel Qi, which flows into Pericardium channel Qi, which flows into Triple Burner channel Qi, and back up to Yin Tang. As the Triple Burrner channel approaches Yin Tang from the ear, it flows deep within, going under the eyebrows. From Yin Tang, the Gallbladder channel Qi flows over the eyebrows and spreads out into a very wide path that covers the side of the head.

There is *no* area on the surface of the body that does not have channel Qi in it. The channels all butt up against each other, and even mingle a bit at the edges. When we refer casually to a channel, however, we are usually referring to that narrower part of the channel that is strong enough to be felt by hand, along which we also find the points of lowered electrical resistance associated with that channel.

Technically, the Urinary Bladder channel goes almost to the lateral side of the body, where its channel Qi mingles with the GB channel Qi. But when we mention the Urinary Bladder channel, we are usually referring to only those portions of the UB channel that have low enough resistance to make a detectable stream, complete with spots of very low resistance that merit named acupoints.

And so on

The Urinary Bladder channel transitions into the Kidney channel, at the feet. The Kidney channel flows into the Pericardium channel, transitioning in the vicinity of the heart. The Pericardium flows over the wrist and fingers while transitioning into the Triple Burner channel. The Triple Burner channel flows to Yin Tang, and then into the Gallbladder channel.

Fun with the Gallbladder channel

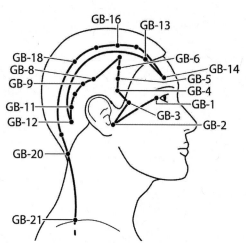

Fig. 5.4 The modern, "Traditional" path of the head portion of the Gallbladder channel. To trace the path of the channel, you must follow-the-dots back and forth over the side of the head.

The Gallbladder channel spreads out over the sides of the head. The point numbering system on the Gallbladder channel suggests that a skinny line of channel Qi zig-zags from point to point, circles behind the ears, and then scampers back to the forehead again to start connecting-the-dots from GB-13 to GB-20. This is incorrect.

By feeling the Gallbladder channel as it courses over the sides of the head, it is obvious that the Gallbladder channel goes wide and shallow as it spans the distance between the middle of the eyebrow and the front of the ear. From there, this wide swath of channel Qi flows in a sheet from the side/front of the face to the side/back of the head. The Gallbladder channel Qi narrows and gathers strength as it approaches GB-20.

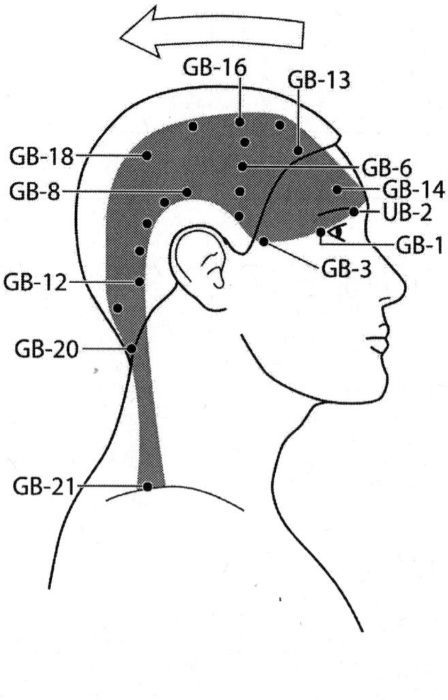

Fig. 5.5 The actual, detectable path of the head portion of the Gallbladder channel.

78

An aside: a Gallbladder channel Qi strength / water-flow analogy

Water in a wide, flat stream seems to move slowly. The exact same amount of water movement picks up speed and power as it flows through a steep narrows. In the same way, the Gallbladder channel Qi movement can barely be felt over the wide areas of the forehead and sides of the head, but it increases in localized strength as it narrows and cascades along the neck and into the shoulder at GB-20 and GB-21, respectively. Even so, the channel Qi can be felt: a slightly stronger sense of the channel Qi can be detected along the *edges* of the swath, where the acupoints are located.

Continuing along the path of the Gallblader channel, on the sides of the torso, the Gallbladder channel is also a wide swath, just as it was on the side of the head. The GB points on the anterior and posterior side of the body are located along the two outer *edges* of this

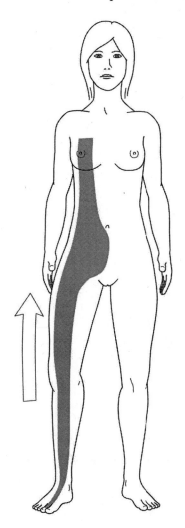

swath. The Gallbladder channel is *not* a thin line of channel Qi that zigs and zags back and forth, "connecting the dots." It is a smooth, wide span of channel Qi that flows in one direction, like a shallow but wide stretch of a river, with acupoints on either side. The channel narrows again, at the knee and at the ankle.

The Gallbladder channel bifurcates at GB-41, on the foot. One branch goes deep (beneath the foot portion of the Stomach channel) and arrives at LIV-3. The other branch goes out to the tips of the lateral toes before moving medially through the foot at the level of the toe webbing, before transitioning into the Liver channel.

Fig. 5.6 The actual path of the Liver channel

The Liver channel "crosses over" the Spleen channel

In several places, a quick glance at the paths of the Liver and Spleen channels suggests that these channels are running in the same place, or you might say, in the same riverbed. The Chinese classics point out that, in these cases, the Liver "crosses over" the Spleen channel. "Cross over" refers to the palpable fact that, in these situations, the Liver channel stays closer to the surface of the skin, while the adjacent Spleen channel flows more deeply inside – going "under" the Liver channel.

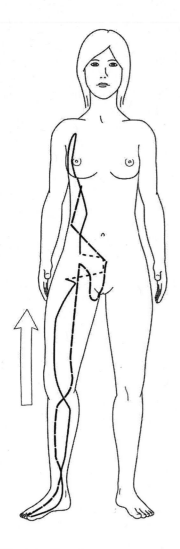

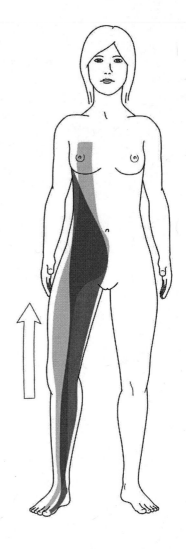

Fig. 5.7 Traditional Liver and Spleen channels. The solid line is Spleen; the dashed line is Liver. They meet and cross at various spots.

Fig. 5.8 Actual Liver and Spleen. The pale swath is the Liver, the darker is the Spleen. The darkest area shows the area of overlap.

A long-standing mistranslation of "cross over" presumes the Liver and Spleen channels are two narrow lines that zigzag back and forth: first, one of the two channels is more anterior and then, after "crossing over," the other is more anterior – creating the effect of shoelaces. This unlucky guess at the meaning of "crosses over," perhaps institutionalized centuries ago by a misguided artist, is *not* borne out by an examination of the paths of the channels.

A better choice of words was used, historically, in describing the exact same type of "cross over" situation, with regard to the Liver and Stomach channel. In the Liver/Stomach section, the author's meaning is clearer: he wrote that the Liver channel goes deep and passes *under* the Stomach channel.

This deeper vs. shallower meaning of "cross over" is the same meaning of "cross over" that occurs in the Liver and Spleen channels. When these two channels traverse the same bit of territory, the Liver channel stays closer to the surface of the skin, which is to say, it goes over the Spleen channel. The Spleen channel goes deep, staying under the Liver channel.

I can only imagine the artistic meanderings and zigzag lines that might today be part of our lore if the writer had ambiguously noted, "On the upper part of the chest, the Stomach channel "crosses over" the Liver channel." We'd probably have something on the pectoral muscles resembling the shoelace-like criss-crosses of the traditional Liver and Spleen channels!

Please, do not take my word for any of this "cross-over" information. Feel the flow of the Liver and Spleen channels on fellow students. Feel it in your own legs and torso.

Getting back to the Liver channel, note that, lower on the torso, the medial edge of the Liver channel touches the Ren channel at Ren-3 and Ren-4, even as its lateral edge extends almost all the way to the Gallbladder channel. In this area, as before, the wide Liver channel is more superficial (closer to the skin) than the equally wide Spleen channel. The Spleen channel, also wide through this area, takes the "underpass" route, relative to the Liver channel.

As an aside, the Kidney channel underlaps the Spleen channel, on the legs, and the Liver *and* Spleen channels, on the torso. The torso portion of the kidney channel only rises up to the surface, where it's accessible for needling (and detection), in a narrow band alongside the Ren channel. In this narrow band, it rises up, like the fin on an orca, from its path deep beneath the other two leg-Yin channels.

An oft used mnemonic device to help students remember which channel is closest to the surface, which is in the middle, and which is deepest, reminds us that, "The Liver is associated with the tendons. The Spleen is associated with the muscles. The Kidney is associated with the bones."

Some tendons are closer to the surface than the muscles, in places such as the back of the knee, and ankle. Bones are deeper inside than both tendons (Liver) and muscles (Spleen). When the three Yin channels of the leg run through similar zones, on the torso and on the leg, the Liver channel stays closer to the surface than the Spleen, and the Kidney goes deepest of all.

Trying, once again, to get back to the subject of the Liver channel, note that, as with the widest parts of the Gallbladder channel, the widest parts of the Liver channel may be somewhat more difficult to discern than the narrow, strongly running areas, for the beginner. Even so, though the channel Qi may be more difficult to detect along the borders of the channel, some channel Qi flow is usually discernable if one holds his hand nearer the "center" of the river – in the midstream part of the channel, along the named points that run up the torso, 4 cun away from the Ren (See Fig. 5.11).

At the end of the Liver channel, the endless loop of primary channel Qi "comes to an end" in name, only. The flowing channel Qi of the Liver channel, the last of the twelve primary channels, comes to LIV-14 and dives "deep into the chest," which is to say, it moves interiorly, diving "under" the pectoral portion of the Stomach channel. (The chest portion of the Stomach channel, running the other direction towards the feet, is closer to the surface of the skin, compared to the Liver channel. We say the Stomach channel crosses "over" the Liver channel.) The Liver channel Qi dives deep, bathing and nourishing the organs of heart, pericardium, and lungs. Meanwhile, the more superficial Stomach channel nourishes the pectoral muscles and the breasts.

After passing through the chest, *most* of the Liver channel Qi re-emerges on the surface of the body at LU-1 – which is where the discussion started!

If a person is not in perfect parasympathetic mode, some portion of the Liver channel Qi is shunted into various divergences, as needed. One of the main divergences is the branch of the Liver channel Qi that flows up to the vertex, communicating vibratory signals from the heart to the brain, and updating the Du with channel Qi information that carries the moment-by-moment Heart-feeling resonances.

When a person is utterly at peace, so that his third eye (just behind Yin Tang) is able to communicate *directly* (via electromagnetic wave signals) with the heart, *no* electrical "messenger" current of Liver channel Qi needs to be sent to the vertex: all of the Liver channel Qi can flow directly into the arms.

Summary of parasympathetic channel paths

The above is a deeply simplified version of the routes of the primary channels.

The details of the many parasympathetic bifurcations, such as the Exit/Entry points and Luo channels, have barely been addressed.

The most important aspect of the bifurcations to remember is this: with all the bifurcations and divergences, how *much* channel Qi flows into which path is determined by many factors, including mood and activity requirements. These factors can change as quickly as a thought.

In every case, the distribution of channel Qi is not random, nor is it automatic. It is directed by consciousness, subconsciousness, and superconsciousness. It can be negatively influenced by harsh weather, pathogens, toxins, wrong food, wrong behavior. It is constantly changing to perfectly accommodate the energetic needs of the moment.

Channels are like rivers

Channels are like rivers of energy. They are wide and shallow in some areas, narrow and deep in others. The named points are like villages that might be located along the riverbanks, or even located in midstream. By looking at an atlas and noticing the cities alongside the blue line that signifies "river," we can discern, somewhat, the course of the river. But this two-dimensional representation will not tell us where the rapids, the shallows, or the waterfalls are.

In the same way, the point system doesn't tell us about the width or depth of a channel: it only gives the overall direction of channel Qi flow and a general idea about the whereabouts of the channel. The modern point numbering system almost does us a disservice, because it makes some people think of the channels as two-dimensional, skinny lines that jerk from point to point.

The original descriptions of the acupuncture points do *not* necessarily describe them as being on a particular channel. The point-naming system that we use in the west is a very new invention. Prior to the twentieth century's new numbering system, the points were recognized as points, and they *happened* to be located more or less along the routes of the channels. Now that we have, in the west, substituted numbers for names, we almost automatically think of the channels as a linearity that connects the numbers.

To understand channels, think of them as three-dimensional rivers, not lines. Channels are not *defined* by the points, any more than the mighty Mississippi is defined as "the connector between St. Louis and New Orleans."

The channels are one thing. The points found in and alongside the channels are something else.

Also, channels can flow under or over other channels, like underground aquifers that follow their own paths, regardless of what the ground-level rivers happen to be doing.

The law of Midnight/Midday

One extremely important aspect of parasympathetic mode channel Qi flow that is *not* always taught or included in the texts is the manner in which a surge of energy, lasting approximately two hours, occurs in each channel, in sequence, every day.

The main variations in channel Qi flow that occur when a person is relaxed and awake, which is to say, in parasympathetic mode, result from the time-of-day variations. Each channel carries, in turn, a larger load of channel Qi for a couple of hours each day. In the classic texts, the charting for the time of day when each channel is dominant is referred to as The Law of Midnight/Midday.

During the time that a given channel is experiencing a surge of energy increase, this surge is not being shunted into the next (sequential) channel. Instead, during this time, more channel Qi than usual is being sent out into the branching channels that flow outward, laterally, from that particular channel. These branches bifurcate repeatedly, into smaller and smaller rivulets, and then trickles, of channel Qi. These streams and streamlets trickle out to the channel's related organs, nerves, blood vessels, and cells – all the ones that are particularly associated with *that* channel.

For example, between 3:00 a.m. and 5:00 a.m., the time of day associated with an increase in energy in the Lung channel, the muscle and bone structures that are overlaid by the Lung channel receive more energy than usual. Also, the lungs themselves, including every cell of the alveoli, receive extra energy and blood supply. During this time, the structures, organs, and cells associated with the Lung channel are best able to perform healing work. If cells need to be replaced, repaired, or re-energized with extra food or structures, this is the time of day when organs and cells that are directed by the Lung channel will perform these tasks.

The "Lung time of day" is *not* the time of day when the lungs work the hardest at *breathing*. The "Lung Time" is when the tissues of the lungs, and all the Lung channel-related physiologies, are repaired and prepared for the upcoming day.

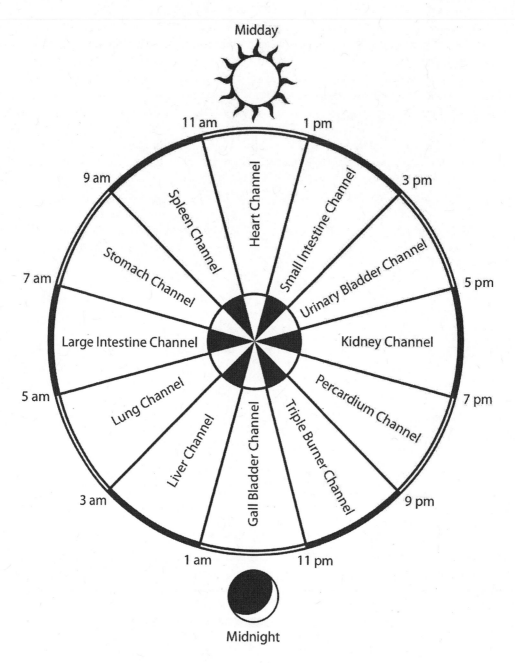

Fig. 5.9 The law of midnight-midday

Performing repairs

Often, if a person has damaged tissues in a particular part of his body, he may feel extremely tired, or more aware of the damage, during the time when his body is doing repair work on that part.

For example, if a person has a leg injury that is predominantly located on the Stomach channel, he may find that he can barely stay awake from 7:00 a.m. to 9:00 a.m. for several days, until the body repairs the damage. Even if he wakes up at six in the morning and is feeling fabulous, he might become woozy and need to lie down when 7:00 o'clock comes around. Then, at around 9:00, he may feel perfectly normal again.

As another example, people who have smoked cigarettes for decades often wake up at 3:00 in the morning and cough for an hour or two. This occurs because, at this time, the body is working hard on the lung damage, trying to perform repairs. The extra stimulation to the alveoli dumps toxins out of these dirty lung cells, out to the inner surface of the lungs. The coughing is the body's way of trying to move those toxins out of the lungs and up into the throat.[1]

The times of day for the Law of Midnight/Midday are not etched in stone. They are more related to the position of the *sun* than they are to the hours of the clock. For a better sense of what the "hours" really mean, consider that "6:00 a.m." actually means "when the sun comes up." Likewise, "6:00 p.m." actually means "when the sun goes down.

This means that, in non-equatorial zones, in the winter, when darkness is longer, more actual time is spent with elevated channel Qi in the Kidney-through-Lung channels. In the summer, the Stomach-through-Bladder channel sequence receives more time with elevated levels of channel Qi energy.

The List of Midnight/Midday
>1. 3:00 a.m. – 5:00 a.m. Lung
>2. 5:00 a.m. – 7:00 a.m. Large Intestine
>3. 7:00 a.m. – 9:00 a.m. Stomach
>4. 9:00 a.m. – 11:00 a.m. Spleen
>5. 11:00 a.m. – 1:00 p.m. Heart
>6. 1:00 p.m. – 3:00 p.m. Small Intestine
>7. 3:00 p.m. – 5:00 p.m. Urinary Bladder
>8. 5:00 p.m. – 7:00 p.m. Kidney
>9. 7:00 p.m. – 9:00 p.m. Pericardium
>10. 9:00 p.m. – 11:00 p.m. Triple Burner
>11. 11:00 p.m. – 1:00 a.m. Gallbladder
>12. 1:00 a.m. – 3:00 a.m. Liver

As an aside, I usually ask my clinical rounds students to memorize the above list: the sequence numbering as well as the hours. Often, when I am treating patients in rounds, I

---

[1] Even western medicine has recognized that certain surgeries have far better results if they are performed at a specific time of day. Despite these well-supported findings, non-emergency surgeries continue to be scheduled first thing in the morning – for the convenience of the doctors and the hospital staff.

mention to the students that I'm noticing a slight blockage in the patient's "twelfth channel" or "possibly a little blocked around noon."

A patient never worries about his liver function or his heart condition when I say that his "twelfth channel is a little squiggly" or "Do you feel tired between 11:00 a.m. and 1:00 p.m.?"If my students know the channels by number and hour as well as name, we can cheerfully, if obscurely, discuss channel flow in front of a patient without getting the patient mistakenly worried – which he might if he heard us speak casually about "Liver" and "Heart" problems.

(Then again, some patients are mildly familiar with Asian medicine vocabulary, are keen to know what their Asian diagnosis is, and speak proudly, even possessively, of "*always having Liver Qi Stagnation*.")

Corrections to the books

Do not pay any attention to the material below while taking your licensing exams. The following information is only provided to keep you from being puzzled when your assessments of channel Qi don't match what the channels are "supposed" to do.

Introduction

Our western idea that, for example, the Spleen channel is made up of the lines connecting those points whose names start with "Spleen," is a completely western, and erroneous, concept.

Only recently did the points receive their modern, western-language names, consisting of a channel name plus a sequential number. These western-language names are often misleading. The channel attribution is often wrong.

Even so, gratitude, and even compassion, is owed to whomever in modern China was assigned the thankless task of re-christening the poetically named points by linking them, via guesswork, with specific channels and numbers. The person who assigned the western names to the points probably wasn't feeling the channel Qi: for some time, in China, the actual *existence* of channels has been denied, for political reasons. Making it harder still, whoever assigned the western names was probably working with a committee! We must be grateful for the effort. Still, it's time to make some corrections.

Maps of the channels, showing the actual, physically detectable paths of the channels, side by side with the "traditional" maps that include the inaccurate numberings and incorrect channel routes (the paths we are currently taught in school), are included at the back of the book.

These maps, and this book, do not include information about the internal paths of the channels. That is a subject worthy of another book!

Gallbladder channel

LIV-13, on the side of the abdomen, at the end of the 11th rib, is on the Gallbladder channel, not the Liver channel. You can feel the channel Qi flowing downward, towards the feet, as it flows past this point. (See the back of the book for a map of the actual Gallbladder channel. For a quick look at the points that actually *are* on the Liver channel, see Fig. 5.10, on the next page.)

Yes, LIV-13 is an Influential point for all the Yin organs. This may be why the decision was made to relegate it to the Liver channel. But this point, even though on the Gallbladder channel, can still influence all the Yin channels: it wields its influence over the Yin organs by virtue of being on the Dai (Belt) channel.

Liver channel

After LIV-6, the Liver channel can be felt continuing along the anterior-medial upper leg, into SP-10. The upper leg portion of the Liver channel flows in what we usually call the path of the Spleen channel, touching SP-11, -12, -13, -14, -15, -16, -17, -18, -19, and GB-24. In the torso, these Liver channel points travel in a fairly straight line, 4 cun lateral to the Ren channel, from SP-13 to GB-24, and finally arrive, still 4 cun lateral to the Ren, at LIV-14.

Isn't that great? The Liver channel actually flows in a direct, powerful line, all the way up the torso. The Liver channel's most feel-able torso points are *all located 4 cun from the midline*. So simple! And easy to feel.

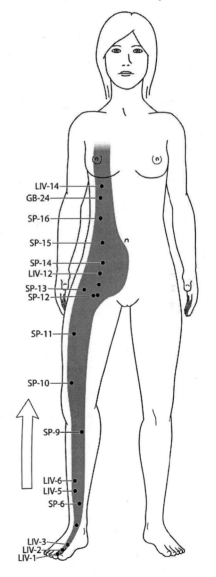

Fig. 5.10   The actual path of the Liver channel, including acupoints.

GB-24, just below LIV-14, may have been assigned to the Gallbladder channel because it is the Front Mu point of the Gallbladder. Also, it sits near the anatomical gall bladder. Still, it is clearly on the Liver channel. This point is actually a common jumping off point for stagnant Liver channel Qi to attack the Stomach channel.

As an aside, I still refer to the modern "traditional," or "classic," path of the zigzagging Liver channel that we are taught in school as "The Liver channel." When speaking with colleagues who are *aware* of the actual path of the channel, if I want to refer to the actual path of the Liver channel, I call it "The 12ᵗʰ channel" or "the *actual* Liver channel."

Stomach channel

ST-8 is not a part of the normal path of the Stomach channel. Stomach channel Qi is only shunted up to this point if dangerous, backwards-flowing (aka Rebellious) Stomach channel Qi makes it all the way up the torso and neck, and arrives at ST-6. If this does occur, the backwards-flowing Stomach channel Qi at ST-6 is shunted up to ST-8, where it does far less harm than it would if it were able to flow backwards across the face, backwards into Yin Tang, and backwards through the brain.

UB-1 is the first acupoint of the Stomach channel. As noted in the classics, the Stomach channel starts at the end of the Large Intestine channel, and traverses Jing Ming (now named UB-1), prior to traversing ST-1.

SI-18 is located on the Stomach channel

Urinary Bladder channel

The incorrect decision that the Urinary Bladder channel must begin at Jing Ming (UB-1) probably derives from misinformation about a branch of the Urinary Bladder channel through which channel Qi flows only during sympathetic mode. This branch is located inside the head (behind the eyes), and travels to the vertex. This branch is discussed in chapter 6 of this book.

As noted above, UB-1 is on the *Stomach* channel. UB-2 is on the *Gallbladder channel*. The first acupoint on the external, primary path of the Urinary Bladder channel is UB-3.

Spleen channel

The Spleen channel travels from SP-9 to LIV-8, and continues along what we usually call the path of the Liver channel. LIV-9, -10, -11, and -12 are all on the Spleen channel. (As already noted, LIV-13, the next in the Liver sequence, is on the Gallbladder channel.) The Spleen channel flows from LIV-12 through the groin. In this area, it flows deeper under the skin than the Liver channel. As the Spleen channel flows deeply, through the trunk, it widens out until its medial edge touches Ren-3 and Ren-4. Then, still wide, and traveling deeper inside the trunk than the Liver channel, it curves over to the side of the torso. The channel narrows again as it approaches SP-21. At first glance, SP-21 might appear to be on the path of the Gallbladder channel. However, where these two channels pass through the same general area, the Spleen channel runs deeper inside than the closer-to-the-skin Gallbladder channel.

Discerning the torso portion of the Spleen channel that flows beneath the Liver and Gallbladder channels can be difficult, for beginners.

I refer to the modern, "traditional" path of the Spleen channel as "the Spleen channel." I refer to the actual path of the Spleen channel Qi as "the actual Spleen channel," or "the 4ᵗʰ channel."[1]

---

[1] After reading an early version of this book, a visiting east coast colleague, a professor at an acupuncture college, questioned the need to teach students about the relative depths of the Liver and

Spleen channels: the Liver running more superficial, the Spleen running more deeply. He was visiting my office, and mentioned this as he was getting ready to lie down for a treatment for his worsening, chronic groin pain from a very old injury. He could feel and visualize that the worst part of the problem was a knot of energy right along the groin. He'd already received many Asian medicine treatments, of various types, for this problem, from other colleagues. He thought the problem seemed to ease up a little, for awhile, in response to each treatment, but overall, it was slowly worsening: the pain area was becoming visibly red on the skin, and the pain was spreading into the testicle.

I felt the flow of channel Qi on his legs, and noticed a blockage a few inches proximal to LIV-8, on the upper leg (on the actual Spleen channel). Stimulating this point with acupressure didn't seem to get the channel Qi moving past this point. I wondered if he had a blockage in his groin at the depth of the Spleen channel. If this were the case, possibly his (actual) Spleen channel Qi, being stymied, was shunting into his (actual) Liver channel. If so, mere stimulation of this actual Spleen channel point would only send more Spleen channel energy into the Liver channel. The pain was in the groin. The blockage was probably in the groin. I wanted to make sure that the channels were flowing at their correct levels through the groin.

First, I asked him to mentally get energy flowing up his 12th channel (the actual Liver channel), from the knee to LIV-14, and keep the energy close to the surface of the skin.

That didn't seem to resolve anything at the blocked place on the leg, so I asked him to mentally get energy flowing up his 4th channel (actual Spleen channel). I reminded him to keep that Spleen Qi running *deep*, below the Liver channel, creating a wide swath of energy that flowed from LIV-8 (on the actual Spleen channel) up to *deep inside* the inguinal groove. From there, the channel Qi should spread out very wide, staying deep, *under* the Liver channel Qi, as it spans medially from Ren-3 and Ren-4 all the way over to SP-15, and then narrows sharply, collecting itself as it veers laterally, still staying deep, supporting the oblique muscles, moving towards SP-21.

As he did this, he could feel a loosening in the tightness and constriction of his long-term groin pain. The heat in the area dispersed. His abdomen and even the muscles of his midback, the ones that connect near SP-21, relaxed. The channel Qi blockage ceased. Channel Qi began to flow correctly.

Evidently, years ago, in response to his groin-area injury, the channel Qi of the 4th channel had gotten blocked, and the 4th channel (actual Spleen) had to use the nearest available area of least electrical resistance – in this case, the path of the 12th channel. Since that time, the channel Qi in the 4th channel wasn't flowing in the correct pathway from the groin over to the side of his body – the 4th channel Qi was diverting into the path of the 12th channel – joining together with the channel Qi of the 12th channel. By mentally replacing the 4th channel Qi in the correct position, the groin problem was instantly assuaged. He also exclaimed, "That's it! I can feel energy going to this place on my side [near SP-21] that's been a problem for *years*!"

The next day, he called to tell me that the groin problem was about 95% healed. I reminded him that he'd asked me why students should have to learn if one channel runs more superficial than another. He laughed.

Several months later he wrote to me. "The condition of the problem area is better than it was before the treatment, but has fluctuated several times since that treatment…The treatment *did* have remarkable results, but my sense is that the "entire" blockage simply wasn't metabolized by it, and therefore was unable to "hold," as there was still too much silt in the riverbed, so to speak. [My ongoing] visualization and sensing of the areas of the meridians involved with the groin pain has continued to help immensely. That's my main form of "treatment," albeit self-administered. …the way I see it is that I'm treating it almost constantly, in the way in which I align and move throughout the day, in a way that encourages, invites, and allows both the dissolution of old patterns and the return of simple alignment."

Another case study in this book will show the opposite situation, in which the 12th channel, traversing the groin, drops down into the deeper, 4th channel, and stays there. The absence of the

Wrong attribution of Sp-17 to SP-20

The points located 6 cun lateral to the Ren channel, on the upper chest, are currently attributed to the Spleen channel. However, by feeling the channel Qi, it becomes apparent that the flow of channel Qi at SP-17, SP-18, and SP-19, is downward. These points are on the Stomach channel, which flows wide through this area.

Even the point names are references to the Stomach channel Qi: when in sympathetic mode, the Stomach channel Qi diverts interiorly, flowing into the chest (towards the heart, from SP-19 ("Chest Home"). Oppositely, when in parasympathetic mode, when the Stomach channel does *not* veer interiorly, the joy of parasympathetic mode (Heaven) streams over the breast at SP-18 ("Heaven's Stream"). The name of SP-17 ("Food's Cavity") is a clear reference to the stomach organ itself.

SP-20 ("Encircling Glory") is on the laterally-flowing beginning of the Lung channel; channel Qi at this location can be felt flowing towards the arm. This point's name is a reference possibly to the thoracic diaphragm, the muscles that open the upper part of the lung.

Du channel

The main branch of the Du channel, in classic literature, is described as going inside the head, to the vertex, and winding to the forehead.

In truth, the inside-the-head, main path of the Du channel goes to the vertex – and stays there – only during deep meditation, when breathing and heartbeat have been consciously stopped – what you might call extreme parasympathetic mode.

In most people, the inside-the-head, main branch of the Du channel does *not* go to the vertex after it travels inside the head. Instead, it meanders up the brain stem and then wanders back and forth, from one side of the brain to the other, and back again, as it "winds its way" (as it says in the classics) towards the forehead, before emerging at Yin Tang.

In a person with high focus and concentration, this main branch of the Du channel travels up the brain stem and then flows directly to the centerline of the frontal lobe, emerging at Yin Tang. This straight path is present in a person who is alert, who is mentally and emotionally healthy, and who is consciously controlling his ego. The straight path may also manifest, temporarily, in a person who is concentrating intently upon some thought or activity.

The portion of the Du channel that connects the acupoints over the surface of the scalp is only a branch, and is influenced by the inside-the-head, main path of the Du. This over-the-head branch meets, and joins with, the main channel at Yin Tang.

Yin Tang

Yin Tang is on the Du channel: the point between the eyebrows.

In 1989, when I was in acupuncture school, the official word from the People's Republic of China was that no channels touched Yin Tang. Yin Tang floated in a zone of its own, untouched by any channel Qi.

I asked several of my China-trained teachers, and despite the illogic of it, they were in utter agreement with the official position: Yin Tang, "the *meeting* place on the Yin side of

---

superficial, 12th channel Qi in this area was allowing the growth of a very large uterine fibroid on the anterior surface of the uterus.

90

the body," did not *meet* with any other channels. Not only that, defying all logic, it was no longer on the path of the Du channel, even though it is located at one of the most important positions of the Du channel – where the *main* (midbrain) path of the Du channel meets back up with the over-the-top-of-the head *branch* of the Du channel.

I suspect that the modern removal of all channel connections from Yin Tang, even the Du channel connections, was a response to the atheism promoted by the mid-twentieth century Chinese government. Yin Tang, a very powerful and frequently used point, is located at the site of the "spiritual eye," or "third eye." These spiritual connections might have been seen as too suggestive of the banned religions. At any rate, Yin Tang was relegated to mere "extra point" status, the name given to peripheral points that aren't clearly associated with any given channel system.

Happily, in 2007, an international congress determined, with the blessings of the Chinese authorities, that Yin Tang could be (once again) on the Du channel. If the points are ever renumbered, Yin Tang might receive the name "Du-25." The subsequent Du points will then also need to be renumbered.

Whether or not Yin Tang, the "meeting place," will, in our lifetimes, once again *officially* meet and marry the arm and leg Yang channels is anybody's guess.

Why learn about the four "seasons:" the four main routes of channel Qi?

When first learning to feel Qi, some practitioners of Asian medicine are especially susceptible to self-doubt if the channel Qi varies too far from what they think of as "normal." What many acupuncturists think of as "normal" are the channel routes that are usually portrayed in the traditional texts.

In fact, these routes are not necessarily the "normal" paths, the only paths, or the correct paths. The routes that are portrayed in traditional texts merely portray the (often incorrect) routing of channel Qi in a person who happens to be relaxing in parasympathetic (awake, not fearful) mode.

Also, predictable, significant channel flow variations in the actual paths of the channels necessarily occur, in a healthy person, if the person is *not* in parasympathetic mode.

An easy way to attain channel Qi-feeling confidence, so that one isn't filled with doubt when coming across channel Qi that's a far cry from "normal," is to learn the actual paths of the channels, and to work a bit with people who are in modes other than parasympathetic. As instructed in the upcoming chapters, by having a practice buddy imagine himself in the fearful or near-death situations that evoke these divergences, one can practice feeling these normal, though highly altered, variations in channel Qi flow. Thus, one can greatly increase his confidence in feeling channel Qi across the spectrum of possible channel manifestations.

Learning to feel the divergences has other diagnostic benefits as well. Some pathologies arise because channel Qi has become "stuck" in one of the divergent pathways even after the need for the divergence has passed.

By studying the healthy divergences, you can learn to quickly recognize when such a "stuck" pattern is present.

In some cases, subsequent to an injury, illness, or emotional trauma, a person fails to snap out of what should have been a short-term neurological shift and the matching short-term channel Qi divergence pattern. In these cases, by correcting the stuck pattern of channel Qi with needle, herb, magnet, laser, or moxa, the patient's health may be restored.

Then again, some "stuck" flow patterns occur when the original danger has passed, but the patient has *decided* he can't or doesn't want to let go of an emotional attachment to the event. In some of these cases, the problem of stuck channel Qi has its roots in a decision to wallow in anger, self-pity, or any of what the classic literature describes as pernicious, "internally" created emotionalism. Diagnostically, the root of these stuck channel Qi aberrations must be classified as Shen (mental/spiritual) disturbance. Treatment in these cases may require counseling, or some manner of helping the patient recognize that his own thoughts and decisions, more powerful than any needles or herbs, are at the root of the problem.

In such cases as these, one can sometimes feel the channel Qi changing from moment to moment, as the patient talks about the trigger events: the channel Qi might be running perfectly well when the patient talks about the weather, but if the subject of the trauma arises, the channel Qi can be felt shifting into some portions of a divergent pattern.

If *you* can feel channel Qi shifting in and out of an inappropriate divergence in response to negative thoughts, you can direct the patient's attention to that body part that is unnecessarily shifting into a trauma-related channel mode in response to thoughts. You might even teach the patient medical Qi gong exercises directed specifically at conquering this shift, controlling his own channel Qi flow, *and* have him practice them while letting his mind dwell on the trauma. In this manner, the patient can retrain himself to be able to think about the trauma while holding his own channel Qi in parasympathetic (not fearful) mode. This retraining can sometimes help a patient let go of a pernicious emotional attachment to the trauma, thus healing the Shen disturbance.

By becoming confident in channel detection skills, you can support the patient by giving him channel location feedback as he works at mentally modifying his own channel responses (medical Qi gong).

This is one of the highest forms of medicine – using non-invasive technical skills to help guide the patient as he heals himself.

Summary

The actual paths of the primary channels are the routes of channel Qi when a person is in parasympathetic mode. As long as a person's channel Qi flows in these pathways, we say his Qi is "going through." This patient will have "no pain."

If a person's channel Qi becomes lodged in patterns other than the primary pathways, the parasympathetic pathways, his Qi no longer "goes through." He will have "pain." This pain takes the form of any of the myriad patterns that we learn in school: the organs become deficient or excess in terms of Qi, Blood, Yin or Yang; internal Wind might arise; Blood stagnation pain can develop; one Element's channel might be attacking some other Element's channel. Each of these "pattern" diagnoses is the result of channel Qi running in some incorrect pattern for an extended period of time.

All of the "patterns" that we learn in school are *pathologies*, meaning "patterns that are not parasympathetic." They are all initiated, originally, either by external causes or internal ones.

The *Nei Jing* includes in the list of the "external" causes: injury; pathogens; poor nutrition; wrong exercise; toxins; and weather-related damage, among others. *All of these external triggers lead* quickly *to alterations in channel Qi flow*. The alterations in channel Qi then, or over a period of time, cause the physiological problems and pain.

The internal problems, also known as the Seven Pernicious influences, are various forms of wrong thinking and emotions: anger, hysteria (sometimes translated as joy), melancholy, worry, grief, fear, and fright (panic). Genetic problems, being the result of emotional negativity retained from past-life attitudes, are also internal problems.[1] All of the ego-based mental patterns create brain-based electromagnetic waves, *signals* that *directly* alter the flow of channel Qi away from the primary pathways – away from parasympathetic routes of channel Qi. These alterations in channel Qi then cause physiological problems and pain.

In either case, whether the problem is externally caused or internally generated, it will quickly manifest in an incorrect (not parasympathetic) channel Qi problem. If the incorrect flow of channel Qi lasts long enough, it will cause pain. By knowing where the channel Qi is going wrong, we can most quickly restore it to the parasympathetic path. When it returns to the correct channel flow patterns of parasympathetic mode, the channel Qi is once again "going through."

After the treatment is over, and channel Qi is going through, so long as there are no *mental* aberrations forcing the channel Qi back into a warped flow pattern, the pathological patterns will then be able to clear up on their own. Then, there will be "no pain."

To paraphrase Leo Tolstoy, "All healthy people are healthy in the same way. All unhealthy people are unhealthy in their own way."[2]

All healthy people *are* healthy in the same way: when awake, their channel Qi flows in the pathways of parasympathetic mode. All unhealthy people have channel Qi flow that varies from the ideal: the possibilities are infinite.

---

[1] Not *all* genetic problems are the result of wrong attitude in past lives. Some highly advanced souls choose to be born with a particular genetic challenge, to demonstrate a spiritual principle. Others take advantage of genetic "problems" in order to take on problematic karma of their loved ones, or spiritual disciples. The possibilities are infinite. However, many, if not most, genetic predispositions to health problems are carried over from attachment to wrong attitudes and emotions in lifetimes past.

[2] A take-off from the opening line of Tolstoy's *Anna Karenina*.

Change of colors ... is valued by gods because it enables us to flee from death...[1]

Chapter six

The healthy paths of the channels: part II

Sympathetic mode

Some of the *Nei Jing*'s divergent channels describe sympathetic mode channel flow: these are the variant routes of channel Qi that help shunt extra energy into the heart and adrenal glands during times of emergency. This "extra" energy is acquired by diverting channel Qi that normally supports digestion, and by diverting channel Qi that would otherwise be released at the tips of the fingers and toes.

In the *Nei Jing*, however, words explaining the purpose and logic of the sympathetic divergences are utterly absent.[2]

By learning how to feel the flow of channel Qi, you will be able to solve, for yourself, many of the *Nei Jing*'s otherwise baffling references to "divergent channels."

Don't take my word for it

Using a practice buddy, you can discover for yourself the pathways of the sympathetic divergent channels. Have your buddy imagine that he is defending himself or a loved one from danger. As soon as his mind really begins to imagine danger, you will feel the channel Qi patterns shift instantly. And voila! Some of these shifts will correspond to the classical text descriptions of the divergent channels.

---

[1] Su Wen, 13-9, from *A Complete Translation of the Yellow Emperor's Classics of Internal Medicine and the Difficult Classic*, by Henry C. Lu, PhD, published by the International College of Traditional Chinese Medicine, Vancouver, BC, Canada, 2004.

The sympathetic mode, sometimes called "fight or flight," enables us "to flee from death."

[2] Much of the *Nei Jing*, and especially the cryptic (lack of) explanations of the divergent channels, brings to mind this plaint: "... classical Chinese really consists of several centuries of esoteric anecdotes and in-jokes written in a kind of terse, miserly code for dissemination among a small, elite group of intellectually-inbred bookworms who already knew the whole literature backwards and forwards," as noted by David Moser, in "Why Is Chinese So Damn Hard," *Sino Platonic Papers* 27, 1991, pp. 59-69.

As mentioned earlier, despite the gradual development of the idea that the *Nei Jing* was written by the Great Emperor, in 221 BC, good research suggests that it was compiled over many years, consists of the work of many authors, and was most likely assembled in something like its present form in 260 AD – nearly four hundred years after the Emperor had died.

This chapter contains *lots* of details. You may just wish to skim the material. The main point to get from an initial perusal is the amazing extent to which channel Qi *doesn't* just flow the same way all the time. Later, you may recall some of these details while helping an individual whose channel Qi is stuck in one of these sympathetic patterns.

Divergent paths of the Urinary Bladder channel

The first divergent channels mentioned in the *Nei Jing* are those of the Urinary Bladder channel, also known as UB channel, or Foot Tai Yang. These are probably mentioned first because this channel is the first to surge into altered mode when fear or stress occurs. Many of us have even felt a "chill" run down the spine when something fearsome crossed our paths.

This surge in Bladder channel Qi helps increase the signal in all the spinal nerves that flow out from the base of each vertebra. These nerves send signals saying "Danger," to all of the organs and muscles.

Increased UB channel Qi causes increased stimulation of *all* the spinal nerves. The organs served by the spinal nerves have one of two possible responses to the increase in UB channel Qi. The heart and other breathing-related structures *increase* their rate and power in response to increased stimulation of their spinal nerves.

Oppositely, the stomach and other gastrointestinal organs *decrease* their rate of function in response to increased stimulation of their spinal nerves.

The *degree* to which the signals indicate either "speed up" and "slow down," to heart and gut, respectively, is related to the *strength* of the signal coming from the spinal nerves. The strength of the nerve signal is related to the *amount* of channel Qi coursing through the Bladder channel. The strength in the Bladder channel is related to the mind's assessment of danger: the greater the danger, the greater the channel Qi in the Bladder channel.

The vagus nerve – opponent of the spinal nerves

All of the internal organs also have another rate-determining nerve. The vagus nerve, one of the cranial nerves, has branches that go to each of the internal organs. The strength of the signals of the vagus nerve is indicative of how relaxed and/or joyful (*not* fearful or stressed) a person is. The vagus nerve signals activate the opposite response of the spinal nerves: increased stimulation from the vagus nerve tells the heart and lung function to *decrease*, and tells the gastrointestinal organ functions to *increase*.

During fear or stress, the spinal nerves are *activated*. The *degree* of activation is determined by the degree of fear or stress. During fear or stress, the vagus nerve is *inhibited*. The degree of inhibition is determined by the degree of the fear or stress. When the fear *ceases*, the spinal nerve signals decrease, and the vagus nerve signals increase.

This jolly give and take is a feature of the nervous system, *when one is awake*. During healthy sleep, *both* of these systems, the spinal nerves and the vagus nerve, are inhibited to a large degree.[1]

---

[1] "Vagus" means "wanderer," from the Latin: it uses the same root word that gives us "vagrant." The lengthy vagus nerve is so named because it "wanders" all through the torso, stimulating or inhibiting all the various internal organs. In millenniums past, there was much communication

Returning to the discussion of divergent channels, when fear leads to an increase in energy in the Bladder channel, it automatically causes an increase in energy in the spinal nerves. The mechanism is simple: the Bladder channel overlies these spinal nerves at the point where they emerge from the spinal column. When the Bladder channel receives a surge of fear-based energy increasing its electromagnetic signal, electrical impulses in those underlying nerves are increased.

Experiencing the channel Qi shift in the Bladder channel

Using your hands to feel the channel Qi on your study partner who is imagining himself responding to great fear, you can *feel* an increase in the amount of medial-side Bladder channel Qi streaming down his back. Following the Bladder channel further down the legs, notice what happens at the back of the knee. At the back of the knee, *some* of the extra UB channel Qi diverges from its normal path (the *amount* that diverges depends on the severity of the fear). The divergent portion flows medially for a moment, towards the Kidney channel. It then merges with the Kidney channel, *ascending*, up the leg. This Bladder channel Qi flows into the Kidney channel, moving toward the kidneys and the adrenal glands.

(When a person's fear is *finished* the Bladder channel Qi ceases to diverge into the Kidney channel. This fleeting shift in channel Qi at the back of the knees, just before the

---

between the east and west. It would not surprise me in the least to learn that the herb formula Xiao Yao Wan, which is translated as "Relaxed Wanderer," takes its name from its strong influence on "The Wanderer," also known as the vagus nerve.

Through constant stress or lack of internal serenity, a person can become "stuck" in the sympathetic mode – the mode that inhibits The Wanderer. When the Relaxed Wanderer herb formula "harmonizes" the Qi, it does so in large part by increasing activity in the vagus nerve, thus returning a person's body closer to the parasympathetic state. Thus, this formula does not tonify or reduce overall Qi levels, but "harmonizes" the channel Qi: the formula returns the vagus nerve back to a parasympathetic-dominant, or "harmonious" condition.

Sometime, try feeling the Stomach and Liver channels in a person whose complaint corresponds to the type of Liver Qi stagnation that typically responds well to this formula. Then, place a bottle of Relax the Wanderer, Xiao Yao Wan, on his stomach, and see how the pulses *and* the flow in the channels change. Never take anything I say for granted: test everything in this book by using your ability to feel channel Qi.

As for testing herbs by merely placing them on a person's skin, this was the ancient method of *using* herbs, let alone testing them. In the *Nei Jing*, the author despairs of his present day (two thousand years ago, more or less) practice of medicine. Prior to his day, when men had been more attuned to spirit, patients merely held herbs in their hand, noted the channel Qi changes thus wrought, and made whatever mental adjustments necessary to keep the channel Qi in the corrected position. The author bemoans his present day, in which people have become so insensitive to the perception of energy and so lacking in the mental focus required to control it, that they have to actually *drink* the herbs, in order to get the desired effect.

As it says in the Su Wen, chapter 13-1, "Nowadays, physicians treat a disease by herbs internally and with acupuncture externally, and the disease is sometimes cured and sometimes not cured. Why is that? In ancient times, people lived with no internal burden of wishes nor external burden of chasing after fame and profit. It was a life of tranquility, consequently, there was no need for them to be treated by toxic herbs nor by [magnetically charged] stone needle. Treatment was designed only to modify patient's thought, in order to alter organ energy and root out the cause of disease."

channel Qi becomes firmly re-established in the parasympathetic pattern, can cause the brief, post-fear sensation of "weak in the knees.")

After the shift at the back of the knee, other aspects of the sympathetic divergent system start to occur, Farther down the leg. Bladder channel Qi flows directly from UB-63 into KI-1, instead of flowing out to the tips of the toes, which would occur if the person were relaxed.[1]

While all this is going on, we might notice some overt physiological effects of the increase in Bladder channel energy in the study partner's upper back: the increased channel Qi running over the muscles between the shoulder blades causes an invigorating tightening between the shoulder blades that pulls the shoulder blades back, opening the front of the chest to more fully facilitate deep, powerful breathing. At the same time, we might be able to feel the increase in rate and strength of the heartbeat.

Finally, the increase in the UB channel Qi causes a diminution of channel Qi in the Du channel. The proximity of these two channels allows them to have an electromagnetic effect on each other.
The UB channel runs in the *opposite* direction as the Du. When the UB channel increases in amplitude, the increase serves to diminish the amplitude of any nearby current running in the opposite-direction: in this case, the Du. This is a basic principle of physics.

When one is attacked by fear or stress, his brain and thought processes rely more on channel Qi brought to the head via a specific Kidney channel divergence, and rely less on the Du channel. The main branch of the Du channel runs on the posterior surface of the brain stem and through the middle of the brain, emerging on the center of the forehead at Yin Tang.
When a person is calmly focused, he keeps his Du channel flowing straight and narrow through to the frontal lobe, un-swerved by distractions coming from the ego-driven areas at the sides of the brain. Oppositely, when a person is dominated by fear or stress, he is less reliant on the spiritually directed "straight and narrow way," the way of fearlessness.

---

[1] New channel Qi (known as Yuan Qi, or Source Qi) is always being created from the life force that flows into the body at the back of the neck, in the area of the medulla oblongata. Excess channel Qi is constantly being discharged in the form of slight static charge from the fingers and toes. During a shift towards sympathetic mode, this discharge from the digits diminishes or, in severe sympathetic mode, ceases. The channel Qi thus conserved contributes to the increase in adrenal (Kidney), heart and lung organ Qi, and contributes to the overall feeling of "extra energy" that one experiences during times of emergency.

In many acupuncture offices, a heat lamp is automatically positioned over the patient's toes, even if the room is warm. This lamp does not serve to merely warm the toes for the sake of comfort. By heating the toes, more blood, and thus more channel Qi, is diverted to the toes. When the brain detects an increase in channel Qi in the toes, it assumes that the body has shifted further towards parasympathetic mode, and further away from sympathetic mode. The brain is easy to fool. When channel Qi increases in the toes, the brain issues all the instructions that are appropriate for a shift towards more parasympathetic mode, including more physical, mental and emotional relaxation. The real reason for the heat lamp on the toes is to get the patient as close to parasympathetic mode as possible, as quickly as possible. Most healing occurs when a person is predominantly in parasympathetic mode.

Instead, he must fall back on a Kidney-based (fear-based) type of brain energy that is associated with the ego-assessing areas on the sides of the brain (the precuneus area).

Actually, the first step in fear is the brain change. As energy on the left and right sides of the brain increases, the Du channel flow through the midbrain is pulled laterally, and thus its forward momentum is diminished. This creates a decrease in the amount of channel Qi getting to Yin Tang. At the same time, the increase in channel Qi going to the sides of the head amps up the UB channels, which run in the opposite direction of the Du, further reducing its power.[1]

The bladder organ

As an aside, not all channel divergences occur on the surface of the skin. Some occur deeper in the body, along the internal channel paths. For example, in response to fear, some amount of energy that usually flows from the Bladder channel to the bladder, along an internal path, is rerouted to the adrenal glands. The bladder *organ* thus receives a decreased amount of channel Qi when in sympathetic mode. Though you might not be able to feel the more interior channels with your hands, it can be helpful to think of these internal channels when you are up against a baffling condition.

In times of momentary fear or stress, the organ of the bladder doesn't *need* its normal ration of channel Qi: energy that helps open and shut the bladder sphincter. During an emergency, a person shouldn't be distracted by information from the stretch receptors of his bladder, or emptying his bladder. Therefore, it's reasonable to shunt some of that bladder energy to a place where it's more needed: the adrenals, heart, and lungs. Of course, if the fear is severe enough, the bladder organ will lose so much Qi that its sphincter will lose muscle tone: in response to a violent fear, the bladder may empty involuntarily.

Reference to the classics

Now, let's compare what we can feel, using our hands on a study partner *and* using our study partner's perceptions, with what it says about the Urinary Bladder divergences in the *Spiritual Pivot* portion of the *Nei Jing*.

"After diverging from the Primary channel in the popliteal fossa [back of the knee], this divergent channel travels to a point 5 units below the sacrum. It then detours to the anal region, connects with the Bladder and disperses in the Kidneys. From here it follows the

---

[1] Recent western research supports this idea that the physiological changes that occur in sympathetic mode are driven by changes in spinal-nerve energy: an extremely new treatment for younger people with uncontrollable (even while taking up to five blood pressure drugs) spurts of very high blood pressure involves damaging the spinal nerves that cause renal arteries to tighten. In younger people, this tightening ordinarily occurs during sympathetic mode. The resulting inability to tighten apparently causes a large decrease in adrenaline release, and a lasting, large (up to 40 points) drop in the *upper* number of the blood pressure. This suggests that many of the sympathetic mode behaviors, such as higher blood pressure and adrenaline release are driven by in increase in spinal nerve stimulation. This matches up with the theory that an increase in UB channel Qi is the first step in driving the processes that make up the sympathetic mode. The research was led by the company that makes the kit for purposely damaging the spinal nerves, but even so, the results were substantiated well enough that they were published online by the British journal, *Lancet*, 2010.

spine and disperses in the cardiac region before emerging at the neck where it rejoins the Bladder primary channel."[1]

Another source uses more literal verb translations: "The primary [channel] of the foot Tai Yang [Bladder channel] diverges and enters the guo [popliteal fossa]. It ascends to a point below the coccyx, where it enters the anus. From there, it homes to the urinary bladder and disperses in the kidneys. It then travels along the paravertebral sinews to hit the heart and disperse into it. The direct ascends [sic] along the paravertebral sinews, where it homes to the foot Tai Yang [Bladder] channel."[2]

The last sentence of the above might be more accurately translated from the original if the phrase "direct ascends" were understood more literally. The word "zhi," translated in the above as "direct," is beautifully explained in Miki Shima's book: "This character originally represented an eye, evoking a directness of vision and spirit (shen)."[3]

The UB divergence's classical explanation may be more helpful when understood as "When one's consciousness, his shen, is disturbed by fear, the driver of his consciousness (zhi, "the direct") ascends, which is to say, rises to the head."

The classics make reference to the specific branch of the Bladder channel that initiates the increased flow of channel Qi, when a person shifts into sympathetic mode.

This branch begins at the outer sides of the eyes and flows posteriorly, through the head, towards the back. When this channel is strongly activated, one can sometimes feel the pull on the lateral sides of the sphenoid bone, just posterior to the lateral canthi of the eyes. The sensation can feel as if the lateral surfaces of the left- and right-side sphenoid bones are being pulled medially, closer to the center of the brain. As the fear ceases and sympathetic mode ends, one can sometimes feel the relaxation at the sides of the head, just behind the eyes, as the sphenoid bones move laterally, back into the parasympathetic position. As energy surges into this divergent branch, it causes a surge in the nearby over-the-head aspect of the Urinary Bladder channel. This drives the sympathetic-mode surge that travels down the sides of the spine.

As an aside, this branch is described in the classics as beginning at Jing Ming UB-1 and traveling through the head towards the vertex. The reference to Jing Ming, an on-the-skin acupoint, is incorrect. The actual location for the point of origin of this branch may have (or should have) originally been described as something like "alongside the corner of the eye," meaning the outer corner. A subsequent decision that this branch starts at Jing Ming – at the inner corner of the eye - is a logical mistake – for someone who was not able to actually feel the paths of the channels.

This error led to the further error of assuming that the Urinary Bladder channel must begin at Jing Ming, recently named UB-1. This incorrect idea then had to be reconciled with the statement in the Nei Jing that the first acupoint traversed by the Stomach channel is Jing

---

[1] *Acupuncture, A Comprehensive Text*, Shanghai College of Traditional Medicine, translated by Dan Bensky, Eastland Press, Seattle, 1992, p. 76.

[2] *The Channel Divergences*, Miki Shima and Charles Chase, Blue Poppy Press, 2001, p. 15.

[3] Ibid. p. 12

100

Ming. Someone then diplomatically came to the happy conclusion that the *Bladder* channel begins at Jing Ming, and the Stomach channel happens to "meet" the Bladder channel at this point, thus keeping everyone happy. But in fact, the result is misinformation.

The actual error here may not seem significant. But it helps make the larger point: the *Nei Jing* is riddled with errors and self-contradictions. Mankind is once again competent to study techniques of meditation and intuition. During the dark ages, such techniques were, for the most part, kept secret from the uninitiated layman. These techniques are, once again, widely and freely available. The time has come to apply our inner wisdom to the *Nei Jing*, separating the wheat from the chaff.

Do not passively accept the accumulated errors of millennia. Prove to yourself the abundant, deeper truths of the classics. Restore any jumbled information into its proper place. Discard completely those statements, no matter how assertive, that are obviously incorrect.

Self-examination will show that the description of this branch of the UB channel *should* be in the section of the *Nei Jing* that discusses the divergent channels. However, it currently resides with the description of the *primary* path of the Urinary Bladder channel. Possibly, for reasons unknown, the description of this branch used to be located in the divergent channel section, and was moved to its present chapter. Or maybe this information was placed incorrectly in the original. No matter. But the current placement of this information, in the primary channel section of the *Nei Jing*, gives the false idea that this branch is *always* active. This is *not* the case. This branch is the first pathway activated when a person slips into fear.[1]

In parasympathetic mode, the correct way of living, all instructions, *including* mental instructions that are focused at Yin Tang, originate from the heart. Only when a person becomes fear-oriented does the self-awareness reference point shift to the sides of the brain, particularly the precuneus area (on the sides, behind the frontal lobe: the area associated with ego-based assessments of all things that seem separate from the self). At the same time, heart-based sensory resonance is decreased. The Shen's center of awareness ascends from the heart to the sides of the brain. (This subject will be addressed further in the chapter on dissociation.)

In the *Nei Jing*'s discussion of the UB divergent channels, the reference to "the direct" ascending is a nod to the consciousness's fear-based, brain-oriented shift *away* from the heart that occurs when a person shifts into sympathetic mode. As the consciousness "rises" from the heart to the head, a branch of the UB channel is stimulated. When this branch

---

[1] For a quick experiment to prove to yourself how this sympathetic branch of the Urinary Bladder channel is associated with a *decrease* in calm, heart-oriented focus, sit quietly, performing any sort of single-point, focused meditation. When you feel deeply calm, bring the attention to Yin Tang (if you are not already using Yin Tang as your point of focus). When you are deeply still and have a good sense for the light and/or energy at Yin Tang, mentally induce a strong current flowing from the outer canthi of the eyes, past the lateral edges of the sphenoid bones, and back to UB-8. Imagine that this tension is accompanied by anxiety or fear. As the mental fear increases and the physical tension increases in the bones behind the sides of the eyes, notice what happens to the focus at Yin Tang: the energy becomes dispersed, unfocused. When fear is allowed to enter the body, consciousness *cannot* maintain a focus on calmness – or on Yin Tang.

is activated, via fear, one cannot hold onto the internal image of a motionless third eye; the energy of the inner (third) eye becomes scattered.

When fear attacks, the surge in energy in this inside-the-head branch of the UB channel, which is to say, in the ego-oriented, relatively more lateral areas of the brain, in turn, shunts more energy into the electromagnetic system that we call the primary UB channel. From there, more energy is delivered to the physical structures that lie just under the UB channel. On the back, these physical structures are the spinal nerves and the muscles of the paravertebral area.

Since this is what actually happens when a person becomes fear-oriented, it makes sense that the classics would have described it that way. However, without an understanding of the physiology of fear, including the heart/brain shift, and without direct experience of the alterations that occur in channel Qi flow, scholars of the dark ages may have only been able to guess at the meaning of the original characters. Certainly, even though activation of these particular branchings of the UB divergent channels is a response to fear, the sympathetic mode association with these divergences was lost, somewhere along the way.

As an aside, at least one translation states that after the "direct" ascends, UB channel Qi goes to the root of the tongue. *Many* of the divergent channels mentioned in the *Nei Jing* are said to go to the throat or root of the tongue. This may well be a reference to the bronchodilation that occurs in sympathetic mode, or it may refer to the involuntary gasp that often occurs at the moment when the fear-based heart/brain shift first occurs.

Certainly, as it stands now in most translations, the description of the Bladder channel divergences makes little obvious sense: some translations even suggest, circuitously, that *Zhi* refers to the Bladder channel Qi! With this understanding, the Bladder channel Qi *ascends* (from where?) to the Bladder channel, then *descends*, following the path of the Bladder channel, and then *ascends* again, to the Bladder channel. This doesn't even make sense. But if one has no idea what the channel Qi is actually doing, one explanation is as good as another.[1]

Verb clarity

Looking into the rest of the classic divergence explanation, notice that highly specific verbs, such as "enter," "disperse," and "hit" are used in describing the workings of the divergent channels. The word "enter" as used here means "merge," as in the "merging" of two freeways. The divergent UB channel Qi can be felt "entering", merging into the Kidney channel, flowing up to the area of the coccyx, and then *merging* into another channel: the branch of the Kidney that goes to the lumbar region.

Although one of the above translations states that the merging goes *into* the anus (and the translator continues in the next paragraph to admit that "this passage is relatively opaque"), *no* one is certain what the original preposition actually was, if any. The palpable increase in channel Qi *actually* occurs in the branch of the Kidney channel that flows to the coccyx and thence to the adrenals: close to the anus, but not *in* the anus. For that matter,

---

[1] As Johann Goethe noticed, "Everyone hears only what he understands."

people beset by extreme fear are more likely to *lose* control of the bowel sphincter, indicating a *deficiency* of anus Qi in times of great fear, and not an *increase*.

Continuing with the *Nei Jing*, the word "disperse," as in "disperse into the kidneys and heart," refers to the transformation of the moving channel Qi into Qi that can power the *organ* into which it is dispersing. It is like saying "electricity travels through the wires of my house until it *disperses* into my light bulbs or my washing machine."

The diverging Bladder channel Qi *disperses* into the kidney and the heart, where it supports increased adrenal gland function and increased heart rate.

The word "hit," also translated as "strike," is used to describe an intense surge of *pounding* power that disperses in the heart. In this case, the word "strike," describing the walloping bang delivered to the gong-like heart by this divergent channel Qi, is poetically exact.

To sum up and *paraphrase* the *Nei Jing*'s description of Bladder channel divergence, "Much of the extra (fear-driven) Bladder channel Qi merges into the Kidney channel at the knee and heads upwards (which is to say, proximally, or *towards* the anus), and flows into the adrenals. The channel Qi *disperses* in the kidneys (adrenal glands) and heart, and *hits* the heart. This set of divergences is triggered by fear. Fear sends the center of consciousness (the "primary energy") away from the heart and up into the brain, thus triggering the extra surge of energy into the paravertebral muscles and the UB channel."

What an accurate description of the manner in which Bladder channel Qi is actually amped up and rearranged – in response to fear – so that it can increase the signals to the spinal nerves (triggering sympathetic mode organ behaviors) *and* be diverted to the adrenal glands and heart![1]

---

[1] As an aside, in the *Spiritual Pivot*, the discussion of divergent channels is immediately preceded by a query as to the relationship between man and the heavens. The reason for this sequence becomes evident when we consider the first divergent channel discussed in the *Nei Jing* is also the first one that kicks in when a person is fearful. When a man is in tune with the cosmos, he is in parasympathetic mode. His channels flow in the primary channel routes when he is attuned with the heavens via his heart.

The *Nei Jing* suggests that, when man feels fear, he ceases to be in tune with the cosmos. He then shifts into sympathetic mode. In this sense, sympathetic mode is seen as somewhat unnatural: out of tune with Man's capacity to live on a spiritual plane: a throwback to man's animal nature.

When we study the implacable calm and joy that permeates the lives of the saints and sages, we see that they have no use for the sympathetic mode. The *eastern* understanding of medicine includes the spiritual implication that considers use of the sympathetic mode to be a divergence from correct living, a step backwards, a step into fear-based living. The *western* understanding of this mode is limited to "fight or flight, or "fight, flight, or freeze": the purely physical functions that occur in this mode, with no reference to spiritual associations.

A person of great spiritual wisdom *is* still able to fight. But he needn't shift into sympathetic mode to do so. The entire *Bhagavad Gita*, a sacred Hindu scripture, might be seen as an explanation of how spiritual training enables us to wage war against even our *most* fearful enemies – our own moral shortfalls, and even death – *without* becoming prey to fear. By union with God and Truth, we can fight all battles, including spiritual battles, even while staying in the neurological mode that is correct for humans: parasympathetic.

As an aside, in sympathetic mode the actual senses of hearing, vision, and smell are altered. Some sympathetic divergent channels go to various locations in the head to facilitate adrenaline-based sensory perceptions.

When relaxed, the brain receives sensory information via a different path: vibrations of sensory information resonate first with the pericardium. The type and degree of resonance thus generated then conveys to the brain the *manner* in which to enjoy and employ the incoming sensory information.

In a state of fear, the pericardium/somatic sensitivity connection is deactivated. In an emergency, sensory input goes *directly* to the brain, where it is assessed only in terms of risk, never in terms of beauty or resonance. In sympathetic mode, certain divergent channels carry an increase in channel Qi flow to the parts of the brain that are used to enhance fear-based sensory perception.

In sympathetic mode, causing or supporting these changes, Du channel flow is decreased, as noted earlier. A concomitant increase in Kidney channel flow to the head occurs.

The divergent paths of the Stomach channel

In the classics, the *first* discussion of a sympathetic mode divergent channel shift refers to the shifts in the Urinary Bladder channel.

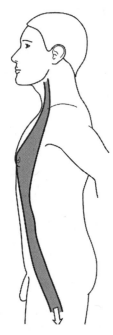

Fig. 6.1 Side view of the torso portion of a healthy Stomach channel in *parasympathetic mode* (review).

However, the sympathetic mode divergences that are *easiest* for some students to detect are the fear-based shifts that occur in the Stomach channel.

Therefore, a student might wish to start his buddy-imagining-fear experiments while detecting channel divergences in the Stomach channel.

The following Stomach channel divergences are not included in the classics, or at least not in the version that has been passed down to us. However, they are easy to feel and diagnostically

---

In this world, we may find ourselves in situations in which we *must* fight – whether the battles are physical or within our own minds. But we should *choose* to fight from a spiritually superior position of heart-attunement, rather than from fear. The *Nei Jing*, like all world scriptures, repeatedly makes the argument in favor of spiritual attunement and fearlessness. One might even say that use of the sympathetic mode, and its divergent channels, is a form of "falling from grace." Certainly, it is a "falling" from spiritual health.

helpful. The classics do not even begin to describe all the possible channel divergences: the list is nearly infinite.

Chest portion of the Stomach channel

When a person is relaxed and awake, the Stomach channel flows in the eye-to-toe pathway that we learn in school. When the body is in parasympathetic mode, the vagus nerve directs the gastrointestinal tract while following, to some extent, the neck and torso route of the Stomach channel.

When fear or stress strikes, the upper chest portion of Stomach channel Qi (both left- and right-side channels) shunts into the chest, where it provides extra energy directly to the heart. The shunt location is variable from one person to the next, but generally occurs in the vicinity of ST-14, or at least somewhere between ST-13 and ST-15. When this channel diversion kicks in, the Stomach channel Qi is palpably absent over the breast and lower ribs. This divergence into the chest, causing an absence of Stomach channel Qi at ST-17, -18, and -19, is possibly the easiest divergence to feel. It can feel as if the Stomach channel flows from the clavicle to its points along the upper ribs, and suddenly disappears.

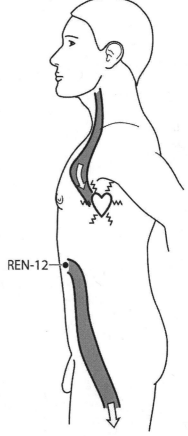

Fig. 6.1 In sympathetic mode, the Stomach channel Qi dives interiorly, supporting the increased energy needs of the fear-driven heart. REN-12— Little or no Stomach channel Qi can be felt from approximately ST-14 to midway down the torso, near Ren 12. Midway down the torso, the Stomach channel Qi can once again be felt. This mid-torso supply of channel Qi derives from the Ren channel.

At the same time that the Stomach channel Qi diverges into the chest, towards the heart, the vagus nerve ceases to send parasympathetic signals to the stomach and digestive organs. Thus, stimulation of the digestive organs is diminished.

But the leg portion of the Stomach channel is still needed, even in an emergency: during times of "fight or flight," the power of the Stomach channel Qi is needed to power the legs. Where will this power come from?

Continue feeling for Stomach channel Qi along the path of the now-missing Stomach channel, while your buddy continues to imagine fear and stress. Notice how, after "disappearing" into the chest, a resumption of Stomach channel Qi can be felt re-emerging a bit farther down the torso, powered by energy emerging from Ren-12. Ren-12 is the front Mu "alarm" point of the Stomach channel.

Channel Qi emerges at Ren-12 and flows into the lower torso path of the Stomach channel. From there, the Stomach channel Qi courses down the torso and into the legs. Thus, Stomach channel Qi flow to the legs is maintained. (And a new appreciation is gained of why some points are referred to as Mu, or "alarm" points: during sympathetic, or "alarm mode," these points can distribute channel Qi to sections of channels or organs that are in need of Qi even while their *usual* sources of channel Qi have been diverted to the heart organ for extra pumping strength. Also, in cases of injury, if the primary channel has become blocked, the Ren "alarm" points can provide a secondary source of channel Qi.)

After the fear or stress has passed, the Stomach channel Qi returns to its "normal" course, moving just under the skin in the breast and upper torso, along the usual path of the Stomach channel. At this point, we can say that a person is back in parasympathetic mode.

The sympathetic/parasympathetic *continuum*, and the ST-14 connection

As an aside, western medicine generalizes the modes as if people are "in" parasympathetic or sympathetic modes. The implication is that people are limited to being exclusively in one mode or in the other. This phraseology doesn't match physiological reality. In truth, there is almost always a bit of *both* modes going on.

For example, heartbeats and breathing *require* stimulation from the sympathetic nervous system. Even when a person is relaxed, his body is operating with enough fear to keep his heart and lungs going. Sympathetic "fear" mode is what keeps the heart beating and keeps air moving in and out of the lungs. No matter how relaxed we are, if we are going to breathe, we must have *some* small amount of sympathetic nervous function.[1]

Oppositely, the parasympathetic system still operates even when we are in a mild state of hyper wariness. For example, we *can* chew, swallow, and digest food even if we are in the moderately "alert and stressful" (sympathetic) condition of driving a car. We are almost *always* using some amount of spinal nerve stimulation, and some amount of parasympathetic.

So it is technically incorrect to speak as if the body must be either in sympathetic *or* parasympathetic.

We are almost always, when awake, in a sort of combination of the two. We can think of the *pure* sympathetic mode and *pure* parasympathetic mode as the two ends of a linear continuum. Most humans, when awake, are in a neural condition that is somewhere in between the two ends. When we are more fearful or stressed, we move towards the

---

[1] Some western researchers have decided that parasympathetic heart rate is around 50 beats per minute, and anything higher comes from sympathetic stimulation. This decision is based on the finding that a beating heart, while removed from a body (such as during a transplant), beats at approximately this rate. This is poor logic. A heart in this condition is *highly* stressed, whether or not it is connected to any nerves. Furthermore, I have an Olympic athlete patient with a heart rate of 36 beats per minute – a steady state multiple of the more common 72 beats per minute. If the lowest resting rate for parasympathetic were actually around 50, my Olympic patient would have to be dead, which she is not. Clearly, these researchers have based their decisions on multiple wrong assumptions, including the idea that a stress response cannot occur in an organ without the assistance of a nerve signal.

sympathetic end of the continuum. When we are *less* fearful or stressed, we move towards the parasympathetic end of the continuum – but we still have some amount of each.[1]

Technically, to be correct, we should describe a person as being, at any given moment, "sympathetic dominant, or "parasympathetic dominant," depending on which end of the continuum a person is *closer* to. But this is wordy and awkward. It will probably never catch on. Instead, using the western terminology, we must proclaim a person to be sympathetic or parasympathetic but, we should remember, when we do so, we are technically incorrect, and are merely generalizing.

But there *is* an objective measure of whether or not a person is far enough into sympathetic mode that he is *significantly* diminishing his vagus nerve function.

The Stomach channel divergence in the upper chest comes close to being an all-or-nothing rerouting of the Stomach channel. Either Stomach channel Qi is *detectable* flowing just under the nipple, or it is not: if Stomach channel Qi can be felt flowing down the neck and over the clavical, but no channel Qi is detectable in the breast area, then one can conclude that much, or even most, of the Stomach channel Qi is flowing internally, deep into the torso, to the heart. This Stomach channel diversion might actually be the most accurate way to determine whether or not a person has shifted into a sympathetic-*dominant* nerve and mind situation.

When the Stomach channel diverts internally, towards the heart, we *can* accurately say that the person is now in sympathetic-dominant mode. He may not think that he is feeling fearful or stressed. He may want to think of himself as cheerful, or even spiritual and unflappable. But if the detectable majority of his Stomach channel Qi is shunting into his heart, instead of flowing just under the nipple, his body is behaving as if he is predominantly fearful or stressed.

A person with this divergence activated may still have quite a bit of control over his digestive system – he might not be throwing up or losing bowel control, both of which can happen during *extreme* sympathetic mode, when the parasympathetic system is almost completely inhibited. But regardless of whether or not his stomach seems OK, *if the detectable-by-hand sensations of Stomach Qi is diverting inward to support the heart*, we can be assured that, to a *significant* extent, the heart *is* speeded up, adrenaline *is* being released in larger measure, and the blood is flowing *increasingly* into the skeletal muscle, and bronchial tubes are *more* dilated, and so on: increases are occurring in all the physiological shifts towards the sympathetic end of the spectrum. And when a significant level of these conditions are active, we *can* say that a person is "in" sympathetic (meaning, sympathetic-dominant) mode.

In trying to decide if a person is in sympathetic mode, or not, the neatest measure, a measure that does not go by degrees, which is to say, along a continuum, is the divergence of

---

[1] Of course, great saints and sages may be able to turn off the body functions of heart and lungs while they enter into conditions of no fear whatsoever, a sort of "pure parasympathetic mode." To attain this state, the energy flow in the Bladder channel and spine must be brought to a halt, or at least brought under conscious control. But for most of us, we always have enough fear of death in our conscious and subconscious minds that we keep our hearts going. Thus, most of us always have *some* amount of sympathetic nerve activity.

the Stomach channel Qi down into the region of the heart. When Stomach channel Qi is diverted to the heart and stops flowing over the breast and stomach, regardless of the *degree* of other *overt* sympathetic symptoms, we can say, "This person *is* currently in sympathetic-dominant mode."

He may still have a considerable degree of parasympathetic function, he may be smiling gently, eating a sandwich, and saying that he never feels fear...but if his Stomach channel is shunting predominantly into his heart instead of flowing over the nipple, his body will be prioritizing, to some degree, fear-based heart function over parasympathetic function, at this point in time.

Using Stomach channel Qi of the chest as a gauge, we have a nice, specific indicator to determine if the mode of "sympathetic-dominant" is operative. This can be very helpful in diagnostics, as some later case studies will show.

For example, very often, a person will present with a calm pulse, but a check of channel Qi will show that his Stomach channel is behaving as if he is in sympathetic mode.

Foot portion of the Stomach channel sympathetic divergences

As you learned in school, the Stomach channel flows from the center of the foot, at ST-42 and fans out over the tips of the second and third toes, flowing over acupoints at ST-44 and ST-45. From the second and third toes, some portion of the channel Qi flows medially over the tips of the toes, and into the beginning of the Spleen channel, at SP-1. But this toe part of the path only happens if a person is predominantly in *parasympathetic* mode. If in parasympathetic mode, *some* Stomach channel Qi shunts from ST-42 over to SP-3, on the side of the foot.

In sympathetic mode, the Stomach channel Qi ceases to flow to the toes. Instead, it *all* diverts from ST-42 into SP-3 and the ball of the foot, preparing the foot for running.

The Stomach channel divergences in the classic texts

The Stomach channel divergence discussed above is *not* mentioned in the classics.

Instead, in the classics, in the extremely short sampling of divergent channel possibilities that have been passed down to us, a different Stomach channel divergence is mentioned. The classical divergence can occur in highly sympathetic mode or mildly sympathetic mode (a beating heart and active lungs means that *some* degree of sympathetic mode is active, however mild). The example of a Stomach channel divergence given to us in the classics describes the divergence that occurs during vigorous exercise involving the quadriceps.

Again, the description of possible Stomach channel divergences given in the classics has nothing to do with fear or frenzy, "fight or fight" level of sympathetic mode, per se. It contains no reference to the "direct ascending" which is to say, the consciousness leaving the heart and rushing to the head, which is the onset of fear. Instead, the classic's example of a possible Stomach channel divergence was probably included as an example of how channel Qi can alter its path in response to moment-to-moment physical need.

In the classics, we learn that the Stomach channel Qi in the upper leg *can* cross over directly into the Spleen channel in the upper leg – when needed.

This specific divergence occurs just above the knee when the upper legs are calling for extra energy – as when bicycling, or when walking uphill. To see the result of *frequent* use of this particular divergence, consider the enlarged quadriceps muscles of a bicyce racer, just above the knee. This enlargement occurs because this muscle is highly developed: some amount of Stomach channel Qi is regularly diverted directly into this muscle in response to need.

Every part of the body can receive more or less energy at any given moment, depending on need and consciousness. The divergences section of the classics gives some *samples* from each channel for just a few of the nearly infinite number of possible divergences. Some samples show divergences for the various neural modes. Other samples, such as this Stomach channel quadriceps example, show use-related divergent possibilities. Considering that the possibilities are nearly infinite, it's reasonable that the *Nei Jing* only included a few divergent examples for each primary channel.

Yang energy in a Yin channel

The Stomach channel-to-Spleen channel divergence described in the classics makes the point that, in some cases, the more Yang energy of a paired group might flow into the path that is usually considered the domain of the Yin channel.

The description of the Stomach divergence into the Spleen channel, just above the knee, shows how Stomach channel Qi, a *Yang* energy, is able, when *needed*, to flow into the Spleen channel's route (a *Yin* pathway) in the area of the quadriceps, and from there, continue flowing in the path of the Spleen channel (running wide through the abdomen, dispersing into the spleen).[1]

Having Stomach channel Qi (the more Yang form, which is to say, the form with greater potential energy, as opposed to the kinetic, or more Yin form) running in the Spleen (Yin) channel can be helpful when certain situations call for a more dynamic kind of energy. For example, when bicycling, the quadriceps might require more dynamic (convertible, potential) energy than they need when, say, sitting in a chair. When sitting in a chair, one doesn't need this divergence, which supplies extra Yang energy to the quadriceps.

Also, this particular divergence, as noted in the classics, goes on to send Yang energy directly into the spleen and pancreas via the (ordinarily Yin) Spleen pathway. Having a bit of Yang energy dispersing into these organs, now and then, is *extremely* important for healthy function of these organs. In English, we might refer to this benefit by saying: "regular exercise is good for the internal organs."

The digestion organs, including the pancreas and spleen (the spleen is not considered a digestive organ in western medicine, but it *is* in Asian medicine), work far better if a person gets regular weight-bearing exercise – exercise that pulls some *Stomach* channel Qi (Yang-

---

[1] Both Stomach and Spleen channels are considered to be made up of predominantly "Earth" type energy. But the Earth energy in the Stomach channel is considered to be more Yang, or more vibratory, less formed (into electrons). The Spleen's Earth energy is more Yin, or more converted into electrons. When the Stomach channel's Yang-type Earth energy arrives at the mid-foot and begins its flow into the Spleen channel (at either ST-42 or at ST-45), it converts into the more Yin form of Earth energy.

type Earth channel Qi) into divergences that directly feed the leg part of the Spleen channel – and then continues on up the Spleen channel, dispersing Yang-type Earth energy into the Spleen-regulated digestive organs.

The classic's description of the Stomach channel divergence further explains that, when Stomach channel Qi *does* shunt into the Spleen pathway and continues on up to the spleen itself, the Stomach channel Qi *does* not get shunted into the Heart channel at SP-21, along with the more Yin energy of the Spleen channel. Instead, this channel Qi that was "borrowed" from the Stomach channel travels up to the throat and face, and up the nose until it is funneled back into the Stomach channel, near ST-1. This keeps the Earth's *Yang*-type channel Qi away from the Spleen channel-into-Heart channel transition point at SP-21. At SP-21, Earth's *Yin* channel Qi (Spleen) needs to transition into *Fire* element's Yin channel Qi (Heart) – a purely Yin transformation.

Spleen channel divergences

Next, the classic's brief description of one Spleen channel diversion makes the point that the Spleen channel Qi can flow in its normal pathway *at the same time* that Stomach channel Qi is using the path. In other words, two slightly different aspects of Earth energy, one more wave-based (Yang), one more formed (Yin), can coexist in this path.

In addition to this aspect of channel divergences (a channel being able to carry both Yin and Yang energy via the same path, when needed), the classics also make mention, very briefly, of one of the sympathetic mode variations that occurs in the Spleen channel: the Spleen channel Qi can be shunted to the root of the tongue, if *needed*.

As mentioned earlier, many of the divergent channels mention the possibility of energy being shunted to the mouth, or throat, areas. This may be related to the widening of the bronchial and throat passages, when the scales are tipped more heavily toward sympathetic mode.

Summing up the subject of classical divergent channels

The descriptions of divergent channels, in the classics, are there to make the point that an almost infinite number of channel Qi routes are possible. This section of our texts makes the point that there is *nothing* cut and dried about the movement of life-force in the body.

In the classic's description of a possible Bladder divergence, the points are made that higher *amounts* of energy can flow in a given channel, if needed, and the channels can shunt energy in paths that are not used in parasympathetic mode. In the classic's description of one possible Stomach divergence, we see that Yang-type energy can flow in channels that might usually transport Yin-type energy.

Each of the classical divergent descriptions opens our minds to yet another possibility of channel Qi flow.

Depending on one's consciousness and on moment-to-moment physiological need, channel Qi can instantly divert its energy into the areas where it is called for. The channel Qi is able to vary its secondary, and even its primary, paths. The consciousness determines where the need is, and the channel Qi responds.

Where the thought is, there also is the energy.

This book will not describe all of the classic's channel divergences in depth. A complete discussion is beyond the scope of this short text on channel theory. And yet, this is a convenient place to insert some divergent thoughts: the next few paragraphs share some possibilities to keep in mind while exploring on your own the *Spiritual Pivot*'s explanations of the divergent channels.

Although not *all* the divergences mentioned in the classic relate to the sympathetic mode, most of them do. As one proceeds through the classic descriptions of the divergences, starting with the Urinary Bladder, the greatest commonality is that most channels, if needed, are able to divert to, home to, disperse into, strike, or even hit the heart. This makes sense in terms of the varying energetic needs of the heart – needs that increase as a person moves closer to the sympathetic end of the mode continuum.

When a person slides towards increased sympathetic mode, the heart gets first crack at channel Qi that would otherwise have gone towards digestion. How *much* it gets, whether it gets a dispersion, a hit, or a bang, depends on the *degree* of fear.

Next, when it says in the classics that a divergent channel Qi can enter the chest and follows the throat, in many cases it makes sense in terms of adrenaline opening up the chest and dilating the bronchia.

As for the hand Shao Yang (Triple Burner) divergence "pointing to heaven," that is meant very literally, and is characteristic of a divergence that occurs during sympathetic mode.

The Triple Burner channel integrates the three energetic levels of one's existence: causal, astral, and physical. To live correctly, in tune with our souls, we must keep our attention on our spiritual compass. Even when we take a spiritual step backwards, into fear, and land in sympathetic mode, the divergent channel of the Triple Burner helps pull us back towards our higher, fearless, consciousness: during sympathetic mode, this divergent channel travels to the vertex, the site of the 7th, highest chakra, "pointing to heaven." By sending energy to the vertex, and thus, energy to the Du, even when fear and anguish are pulling energy *towards* the precuneus area of the brain and *away* from the Du, this Triple Burner divergence helps draw us back towards parasympathetic mode, bringing us back to our higher awareness, during and after the fear-triggered crisis.

Rates of change in channel Qi and physiology

As you work with patients, bear in mind that, in *general*, Channel Qi can shift faster than body chemistry can change. For example, when we are awakened in the night by a loud crashing sound, we are jerked into a sitting up position and our heart starts pounding. Our channel Qi has shunted in sympathetic mode, and the physical body is already on red-alert.

As soon as we realize it is just raccoons getting into the garbage, again, we relax. At this point, the channel Qi resumes its parasympathetic flow pattern. Even though neutralization of the adrenaline might take ten minutes, during which time the heart rate and air exchange rate will remain elevated, the body's channel Qi system has already returned to parasympathetic.

In other words, the channel Qi system is a much faster and more accurate indicator than heart rate or other physiological behavior as to whether or not a person is in sympathetic or parasympathetic mode at any given moment. A person's channel Qi can flip from one mode to another in less than a second – as quickly as a thought.

For another example, a person can be feeling just fine until he remembers his upcoming thesis presentation – at which point, he soon develops "butterflies" (or "running piglets") in his stomach. Even if he calms himself by changing his thoughts or munching on something (thus immediately stimulating the vagus nerve and sedating his spinal nerves somewhat), his body will have to deal with the residual chemistry of his panic. Several minutes may be needed to clean up the chemistry of fear, even though the electrical system reverts back to calm as quickly as the speed of thought.

An important clinical corollary is that channel Qi may appear to have become quickly corrected as a result of clinical manipulations. However, it is also very possible that these corrections will revert back to their pathological patterns soon after the treatment ends.

If the underlying causative forces, including incorrect or negative thoughts, have not been corrected, the channel Qi will, sooner or later, revert to its pain-causing, non-parasympathetic flow patterns.

Study

There are two very good ways to experience tangible paths of the divergent channels. First, work with a study partner to feel what happens to his channels during fear mode. Second, and possibly more important, take some time to sit very still and feel within your self the classical routes of the divergent channels. Then, imagine sending increased energy and awareness to various body parts. Notice the increase in channel Qi that flows into these areas as awareness shifts. This increase comes from channel Qi that is *diverging* away from its resting flow patterns.

In this manner, you will become familiar with both the sympathetic mode and the other, event-specific, possibilities of channel Qi variation.

A practice scenario: a day at the beach

Have a fellow student lay down on his back, looking at the ceiling. Start with parasympathetic mode. Ask him to imagine that he is resting on a sunny beach; the warm air is gently caressing his toes. When he starts to smile gently, run your hand over his Stomach channel on his left side. (The sympathetic channel shift occurs on both sides, but is sometimes easier to feel on the left side.)

If he has no leg or torso injuries or scars that bisect the Stomach channel, you should be able to feel the Stomach channel Qi flowing in the exact pathway that you are taught in school. Let his channel Qi guide your hand.

Notice that the channel *does* actually move medially for a bit, below the rib cage, before it moves laterally over to the side of the leg. Also note the amount of Qi flowing to his second and third toes, the amount flowing to the side of his foot at SP-3, and the amount of channel Qi flowing along the balls of his feet in the vicinity of SP-3 and the energy at KI-1.

Next, ask your practice-buddy to notice how his feet *feel*. Ask him to commit to memory the sensations inside his feet and toes, as he imagines the warm, sunny, beach air moving over his toes.

Then, tell your practice-buddy to daydream (imagine) the following: a few feet farther down the beach, a curly-headed toddler, his god-daughter, is playing with her sand bucket. And horribly, a cruel-eyed, but scrawny and short, hoodlum has just emerged from the shrubberies, carrying a baseball bat. He is creeping up on the toddler, intending to smash her in the head! Your buddy must rescue the poor child! He must jump up and overpower the creep!

As your buddy imagines this scenario, feel what happens to his Stomach channel Qi. You will not be able to feel any Stomach channel Qi past ST-14, or possibly ST-15 or ST-16. It will seem as if the Stomach channel Qi has disappeared. But feel lower down on his torso. You will be able to feel Stomach channel Qi flowing into his legs. But even farther down, by his toe tips, you can feel that the flow of channel Qi in his toes has become inhibited.

And the flow of energy on the sole of the foot will be increased in the area of SP-3, as well as the area of KI-1.

Now, ask the daydreamer how his feet feel. Ask him if they *feel* different, now that he is ready to rescue the toddler.

Most of the people with whom I've done this have reported that, during the rescue-the-toddler phase, they feel an increase of energy on the bottom of their feet. They have variously described it as throbbing, or surging, or warmth. Whatever they call it, it is an increase in the channel Qi that flows directly to the bottom of the feet, and a *decrease* in *toe* energy.

Now, change the story. Tell your friend that it was only a dream: he has no goddaughter at the beach. The presumed creep-o is a perfectly nice guy, heading down the beach to play ball with his friends.

Your friend should be once again enjoying himself, lounging on the sand, amused at having had such a curious daydream. Let the idea of warmth return to his toes. See how long it takes for his channel Qi flow to be restored to the parasympathetic, "normal," positions.

If you were to measure his adrenaline levels, you would see that it can take several minutes for the body to neutralize the adrenaline that was released in the above scenario. But the electrical systems of the body can resume parasympathetic patterns quicker than the blink of an eye.

Case study #6

Stuck in sympathetic mode during the night

Male, age 51, troubled by insomnia. Pulse was healthy, and only slightly wiry in the Liver position; his tongue was healthy.

His life was happy and successful; he was deeply content. But he'd been waking every night, at exactly 3:00 a.m., for the last three years. His wake-up was always preceded by violent, horrible dreams from which he would awake thrashing violently, with his heart pounding and heavy sweating – sometimes screaming out loud.

History: he had been his father's caregiver as his father died from cancer. This had been in the 1980s Soviet Union (now Russia), so, because they were Jewish, his father had not been provided *any* treatments *or* medication to assuage the pain. For more than a year, until his father's passing, my patient had been awake much of every *night*, trying to ease his father's terrible pains and fears.

I had only recently been licensed. Insomnia? I treated him with the basic Heart, Pericardium, and Liver points that I'd learned in school for this type of insomnia pattern. He came back the next week: no noticeable benefit whatsoever from the treatment.

Thinking that the 3:00 a.m. timing was significant, and suspecting some blockage preventing Qi from getting into the lungs (the 3:00 a.m. organ), I needled his back in a "Shen circle" (inner and outer UB points for the five Yin organs, plus a few Du channel points, also referred to as "aggressive energy treatment" by Five Element practitioners), with extra emphasis on the Lung-associated points of the Bladder channel.

He returned a week later: no benefit whatsoever from the treatment, but he was happy and excited. He told me, "I know what you are going to do today! I had a dream, and you needled the point on my feet." He beamed at me, expectantly.

I asked, baffled, "Do you remember which point on your feet?"

He smiled as if I was playing with him. "You know. The one on the feet!"

His shoes were already off. I pointed to Liver-3. He shook his head as if I were toying with him. I pointed to Spleen-3. Again, he clucked his tongue as if he wouldn't be fooled. Having no idea what he was talking about, I asked him to show me the point that he'd seen in his dream.

He pointed at GB-41.

I was perplexed. I had no idea what GB-41 had to do with violent dreams, screaming, 3:00 a.m., or profuse sweating.

In my insecurity, I pretended that this was, indeed, the point that I'd planned to needle today. But as I prepared to needle him, my thoughts murmured, "GB-41 is an exit point. It shunts Qi into the Liver channel. If the goal is to get the Qi to flow correctly *throughout* the Liver channel, including from Liver-14 into the Lungs, at LU-1, which it does *in abundance at 3:00 a.m.*, I might need to remind the Liver channel Qi of LU-1, the point into which the Liver channel exits."

Despite the assurance I'd given my patient that I would needle the dream-point on the foot, I found myself inserting the first needles of the treatment into LU-1. I could feel no sensation of channel Qi meeting the needle. I had needled into a Qi-free zone. In an attempt to get some channel Qi flowing into LU-1, I added needles at Liver-14. I checked on the needles in LU-1: still no channel Qi.

And then it dawned on me. With the needles in position at LU-1 and LIV-14, acting as tiny lightening rods, an insertion into GB-41 (the exit point from which Gallbladder channel Qi is able to offer channel Qi to the Liver channel) might cause channel Qi to surge up through the Liver channel and into LU-1. Was that why he'd dreamed of this point?

I inserted GB-41 on both feet. The patient sighed deeply. I felt for channel Qi in the needles at LU-1. The strength of the channel Qi was palpably pouring into the needles.

Explanation: during the stressful months while he tended his father, his body was chronically in sympathetic mode. In highly sympathetic mode, *most* Liver channel Qi flows to the vertex. It does *not* flow into the Lung channel. Instead, the Lung channel receives auxiliary channel Qi from the Lung alarm point at Ren-19. (As an aside, the Lung Alarm (Mu) point is *not* LU-1, as stated in the classics, and in all your texts. The Lung Mu point is

114

Ren-19. (This alarm point error crept into the lore goodness knows when – and is still there. Therefore, on your licensing exams, *be sure to say that LU-1 is the alarm point of the Lungs*.)

Test this for youself. Have a friend pretend to be in sympathetic mode, and run your hand from Ren-19 *inferiorly*, towards Ren-14, while using Qi from your own hand to push your friend's Ren channel inferiorly. This will temporarily reduce the flow in your friend's Ren channel. If your friend has a good imagination and is truly feeling scared, you will now be able to notice a deficiency of channel Qi at LU-1. After noticing this deficiency, stimulate Ren-19 with acupuressure. Notice how LU-1 quickly picks up channel Qi from Ren-19. You can feel the flow of channel Qi moving laterally across the chest from Ren-19 into LU-1. When the normal source of channel Qi for LU-1, the Liver channel, is busy being diverted to the head to deal with the fear-based crisis, the lungs can be supplied with channel Qi from an alternative source – in this case, Ren-19.

Keep in mind that the body has a nearly infinite number of alternative paths to keep channel Qi flowing to those parts of the body that are calling for energy at any given time. We are healthiest when the parasympathetic mode channels are providing the channel Qi, but if, for whatever reason, they cannot, the body will find another way to keep channel Qi flowing to the body parts being called upon.

Getting back to my patient's case study: his Liver channel Qi had become entrenched in using this divergent pattern at night. At night, his Liver channel Qi, from long habit of stress, was no longer flowing in its healthy, parasympathetic course, going deep into the chest and emerging into the lungs. His Liver channel Qi was still behaving as if he was in a dire emergency. Every night at 3:00, the extra surge of Midnight/Midday energy flowed out of the Liver channel *into* the sympathetic divergent pathway – up into the head. This surge of energy into the head was causing nightmares.

His lungs did *not* receive the 3:00 a.m. surge. Instead, the emergency-assessing sectors of his brain were filling up with the surge of Midnight/Midday energy. He would wake up, thrashing and screaming.[1]

After the needle-assisted re-routing, his body was able to function in parasympathetic mode – even at 3:00 a.m.

When his channel Qi levels surged at 3:00 a.m. the next night, he slept like a baby: when the healing/restoring surge in the Liver channel Qi tried to make the 3:00 a.m. transition to a healing/restoring surge into the Lung channel, it was able to do so.

---

[1] As an aside, this patient was not in sympathetic mode while he was awake. This patient was a world-class classical cellist. I have observed, over the years, that my patients who are professional musicians are able usually to get themselves into parasympathetic mode via music, even if there are ongoing stresses in their lives. They need to do this, in order to *feel* the music (rather than just assess the music analytically or by using words). This may contribute to the fact that, of all the professions, music conductors have the longest life expectancy. Many symphonic conductors are still working, vigorously, up into their eighties. Professional-level classical musicians also tend to have a long life expectancy. At any rate, this patient was able to be wonderfully calm and joyful so long as he was awake.

It is easier for the channel Qi to flow in parasympathetic mode than in sympathetic. Think of parasympathetic as having a lower potential energy requirement. It requires work, kinetic energy, to shift the system into sympathetic. Therefore, if the body can be restored, even briefly, to parasympathetic, and if no other situation, such as a wrong mental attitude, arises to jerk the body back into sympathetic, the Qi flow can easily be rerouted to parasympathetic, *and will tend to stay there.*

Then again, negative thought waves carry energy, and can serve to jerk the body back into sympathetic, and return the channel Qi to the sympathetic divergent patterns. But if no further trauma occurs *and* the thoughts are predominantly joyful or calm, the channels, once returned to parasympathetic, will stay in parasympathetic until the next truly fearful event.

The patient had no more nightmares.

I have since used this combination of needles, in this insertion sequence, in many situations in which the Liver Qi has become stuck in a predominantly sympathetic pathway. As noted in an earlier footnote, I have learned that many senior acupuncturists prefer to use GB-41, instead of LIV-3, for providing a temporary increase in Liver channel Qi. As some of my teachers have reminded me, "The Liver doesn't like to be forced into anything."

If there is resistance in the Liver channel, needling LIV-3 can be painful, and the body will not accept the stimulation. The Liver channel can become *more* blocked if it is *forced*. By using GB-41, you are giving the Liver channel a *choice* to either take the extra channel Qi, or not. The Liver channel is more likely to accept the increase in channel Qi if it has a choice in the matter.

Dream points and mis-translations

As an aside, I was so puzzled by my patient's dream choice of GB-41, a point I had never used, that I looked up the point indications in my notes. One of the indications was "breast cancer." I stared at that phrase long and hard. My patient did not have breast cancer. But he had been carrying a metaphorical "lump" in what we would call, poetically, his "breast" (the emotion center of his chest.)

I had to wonder, did the original point indication say that GB-41 could be used if a person had a blockage in his (poetic) breast? And had the Chinese phrase, "breast yong" been mis-translated into medical-ese by some technician who didn't understand the implications of habitual sympathetic mode congestion in the breast? Had this technician mis-translated breast yong, which means "block in the chest," into "breast cancer?" It was a reasonable guess at translation, especially given the mid 20th century communist party policy, which held that *emotional* problems did *not* exist in a *truly* communist country, but cancer *did*.[1]

---

[1] Recent research suggests that the best single point for treating breast cancer is LIV-2, and not GB-41 (which flows into the Liver channel at LIV-3, *downstream* from LIV-2). GB-41 doesn't seem to do much for breast cancer. LIV-2 is approximately the same *energetic* (amount of amperage) distance to the beginning of the Liver channel as the breast is to the end of the Liver channel. Again, physics tells us that a wave aberration at one location along a string can create a matching aberration at a spot equidistant to the other end of the string. A stress that keeps the Liver Qi from flowing in its parasympathetic path deep under the breast *may* create a matching aberration near the toes, in the vicinity of LIV-2. Oppositely, deficiency of Wei Qi in the breast that allows the development of cancerous breast tissue may be set in motion by an aberration in the flow of channel Qi at LIV-2.

116

Pondering over whether or not an historical point indication, "a lump of tension or hardness in the emotion center of the chest," had become grossly mistranslated as "breast cancer" made me suddenly aware that I could not trust any of the translated books that I had lovingly collected, books that were smiling up at me from my office bookshelf.

I knew, from that moment, that I could no longer blindly trust the point indications I had learned in school. I needed to *know* what was going on with the points, and with the channels. Evidently, the books *might* provide guidelines, but they *might* also be dead wrong.

It was this very moment, carried to me on the wings of a patient's dream, that led me down "the road less taken:" inquiries that increasingly relied on tracking a patient's channel Qi. This led to my personal experiences of channel flow patterns and *far* more understanding of the effects of specific acupoints on channel Qi than is provided in the "point indication" lists.

This information is available to *everyone* who takes the time to notice how the flow of channel Qi responds to thoughts, traumas, external and internal "evils", and how the channels respond to herbs, acupuncture needles, and all the other healing modalities.

The redirection of channel Qi into the sympathetic mode-supporting divergent channels in times of stress, danger, or emergency, and the ability of these divergent patterns to become habitual unless redirected by a somewhat fearless consciousness, can be hugely important to understanding the physiology of chronic illness. The subject merits a second case study.

Case study #7

The "painful point"

Female, age 43, lack of appetite, "not feeling right: mildly agitated all the time." Her athlete's pulses were harmonized, as well as being very slow, steady, deep and strong, as always. Her tongue looked healthy.

An otherwise *very* healthy patient, with a good marriage, a beautiful child, and a gratifying job, she was puzzled by these symptoms. She wondered if they might be coming from the recent re-surfacing in her life of "an old boyfriend, from a decade ago, who always brings bad luck to everyone, especially himself." Even though she'd quickly told him to move along, and was not planning to ever meet up with him again, she'd been feeling funny ever since he'd called her, one week ago.

A quick assessment of her channel Qi showed that her Stomach channel was not flowing past ST-14. I explained to her the correct path of the Stomach channel: just under the skin of the breast, passing just under the nipple.

(As an aside, the channel Qi is very easy to detect in this area, so I am able to hold my hand two, or even three inches away from the skin. Because of our culture's puerile hyperawareness of breasts and nipples, I recommend that, in this part of the body, keep your hand as far away as you can while still being close enough to feel the channel Qi.)

I asked her to get her Stomach channel energy up out of her heart, and let it flow over her chest again.

As soon as she did this, she felt more relaxed. I asked her to keep that energy pattern going for several minutes. She felt her stomach begin to move, and she suddenly felt hungry.

(Several times, I have seen this sudden appearance of healthy hunger, upon correction of the Stomach channel in the vicinity of ST-14.)

I didn't bother to insert any needles for her Stomach channel diversion. It was healed. Instead, I needled the site of the ankle injury for which she'd originally made the appointment.

I told her to keep tabs on the energy in her Stomach channel. If she caught herself indulging in thoughts that caused the energy in that channel to go inwards, instead of staying up on the surface and moving over the breast, she needed to mentally restore the channel to its correct place.

She reported back to me, a week later, there had been no return of the poor appetite or the agitation. She was enjoying "checking in" with the energy flow over her chest. It was always running just right, and she felt good knowing that it was.

In this case study, I have included seemingly extraneous details about the patient's emotional life, because, in her case, the "fear or stress" that was forcing her Stomach channel Qi to diverge into sympathetic posture was a purely emotional factor. There was no physical channel Qi blockage. There was only a mental force being exerted that was altering the course of the channel Qi. The treatment reflected this. She did not need acupuncture needles – she needed to know that her thought patterns were causing a problem, and that her thought patterns could also resolve the problem.

Disappearing Stomach channel Qi in association with negative thoughts

I have seen Stomach channel Qi "stuck" in a divergent pattern – flowing deep into the chest from approximately ST-14 – many, many times. In these cases, the Stomach channel is palpable, from the face, down to around ST-14 or ST-15, and then "poof:" it disappears. It *cannot* be felt by hand as it drops deep down into the region of the heart.

Instead of automatically needling the Stomach channel at ST-16 or ST-18 to try to pull Stomach channel Qi back to the surface, and thus redirect the channel Qi, I usually just tell the patient what is going on, and ask him to mentally bring that energy back up to the surface, to the skin level, and let it course down the breast, over the nipple. It usually works just fine, and lets the patient take responsibility for his own neural mode status.[1]

---

[1] A few years ago, a technique for dealing with habits of stress, called EFT, or Emotional Freedom Technique, was very popular. One of the instructions for the EFT protocol was something along the lines of "think about the troublesome issue and massage the *Painful Place* on the chest." A diagram showed the location of the Painful Place: ST-14.

In people who feel upset about a particular issue, just thinking about the issue can cause a mild shift towards sympathetic mode: the Stomach channel will divert into the heart in the vicinity of ST-14 *whenever they think about the thing that causes them pain*. If the Stomach channel stays in this position for more than a short while, the St-14 area becomes slightly painful, when rubbed. (The famous Asian medicine adage, Go Through, No Pain, refers to channel Qi going through in the *parasympathetic* mode. Anything other than that eventually causes pain – either physical or metaphoric.)

The point of the EFT program was that one *can* train the body to stay in parasympathetic mode even while thinking of specific negative experiences. By mentally keeping the Stomach channel in parasympathetic mode while simultaneously dwelling on the negative experience, one can retrain

Application

After detecting that a patient's channel Qi is using a sympathetic channel flow pattern instead of the Primary path, you should then determine if a physical or chemical impediment is causing the aberrant flow, or if some part of the patient's mind or body is stuck in a deleterious sympathetic mode pattern.

Either way, healing occurs most easily in parasympathetic mode. If someone is *stuck* in sympathetic mode with regard to some physical injury or some emotional blockage, healing will not occur, at least not at the normal pace. Also, variants of "pain" will be able to develop.

By rerouting channel Qi back into the parasympathetic, "normal" path of the channel, you can often bring the person back to a much healthier position, very quickly.

The body was never designed to be in sympathetic mode for more than about ten minutes at a time, and not more than a few times a day, at most. If a person has developed a holding pattern that is *keeping* him in sympathetic mode in some part of his body, you can be certain that this holding pattern is contributing to some health problem, either now, or down the road.

By helping reroute sympathetic mode channel divergences back to parasympathetic mode, into "normal" channel pathways, you may be doing a profound service. You are helping alter something at the root level, rather than just treating a symptom – if the patient is able to maintain the restoration.

Then again, if the channel Qi spontaneously *returns* to the sympathetic mode even after you've returned it to parasympathetic, then you can be certain that there is an *ongoing* fear, stress or Shen disturbance (mental/emotional problem). In such a case, you will be able to provide only palliative, temporary-benefit treatments until such time as the patient *removes* himself from vulnerability to ongoing fear or stress, or processes the mental/emotional blockage that he is hanging on to.

Of course, even if our treatments are only palliative, we should still do them: they reduce pain. This is compassionate. This is our job.

But it is best if we are clear on what we can and cannot fix. As the *Nei Jing* makes abundantly clear, we *cannot* permanently resolve a patient's "pain" so long as that patient is susceptible to stress, or, to put it into old fashioned words, is not in tune with Spirit. On the other hand, if a patient *is* in tune with Spirit, the conditions of his life, no matter how dire, will not be able to sway him from attunement with joy, truth, and attunement with the attitudes that keep the channel Qi running in parasympathetic mode.[1]

---

the brain – shifting the memory of the experience out of the "Oh NO!" (sympathetic part) of the memory bank into the "Huh, whaddya know, that was interesting" (parasympathetic part) of the memory bank. When this brain shift occurs, a person can then think about the experience as a mere memory, without becoming physically re-traumatized and plopping himself into the relative discomforts of sympathetic mode every time the memory is stimulated.

[1] For a stirring testimonial to the human ability to attune with joy regardless of externals, an ability often disdained in our culture, I highly recommend *And There Was Light*, by Jacques Lusseyran. Lusseyran was physically blinded in an accident at eight years of age. Nevertheless, light and joy sometimes permeated his body. By training himself to stay always attuned with the light, he

became able to perceive, in his heart, ambient light wave energy, which he learned to translate into a unique sense of "vision." For example, he could discern the energetic difference between distant mountains, spreading farmland, and individual trees. He could also "see" whether or not a person was telling the truth, based on the radiance that the person emitted. He was a political activist during World War II. His unique ability to detect honesty – or treachery – made him a crucial member of the recruitment branch of the French resistance. After the Germans invaded Paris, he was captured and sent to the Buchenwald concentration camp.

After that, he succumbed to fear. When this happened, he was unable to fill himself with light. He lost his ability to "see." His comrades died, his body was tortured, starved, and unprotected from the freezing winter. When he was dying with a high fever, he decided that he did not want to die in that manner. He wanted to fill himself with light, despite the horrors around him. As he lay dying, he forced himself to attune with the light, instead of with his feverish, emaciated body. As he refocused his heart on the immutable, unchanging love and light that is always just behind our seeming physical reality, he felt his fever pass. His unique form of "vision" was restored. He realized that his inability to be filled with light, in the camp, had been a *choice*, a wrong choice.

He quickly recovered, and began work on a resistance effort from within the camp. Because he was blind, his captors ignored his movements, never suspecting him capable of anything. Using a forgotten radio in the kitchen basement, he was able to send radio transmissions to the Allies, sending inside information about German troop movements. He was also able to encourage and provide some degree of support for the others in the camp who, like him, were in the "unfit to live" group. Although those "unfit to live" were not given food or health care, Lusseyran was one of the few prisoners who survived to be rescued by the Allies.

He never again chose to lose his ability to "see."

I highly recommend this book. Although it gives the most graphic details of life in camp of any book I have read, he emphasizes that he includes these details not to horrify, but to help the reader understand that one *always* has a choice as to whether or not to attune the heart with light and joy, *no matter what the circumstances*.

Heart attunement, no matter what the circumstances, is the key to keeping the channels in parasympathetic mode. Acupuncture, herbs, Tui Na and diet are only feeble tools, useful for pointing the way, for someone whose channel Qi has gotten confused. But it is the patient's job to live and think in such a way as to keep the channel Qi running true, once it has been straightened.

It is good to use acupuncture and other medical tools in order to mechanically correct the errors in a patient's channel Qi. But the more you gently direct the patient to correct his own negative choices and habits, the more you are practicing true, lasting medicine.

120

"Even in a perfectly healthy person, channel Qi flows in the manner that you learn in school, only about seventy percent of the time, at most." [1]

Chapter seven

The healthy paths of the channels: part III

Sleep: "tired nature's sweet restorer" [2]

The Du channel regulates consciousness. In order to fall asleep, a neural mode in which consciousness is diminished, the energy level in the mighty Du channel must be diminished.

The Du channel, not technically a part of the primary channel system, courses up behind the spine, along the posterior surface of the brainstem and midbrain, and right through the center of the brain, emerging out to the forehead at a point between the eyebrows (Yin Tang).

A *branch* of the Du channel travels over the top of the head. This *branch* contains the Du channel points that can be needled, but the mainline of the Du channel goes right through the head. This through-the-head portion of the Du channel provides the energy that directs thought and supports consciousness.

After the main branch of the Du meets the over-the-top branch at Yin Tang, the channel flows down the center of the face to the upper lip. From the upper lip, it flows into the mouth, down through the gut, out the anus and, voila! it is once again flowing posterior to the spine, where it begins anew its ascent up to the head.

In order to induce sleep, the power, or amperage, of this channel must be diminished. This power-reduction job belongs to the Gallbladder channel.

Falling asleep

At 11:00 p.m, approximately, the Gallbladder channel experiences a surge in energy level. The Gallbladder channel runs in the *opposite* direction of the Du channel. The Du channel runs from the back of the head towards the face; the Gallbladder channel runs from the face towards the back of the head. [3]

---

[1] From a 2008 DAOM (doctoral) class lecture by Dr. Wang Ju-Yi, author of the book, *Channel Theory and Diagnosis*, Eastland Press, Seattle, 2008.

[2] Edward Young, English poet (1683-1765).

[3] Of course, a person can override the tendency to fall asleep at 11:00. This override merely requires the use of adrenaline. However, this stay-up-late override is usually not a healthy habit. Also note, in winter, the GB time of day will occur earlier, depending on what time the sun sets.

The changing of the Du

Based on simple principles of high school physics, we can appreciate that a big surge in strength in the Gallbladder channel will cause a *decrease* in the strength of any nearby channel running in the opposite direction: in this case, the Du.

Restating the above, the big surge of energy running in the Gallbladder channel, which occurs at approximately 11:00 p.m., diminishes the relative strength of the head and neck portion of the Du channel – the channel that powers consciousness. The surge in Gallbladder channel Qi allows a person's consciousness to diminish, or drop off: sleep ensues.

This moderate inhibition of the Du channel triggers other changes as well. For example, the Yang channels of the arm have branches that connect, briefly, with Du-14, before continuing on their path to the face. When the Du channel is inhibited, these Yang channels of the arm pick up on the sleep-time inhibition at Du-14. When a person is awake, his Yang channels get a bit of a boost at Du-14. During sleep, they do not. The decrease in Du channel Qi causes a decrease in the level of activity in the portions of the arm Yang channels that are downstream from Du-14: the portions on the neck and head.

Slowing of the Triple Burner

Because it runs in the opposite direction of the Gallbladder channel in the vicinity of the ears, the Triple Burner channel also is slowed at 11:00.

The TB channel regulates the relationship between the crude physical (chemical and electrical) body, the more purely energetic (astral) body, and the subtle, causal body, made up of thought waves that maintain the idea of our existence – with or without a body.

In the *Nei Jing*, the three planes of existence, physical, astral, and causal, are described metaphorically. The physical body is compared to a sewage plant. The astral body is energetic: fluid and vibratory. The *Nei Jing* gives an analogy for the astral, energetic realm by comparing it to the form-shifting that occurs in water: water can exist as rain, when it falls in the mountains and flows down into the ocean. Water changes state, which is to say, becomes gaseous, as it evaporates up to the clouds. The airy moisture changes state again when it condenses again into liquid and falls again, as rain. The causal vibrations are physically imperceptible, and are compared to the physically imperceptible heaven.

Again, the three "burners," or you might say the three types of energy, are the physical, astral, and causal body. The Triple Burner provides the energy that *integrates* these three levels of energy, forcing them to work together.

The head portion of the Triple Burner flows around the ears: the sides of the brain, which are stimulated by the Triple Burner, contain the brain's precuneus area that regulates ego-based self-image and negative thinking.

The precuneus, in animals, is designed to override seeking behaviors during times of danger. In humans, the precuneus can override the information of the central frontal lobe, the universe-attunement area of the "third eye," at Yin Tang. The degree to which it does this is related to bad habits and ego-based will.[1]

---

[1] The ability of the precuneus to override Yin Tang in animals allows non-rational animals to learn life-preserving fears, fears that are able to override their innate curiosity. In man, this part of the brain is often used to excess. A poorly-disciplined mind may excessively anticipate problems and

Thus, the Triple Burner, by integrating our physical, astral, and causal energy *and* by stimulating the ego-driving areas on the sides of the brain, just posterior to the frontal lobe, pushes us to imagine ourselves as being physical bodies, instead of knowing ourselves to be, in truth, immortal, wise, conscious vibrations of love. Only regular spiritual discipline can keep the truth-aligned frontal lobe signals that should direct behavior from being overridden by the delusions put forth by the ego-assessing, precuneus area – the area supported by the Triple Burner channel.

In sleep, the head portion of the TB channel, which runs from the back of the head towards the front, is moderately inhibited in two ways: 1) via directional opposition from the Gallbladder channel and 2) via contact with the diminished Du at Du-14.

When the energy in the Triple Burner channel decreases enough, during sleep, the delusive burden of body and ego awareness also decreases. We can then sleep, free from bodily pain, and can create causal and astral dream universes of our own, as is our soul-right.

In review, the Gallbladder surge does more than shut down consciousness: it inhibits the Du, which then inhibits the head portions of the arm Yang channels, Large and Small Intestines and the Triple Burner. The diminished channel Qi in the head portion of the Large Intestine channel is not then strong enough to activate either Ren-24 or Du-26. Thus, the Ren channel is somewhat inhibited as well. With less LI channel Qi getting to the face, the energy in the Stomach channel Qi is greatly decreased. (The Large Intestine channel flows into, and supplies, the Stomach channel.) With the energy in the Stomach channel decreased, vagus nerve function is decreased.

With all these channels somewhat inhibited, we sleep: the face, gut, and body awareness have some time off.

Facial Du connections

At Yin Tang, the Du channel also connects with and energizes the beginnings of all the Yang *leg* channels. During sleep, when the power level in the Du channel drops, the channel-driving power to the Yang leg channels that is provided by this connection is diminished.

The Du channel also connects to the Large Intestine and Stomach channels at Yin Tang *and* at Du-26 and helps power those two channels. During sleep, the Du-driven power at these *two* facial intersections is diminished: the Large Intestine and Stomach channels are thus *doubly* inhibited, contributing further to a stilling of the gut.

In review, when the Gallbladder channel surges, the Du channel Qi flow is altered and diminished. Consciousness is directly inhibited. Via all the above connections and intersections with the "sleeping" Du channel, gastrointestinal activity, and self-limiting ego-based fears and pain awareness are also greatly diminished. Yang leg channels, all of which begin at Yin Tang, receive less energy.

---

enjoy dwelling on the problems of the past. These processes, nurtured in the precuneus area, can be incorrectly used for self-tormenting negative self-images and near-constant inhibition of information from Yin Tang.

Waking up

At 1:00 a.m., the Liver channel in the sleeper starts to surge. This surge will not wake the sleeper. The Liver channel surge, in an emotionally serene, healthy person, stays in the legs and chest, and doesn't go to the head.[1]

Two hours later, at 3:00 a.m., the "surge" level of channel Qi will manifest in the next channel: the Lung channel. This surge will not wake the sleeper. The increase in channel Qi in the Lung channel, like the surge into the Liver channel, doesn't go anywhere near the head. It will *not* disturb the diminished level of energy in the head portion of the Du channel. The Du channel can remain in its lowered-energy condition even while channel Qi surges in the Lung channel.

From 5:00 a.m. to 7:00 a.m., the channel Qi surges in the Large Intestine channel. *This* channel is going to slam the Du channel *twice* – and wake it up. The Large Intestine channel intersects the Du channel at the upper lip, at Du-26, and again at Yin Tang.

When the Large Intestine channel skirts the lips, slapping Du-26, it provides a jolt to the Du channel.

The right-side Large Intestine channel flows over to the left side of the face. A split second later, the left-side Large Intestine channel flows over to the right side of the face. They steadily take turns, flowing first from the right side and then from the left.

This side-to-side switching of the Large Intestine channel Qi alternates rapidly: first it hits Du-26 from the right, then it hits Du-26 from the left, then from the right, then from left, and so on, for two hours – from 5:00 to 7:00 a.m.

Meanwhile, the left and right Large Intestine channels flow up to Yin Tang, striking it over and over: bing, bing, bing. The Du channel is stimulated by this incessant activity at the frontal lobe and at Du-26. The main path of the Du channel begins to flow with more power through the middle of the brain. A person may or may not experience strong dreams at this point, just before waking up.

When the Du channel finally attains enough strength to initiate consciousness, wakefulness occurs. At this point, the increase in Du channel energy leads to an increase in energy in all the Yang channels of the arms and legs. The body stirs. Consciousness resumes full alertness. The Wake-Up is underway.

As the Large Intestine channel Qi surges, peristalsis resumes. The lower gut starts gently heaving its contents along. Gas may be expelled, and the bowels may want to move.

---

[1] Then again, if the pericardium is producing a signal of emotional distress even during sleep, some portion of the Liver channel Qi, after passing the pericardium and picking up the distress signal from this central organ, will divert into the Liver channel branch that travels to the very top of the head, to assist with the mental processes needed to deal with the stressor. If Liver channel Qi is being sent to the vertex in the night, the Du channel may become stimulated enough to rouse one to consciousness in the middle of the night: stress-triggered insomnia.

Ideally, if this Liver Qi-to-the-vertex pattern occurs during the day, a person might feel more mentally focused. He might *also* have a mild headache, or tension in the head from excess Qi being diverted to the vertex. This headache and/or tension is helpful: a person who is listening to his body will use this tension as a cue that he needs to rest for a bit, maybe even meditate for a while, and thus productively process whatever is stressing his heart or pericardium.

124

Next, from 7:00 to 9:00 a.m., the surge of channel Qi shifts over into the Stomach channel. The Stomach channel, like the Large Intestine channel, skirts the lips, also hitting the Du at Yin Tang *and* Du-26. This continuing double stimulation of the Du channel ensures that a person becomes fully roused to consciousness.

Also, the surge of channel Qi in the Stomach channels triggers movement in the stomach. With these movements, sensations of hunger arise. Fortunately, the large intestine has already been moving for two hours, getting the peristalsis moving and making way for the incoming rush of business: breakfast.

From 9:00 to 11:00 a.m., the Spleen channel surges, and two hours later, from 11:00 a.m. to 1:00 p.m., the Heart channel surges, and so on, throughout the day.

The main point here is that, during sleep, the Du channel is inhibited. The flow of channel Qi in the Du, Large Intestine, Small Intestine, and Triple Burner channels are *all* inhibited. Further inhibition also occurs in the Stomach, Urinary Bladder, and Gallbladder channels, all of which originate at Yin Tang. (Of course, the Gallbladder is enjoying its surge during part of this time, and so is far less inhibited than the other Yang channels.)

This inhibition helps us understand why we do not have bowel movements, hunger, or bladder activity while we are sleeping. If we *do* need to experience these actions, we are able to rouse ourselves briefly, using adrenaline (which can override any other neural mode), but we can usually fall back into somnolence as soon as we get back into bed and the adrenaline is neutralized.

An aside – an historical interlude about the neural mode nomenclature

Western scientists consider sleep to be a form of parasympathetic mode even though the digestion – the system most characteristic of parasympathetic mode – is turned way down, even turned off, during sleep. (For example, one does not have bowel movements in his sleep, nor does his stomach process food except in a minimal, inefficient fashion.) Just as significantly, heart rate and breathing are different during sleep than they are during curiosity and relaxation mode. Even consciousness is highly altered during sleep. To blindly insist that neural stimulation of consciousness, gastrointestinal and respiratory organ function, and sense perceptions are the same during sleep as they are when awake is ludicrous. [1]

Galvani's frogs

The reason for the western idea of only two modes, sympathetic and parasympathetic, goes all the way back to Galvani and his electrical-shock experiments on frogs. He named those nerves that respond to electrical shock "sympathetic," meaning "responsive." He decided that all other nerves were "neutral" or "automatic": they just ran all the time and didn't respond to anything.

Years later, researchers discovered that some non-sympathetic nerves weren't "automatic" after all. They turned on and off. Not only that, all organs seemed to have two sets of nerves, one set that was triggered by the "sympathetic" spinal nerves and the other

---

[1] This is glaringly obvious. In the immortal words of Yogi Berra, baseball great, "You can see a lot by looking."

triggered via certain cranial nerves, and in particular, the vagus nerve. This second group of nerves was named the parasympathetic group.

At that time, the hypothesis of nerves was modified: there were *two* active neural modes, sympathetic and parasympathetic, and all *other* nerves were still automatic. Researchers then assumed, based on nothing in particular, that animals were always using either the sympathetic set of nerves *or* the parasympathetic set. The theory of the day held that usage of these nerve systems was a clear-cut case of one-or-the-other, black or white, with no gradations of grey: all sympathetic, or all parasympathetic – a person could either be perfectly at peace, or in a state of pure panic. This aspect of the theory is still adhered to by some MDs, even though it should be obvious to the meanest intelligence that most people are, at any given moment, partly relaxed, and partly fearful.

Over the years various modifications were inserted into the system. In the 1920s, some nerves that had once been deemed "automatic" were declared to be gland-regulated. In the 1940s and 1950s, glands declined in popularity and hormones were said to control many "automatic" nerves. During the twentieth century, the nerve system theories constantly changed in response to new discoveries. Currently, neurotransmitters are popular "other nerve" regulators.

And yet, according to basic, western medical theory, the only nerve systems that still vary *in response to externals* have remained the sympathetic and parasympathetic. We now know that this entire premise is incorrect: both sympathetic and parasympathetic responses can be triggered by *non*-externals, such as thoughts, hormones, and so on, *and* nerves other than the sympathetic and parasympathetic do respond to external stimulation.

Even so, we still use the highly outdated sympathetic/parasympathetic one-or-the-other nomenclature to describe most "responsive" behaviors.

Increasing the error, there are two other neural modes: sleep and dissociation. In both of these modes, *both* sympathetic *and* parasympathetic nerves are deeply inhibited.

In all four of the modes, Asian medicine, using a channel perspective, is able to show the *mechanisms* that trigger the nerve turn-ons and turn-offs.

Practice feeling channel Qi

If you get the opportunity, please feel the channel Qi flow in someone at nighttime, in someone who is sleeping soundly, and also feel his same channels during the day, when he is awake. Notice the difference in the flow patterns. It almost feels as if the Yang channels are tiptoeing, rather than galloping. They are hushed. They are certainly not moving with the same energy as in the daytime. While falling asleep, the body becomes Gallbladder channel-dominant. When awake, the body is Du channel dominant. The *routes* of the channels are relatively unchanged during sleep, but the *distribution* of the energy in the channels is greatly altered. It is in this sense that, even in a healthy person, the channels only flow in the manner we learn in school, at the most, seventy percent of the time. The other thirty percent of the time, the channels are in sleep mode.

Case study #8

Insomnia due to injury at GB-20

Female, age 57. Utter insomnia following a *severe*, nearly fatal neck injury, from a bad fall while hiking.

Following the post-injury concussion that lasted three days, the patient had not experienced sleep for nearly six weeks. At nighttime, she would lie as motionless as possible. Through self-control, she could make her breathing become very regular, and she could still her thoughts. However, she could not "drop off." She was conscious of being conscious through the entire night.

Due to several weeks of this complete inability to drop off to sleep, she became increasingly exhausted. She could feel somewhat restored by "napping" during the day: during her "naps," she would lie motionless, stilling her thoughts, but even so, her consciousness never turned off.

Both left and right Gallbladder channels were blocked by the swelling and twisted fascia in her neck. I was amazed that she had not broken her neck in this injury, as were her other doctors.

No Gallbladder channel Qi was moving past GB-20, on either side of her neck. An extremely Yin style of Tui Na was applied to the neck. Tissues in the neck relaxed slightly, but not enough to allow a significant amount of Gallbladder channel Qi to move past GB-20.

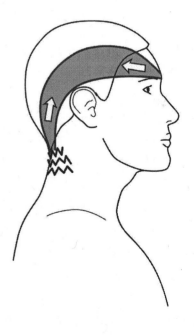

Fig. 7.1 In this patient, the Gallbladder channel Qi was hitting the injury-based blockage at the back of the neck, and was unable to flow past it. Instead, the Qi then flowed backwards, into the head, into any area of lower resistence – and even back into the Gallbladder channel. The result was a detectable jumble of channel Qi at the nape of the neck, and diminished flow of channel Qi into the blocked up Gallbladder channel.

The delicate consciousness-regulating balance between the Du channel and the Gallbladder channel was completely out of order.

In a healthy person, at the nape of the neck, the channel Qi of the Gallbladder channel should flow down to the shoulder, on its way to the feet. From 11:00 p.m to 1:00, an even larger amount of Gallbladder channel Qi should course through this path – exerting a strong inhibitory effect on the Du channel – and consciousness – thus allowing a person to fall asleep.

Needles inserted into GB-20 and other points along the GB channel caused extreme pain and only initiated minimal flow of channel Qi past GB-20. As soon as the needles were removed, the channel Qi resumed its blocked behavior. With the physical blockages in her neck, the channel Qi was not able to move past GB-20. The Gallbladder channel Qi, having no other outlet, was shunting into the nearby UB, TB, and Du channels – creating agitation in the channels that was keeping her awake.

The herbal formula Xiao Chai Hu Tang, which electrically, not chemically, rectifies flow in the torso portion of the Liver channel and Gallbladder channel, was not able to clear up the neck blockage at GB-20.[1] Next, even though her problem did not seem to be heart related, I tested her with several non-opiate based, "Heart pattern" sleep-inducing herbal formulas. I placed the herbal tablets on her abdomen and checked for changes in the channel Qi in the neck portion of her Gallbladder channel. No result.

I was certain that the physical work on her neck would need to proceed with extreme caution. This would take time – possibly weeks. But she already was starting to feel rumblings of mental and emotional disturbance from the extended lack of sleep. She had taken a leave from work. She did not want to start on pharmaceutical grade sleeping pills.

I instructed her as to the path of the Gallbladder channel and asked her to move the channel Qi through this channel mentally (medical Qi Gong) whenever she thought of it. At night, she should repeatedly, mentally, move as much energy as she could over the sides of her head, through GB-20, down into her shoulders at GB-21, and down the sides of the torso. She could thus *mentally* contradict the flow of channel Qi in the Du channel.

At bedtime, she performed this mental stimulation over and over. On her first night of practicing moving the Gallbladder channel, she fell into a much-needed sleep within ten minutes, and stayed asleep until 7:00 the next morning.

She needed to perform this Qi Gong treatment on herself every night for the next few weeks. If she did *not* do this, she did not fall asleep. Instead, she remained in a stillness of body and mind with retention of complete consciousness until she did the Qi Gong exercises.

Prior to the accident, she had always fallen asleep easily. Now, she could only fall asleep if she consciously moved channel Qi over the sides of her head, past GB-20, and down into her shoulders and sides of the torso.

Over the next few weeks, after the neck had been very slowly realigned and the swelling slowly went down, she was once again able to fall asleep "at the drop of a hat," or more exactly, "at the drop of energy flow in her Du channel."

I like this study because it shows the value of Qi Gong. In situations where needles and herbs are not effective, or will not work quickly or lastingly enough, the patient may benefit from being shown that he always holds within himself the key to recovery. Our job, by virtue of our training and through accurate diagnosis, is to bring that key to his attention.[2]

---

[1] As for Chai Hu working primarily as an electrical, not chemical, activator, do this experiment: next time your Liver channel feels blocked, try holding a bottle of Xiao Chai Hu Tang against the skin of your abdomen and feel how it immediately straightens your channel Qi. This is an electrical effect. The *subsequent* chemical changes that you can feel slowly occurring in the body are the *result* of the electrical (channel Qi) reconfiguration.

[2] Medical Qi Gong consists of teaching patients how to redirect their thoughts and energy to restore channel Qi and send positive thinking into body areas that have become damaged, distorted, or ignored. Many excellent, simple exercises, ranging from callisthenic-type movements all the way to

Insomnia is a significant problem in our culture. Therefore, I'm including the following insomnia case study in this chapter on sleep to show that *not* all insomnia problems are due to a failure of the Gallbladder channel to sedate the Du.

Case study #9

Violent wake-ups at 5:00 a.m.

Male, age 53, very healthy, thin, athletic, with excellent diet and long-term, regular spiritual disciplines including daily meditation.

The patient sometimes woke up in a heart-pounding panic at 5:00 a.m. instead of waking gradually and peacefully at his usual wake-up time of 7:30. This occurred whenever he experienced work-related "deadline" stress – about three days out of every month. It had been going on for years. He also had an assortment of other issues including mildly high blood sugar levels that did not match his low weight, lean diet, and high exercise profile.

I treated his severe channel blockage at left-side ST-4 (probably from a childhood face injury involving a baseball bat) that was clearly inhibiting the flow of Stomach channel Qi on his left side and which might have been contributing both to his poor tooth roots on his lower left jaw and to his very mild blood sugar problem. Over the next few sessions, I treated various other glaring channel Qi problems. Within five sessions, all of his other mild health problems were gone. All that remained was the 5:00 a.m. panic, which he'd just experienced again the last few days. Tongue and pulse were both in reasonable shape, although Lung pulse seemed *possibly* a little deficient.

I was baffled by this case. Over the course of several visits, his channel Qi had been restored to health, body-wide. His tongue and pulse were now consistently good and his minor health problems had resolved, but he'd just had three consecutive 5:00 a.m. panic wake-ups. I was clearly missing something subtle, something that wasn't even being picked up by tongue and pulse (so I thought). I inserted a needle at Yin Tang in the patient and went in the other room to think things over.

I had examined and/or treated everything that might be related to 5:00 a.m.: the areas around the UB points for the Lungs and Large Intestines, and all the usual suspects: the channel divergences that can signify being stuck in sympathetic system. I decided that the only thing I hadn't checked was the thumb and index fingers. If he had a scar somewhere between the paths of the Lung and Large intestine just past LU-7 or prior to LI-4, then the surge of healing channel Qi into the Large Intestine channel – which occurs at 5:00 a.m. – would be unable to follow the route involving the tip of the thumb and the tips of the index

---

mental movement of channel Qi have been developed and written up. Medical Qi Gong was a required part of my training when I got my Master's degree in Asian medicine.

As an aside, some students have wrongly been taught that medical Qi Gong consists of powerful manipulation of the patient's channel Qi *by the health practitioner*. When a patient submits to this, he is allowing his own will to become subordinate to the will of the practitioner. This is a dangerous practice – for the spiritual well-being of the practitioner. It also provides no *lasting* benefit for the patient.

Of course, great saints and sages often have the ability to heal others with a word or a glance. However, they *never* avail themselves of this ability unless *commanded* by God.

This is a very important subject, but too involved for this book on channel theory.

finger. Instead, most of the surge would have to travel through the Luo of the Lung channel, rather than over the thenar prominence and out to the finger tips.

The *parasympathetic* route of the Lung channel into the Large Intestine travels predominantly over the tips of the fingers. The Luo ("connecting") route is predominant during sympathetic mode.

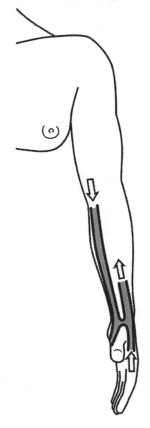

Fig. 7.2 Parasympathetic mode paths of the Lung channel and Large Intestine channel. Note the *small* connection at the wrist, where a small amount of Lung channel Qi flows over to the Large Intestine channel.

In sympathetic mode, the ratio of Lung channel Qi going to the fingers compared to the amount going over the Luo changes: less goes to the fingers, and much more goes directly into the Large Intestine channel.

In sympathetic mode, the amount going to the fingers is determined by the exact need of the fingers at that moment. The rest is able to flow up to the head, then into the Stomach channel, and then into the heart – as needed.

If a significant scar was blocking the channel Qi in this area, even a little, so that the channel Qi had to send more Qi than usual via the Luo, the channel Qi would be traveling in the path that is predominant when in sympathetic mode, instead of using the finger path, which is predominant in parasympathetic.

The Luo channel is active in *both* parasympathetic mode and sympathetic mode. But in sympathetic mode, the Luo becomes the primary path, instead of the secondary path.

When the patient *wasn't* stressed from work, the surge of 5:00 a.m. channel Qi being shunted (because of the scars) into the Luo was *not* enough to force him into sympathetic mode. *But* when, in addition to a finger-route blockage, he was also stressed at work, the *combination* of stressors – work stress sending more Liver Qi than usual to the vertex, *plus* slightly too much Qi being routed through the Luo, making the heart resonate in a more sympathetic-mode pattern – might be shoving him closer to the sympathetic end of the sympathetic/parasympathetic continuum at 5:00 a.m.[1]

---

[1] Just as heart signals influence the directions and amounts of the channel Qi, the directions and amounts of channel Qi can influence the heart signals. Resonance between electromagnetic forces always works both ways.

The *combination* of stress signals might have been enough to push him into a fairly high degree of sympathetic mode, making him wake up in a panic.

I came back in the room and asked him, "You have to have a scar on a thumb or first finger that runs perpendicular to the length of the finger. That's the only thing left that I can think of that would cause that wake-up pattern."

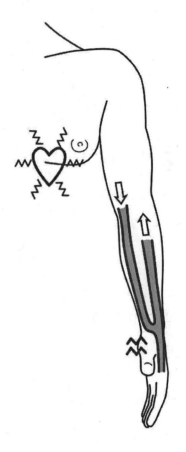

Fig. 7.2 In this case study, scar tissue was somewhat blocking the fingers-path of the Lung channel. (The illustration suggests that the blockage was utter. In fact, the blockage was only partial – but that's harder to draw.)
The semi-blockage forced much of the channel Qi to flow in a pattern that signifies sympathetic mode. When it was time, at 5:00 a.m., for the Lung channel to surge, the surge had to flow primarily in a sympathetic pattern. This flow pattern alerts the heart, causing the heart to respond as if in sympathetic mode. This would cause the patient to be jerked awake in a panic – if he was also feeling a bit of stress from work.

The combination of a pre-existing stress, plus the sympathetic signals triggered in the heart by the channel Qi behavior was able to push him over the edge: from predominantly parasympathetic to predominantly sympathetic.

I was tickled to see the surprised look on his face. "I do have a scar there. I cut myself with a knife and sliced it to the knuckle. It was years ago. I don't remember which thumb."

I found a scar was at the joint of the 1st and 2nd phalanges on the thumb, at the border of "the red and white skin": the exact path of the Lung channel.

He found another scar, on the *other* thumb, closer to the nail. Both scars were perpendicular to the channel, completely blocking the channel, and would have created significant resistance.

So the very slightly diminished lung pulse *might* have been significant! And yet, blindly treating him for Lung deficiency, based on slightly diminished Lung pulse, using any points on his Lung or related channels would never have made any difference – the scars would have continued to exert their influence.

I treated the scars.

So far, he's had no more panicked wake-ups.

I included this case study to show that an understanding of channel Qi, its behavior in fear and in health, can allow you to make *predictions* about what *must* be going on with a patient. It would have taken me a long, long time to cover every inch of his body looking for a blockage. By knowing how the body works, I was able to predict that he must have a scar or emotional trauma traversing an area involved in the 5:00 a.m. surge – the transition from Lung to Large Intestine. The thumb/index finger transition was the only place I hadn't yet looked. Ergo, there must be a blockage between the thumb and index finger.

The above patient was a scientist. He was pleased with my prediction that he must have a scar on his thumb or first finger. He reminded me that one of the credos of scientific thought is, "If it's *really* a science, it will allow you to make useful and accurate *predictions*."

Many patients have problems with insomnia – either inability to fall asleep, or inability to stay asleep. By understanding the channel Qi variations that must take place in order to trigger waking and sleeping, including any variations that inadvertently evoke sympathetic patterns, which override the sleep triggers, one can more easily track down and treat the underlying causes when a patient presents with insomnia.

The four modes are all *healthy* modes – a bit of review

Sleep is a perfectly healthy mode. There is nothing pathological about the channel Qi divergences and changes that occur during sleep.

For that matter, there is nothing unhealthy about the sympathetic and dissociative modes either. Although parasympathetic mode is the ideal that we learn in school, and is the healthiest mode for a person who is awake, at peace, and curious, all the modes in this four-chapter discussion are healthy modes.

Parasympathetic mode, sympathetic mode, sleep, and dissociated mode are associated with four distinct routings of channel Qi flow that might occur in a *healthy* person. (OK, technically, a person with a mortal injury is not "healthy," but that person stands a far better chance of surviving his injury and becoming healthy again *if* his body shunts in dissociation mode for a while.)

Although we might say that parasympathetic mode channel routes best represent an ideal for "health" or "normalcy" or, as we say in Asian medicine, "going through," the divergent modes are also healthy and normal – in the correct context.

Unhealthy divergences

Of course, if a person is *not* healthy, all bets are off: in terms of channel Qi flow, anything can happen. In response to any externally-induced trauma, including injury, illness, emotional shock, toxins, external weather conditions, and so on, channel Qi flow can go off in a potential *infinitude* of *un*healthy directions. Technically, we can call these incorrect routings "divergences," but they are *unhealthy* divergences.

These unhealthy alterations follow physical laws of electricity and magnetism, and are logical. They are specific responses to the *specific* injury, the *specific* nature of the pathogen, the *specific* emotion, the specific toxin, and so on. If these aberrant variations are not corrected over the normal course of an injury or illness, which is to say, if the channel Qi becomes "stuck" in the pattern of illness or injury, the warped flow of channel Qi may sooner or later lead to other problems: pain (excess), weakness (deficiency), poor functioning of body dynamics (both Yin and Yang), including poor immune response or mental state, and may even eventually open the door to body-destroying illnesses such as cancer or organ disease.

In addition, unhealthy patterns of body-wide *or* localized areas of sympathetic or dissociation-type channel Qi flow alterations can be mentally induced and maintained, even when not physiologically needed. By being fearful in general, or fearful of some body part, or by *mentally* separating away from normal consciousness some unpleasant memory or awareness that involves a particular body part, channel Qi can travel in sympathetic or dissociated routes in the over-all body or in an affected body part. For example, a person with anxiety will maintain a body-wide sympathetic-mode channel Qi flow pattern, even though there is nothing to fear. Diagnostically, psychologically maintained channel Qi divergences can be a form of Shen (mental/consciousness) disturbance.

In my limited experience, one of the most difficult-to-treat patterns of ill health occurs when a person chooses to take advantage of the body's healthy paths of dissociation in order to lock in, for the long term, the suppression of some negative memory or emotion.

And this brings us to the most fascinating of all the healthy divergences: dissociation.

"Change of colors ... is valued by gods because it enables us to stay close to life."[1]

Chapter eight

The healthy paths of the channels: part IV

Dissociation: at the edge of death

"Dissociation" is a term that has been adopted by two fields of scientific inquiry.[2]

In psychology, the term refers to a separation of some mental data from normal consciousness.

Animal behavior biology, which is the study of *large-scale* behaviors such as eating, play, assertion and self-defence, as opposed to small-scale behaviors of animal chemistry and physiology, uses the term "dissociation" to refer to the large and small behaviors that occur in the near-death and/or pre-death state. In this chapter, unless specifically stating otherwise, I use the word "dissociation" to refer to this animal-behavior mode.

The state of dissociation occurs naturally during mortal injury, severe blood loss, or other near-death conditions. It can also be induced, in varying degrees ranging from mildly altered consciousness to full-blown heart stoppage, by almost any process that penetrates the skin, including slashing, self-cutting and to a mild degree, excessive acupuncture.

During dissociation one may experience, in varying degrees 1) a decrease in rate and power of heart and lung action, 2) blood leaving the skin and muscles and shunting deeply interiorly to the spine and brain – *not* to the heart and lungs, 3) a release of endorphins and concomitant inability to feel pain and 4) the sensation of one's consciousness being separated from the physical body: as if one is outside of one's own body, *observing* one's own body from outside it, while *feeling* no physical pain.

A fascinating shift in channel Qi flow occurs during animal behavior-type dissociation: the near-death or pre-death experience. In this mode, the channel Qi in *some* channels runs backwards, or rapidly vibrates back-and-forth. In other channels, the channel Qi dives *deep* within, leaving the skin cold, and rendering physiological functions almost inert.

---

[1] Su Wen, chapter 13-9, from *A Complete Translation of the Yellow Emperor's Classics of Internal Medicine and the Difficult Classic*, by Henry C. Lu, PhD, published by the International College of Traditional Chinese Medicine, Vancouver, BC, Canada, 2004.

Dissociated mode, which is a last-ditch attempt at the body to stay alive in the face of mortal wounds, lets us "stay close to life."

[2] Originally, "dissociation" was a social science word. It was used to describe separation from a religious organization.

Dissociation is a *healthy* response to severe danger. It can be a life-saving mechanism.

Dissociation is a healthy, correct response to a dire, life-threatening condition. When a person loses a lot of blood, or the skin is perforated excessively (which occurs, for example, during self-cutting, and even during an acupuncture treatment that employs too many needles), or for some other reason the body assumes that it may be dying, the dissociation response kicks in: the heart rate becomes extremely slow, the breathing becomes very slow. The blood and energy in the body move deeply interior. The extremities may become very cold, and the body may curl in, into a somewhat fetal position. Consciousness may seem absent, or altered, as if it is outside the body.

In a dire situation, some channel Qi will leave the traditional channels completely, and become lodged in the spine and brain.[1]

---

[1] The use of the spine and brain as a holding area for channel Qi that has moved deeply interior and has transformed from moving, particulate (electron) energy into wave energy is referred to, in the classic Asian texts, in the statement: "The Du channel is a reservoir for channel Qi."

During life, channel Qi is constantly generated in the spine. Channel Qi derives from wave energy that pours into the body from outside the body, entering at the medulla oblongata, and converting into currents. These currents, also known as channel Qi, first form in the spine. The various currents are then distributed to the channels via the heart. While coursing through the channels, these moving currents constitute the Dragon that joins Heaven and Earth. During near- and pre-death, channel Qi returns to the spine. In pre-death, during the transition into death, much of the current energy is transformed, or "pivoted" back into wave *energy*, the "heavenly" state of energy.

An ancient Chinese "myth" holds that man is like a carp: a fish swimming in dirty water who doesn't even know that he is a fish, or that he is in water. But if a man can pass through the Dragon Gate, he is transformed from a carp into a dragon. The Dragon Gate is the medulla oblongata. If a person can learn to consciously control his body's energy, return it to the spine, and pass it up to the medulla or to the top of the head and consciously exit the body, he has become like the dragon: able to control the creation and destruction of matter itself, including the matter of his own body.

The title of the ancient Chinese classic, "*The Spiritual Pivot*," is a reference to the life force's ability to "pivot" or transition, back and forth between vibrational energy and moving currents. The word "spiritual" in this case refers to transitions that are controlled via one's consciousness (causal, or "thought" waves), as compared with those energy transitions that occur merely mechanically, throughout the universe. Of course, one might also say that even the mechanical transitions are occurring via the consciousness of God, but in the case of this book, and in *The Spiritual Pivot*, we are considering the role of *human* consciousness on behavior and health. Therefore, we can assume the narrower understanding of "spiritual." Either way, it's a *great* book title. It proclaims right up front that the essence of health is the *consciously*-controlled creation and regulation of channel Qi.

For more information about the energetic centers in the spine and their role in transitioning energy into, and in serving as "reservoir" for, channel Qi, especially during dissociation (near- and pre-death conditions), I recommend study of Vedic texts and personal exploration using methods such as Qi Gong and/or single-focus meditation.

Single-focus meditation, during which all breathing and heart function may cease, is not dissociation: just the opposite. This type of meditation trains a person to bring all the life force energy deep within the body, so that physiological functions cease, while *maintaining* the seat of consciousness and perception in frontal lobe, and heart, respectively. In this manner, a person can perceive himself, and all universal vibrations (sensory heart-input), as and via his true nature: pure vibratory love. The delusion of being defined by the body is thus destroyed. Identification with *all vibrations* in the universe (the Great Om or, in Chinese, Da Om, now pronounced Tao), also known as

When this pattern occurs prior to death, in the seconds, minutes, or hours during which a person's body prepares to die, the channel Qi collects in the spine and mid brain. At the time of death, the crucial portion of this energy exits the body in the form of causal, astral, and some electromagnetic waves.

In summary, dissociation channel-Qi flow occurs in response to extreme loss of blood, excessive perforation of the skin, and/or severe trauma. It is a collection of drastic channel Qi shifts that may save a life or, as it's translated from the *Nei Jing*, it enables a person to "stay close to life" in the face of highly destabilizing events. It also serves as preparation for death.

Many of us have seen dissociation save the life of a mouse, after the mouse is caught by a cat. As the claws of the cat sink into the mouse, the mouse becomes rigid. His body starts to curl up as if death has arrived. If the cat was hunting merely to amuse himself, and not to satisfy hunger, the cat may biff the now-rigid mouse around a few times, seeking a response. If the mouse remains rigid, the cat will soon lose interest, and go off in search of other sport. In about ten minutes, the mouse will come back to alertness, and scamper to safety.

The mouse was not "playing dead." A mouse does not have the intellectual capacity to "play dead." The mouse had entered into an involuntary condition of dissociation brought about by penetration of his skin by the cat's claws. This collapse into dissociation, by rendering him rigid and corpse-like, saved the life of the mouse.

In other situations, such as severe injury with bleeding, dissociation's extreme reduction of heart-force and breathing *greatly* slows the rate at which blood is pumped out of the injured body. By reducing blood loss, the dissociation response may be able to save a life.

Full-blown dissociated mode, a condition in which the patient is motionless, as if "playing possum," is not usually seen in clinic.[1] However, modified forms, in which some *portion* of channel Qi becomes stuck in the weird flow pattern characteristic of this mode, are *not* uncommon in clinic.

As already mentioned in chapter five, the word dissociation is often used to describe a completely different phenomenon: psychological dissociation. This type of dissociation is considered, by western medicine, to be an utterly different event. Psychological dissociation is a process whereby certain thoughts are held separate, or as it says in the texts, "compartmentalized away," from normal consciousness. For example, a person can "blot" out a negative experience so that he has no recall of the terrible event.[2]

"The Way" back to the origin of all vibration, is obtained. This is very different, almost the opposite, from the *ego-identified* sense of self that perceives itself as distinctly apart from the universe *and* outside of its physical body, during dissociation.

[1] A possum's "go-to-sleep" response to being startled is not a "trick." The possum has a hair-trigger, *involuntary*, full-body dissociation response when startled. This is very different from the frozen "deer in the headlights" phenomenon, which is a pre-action part of the sympathetic response.

[2] It has recently become popular, in some circles, to claim to be suffering "dissociation" because of some remembered, negative experience. In most cases, this is not correct. A person might say: "I've dissociated from my ability to trust and be loving because my ex-wife was a selfish, nasty person," but this is not dissociation: this is hard-heartedness due to resentment and sulking. If a person

In another form of psychological dissociation, a person might dissociate from the negative event while it is occurring, so that he feels nothing, including no pain, during the event. In such a case, he may be able to remember the horrific event, but he remembers it in a detached manner, unable to recall any emotional connection to the event – because there was none, at the time.

In yet another form of psychological dissociation, a person might have a negative experience with a specific part of his body, during which, or after, the person may no longer have proprioceptive awareness of that body part. He might be able to see the particular body part, and he might be able to use that body part, but he might have no *physical* awareness of the body part if, for example, his eyes are closed. This type of mental dissociation from a badly injured body part is *not* uncommon.

Does dissociation describe two different phenomena – or are they related?

Officially, western medicine recognizes two, distinct, *utterly unrelated* sets of behaviors, both of which are, confusingly, referred to as dissociation: psychological dissociation and animal behavior-type dissociation.

The first, psychological dissociation, is considered to occur only in the mind. The second, animal behavior-type dissociation, is considered to occur primarily as a shunt of blood moving away from the heart, lungs, and skin – and is thought to be activated *only* in response to a pre-death trauma or loss of blood.

The shared use of the word "dissociation" is considered to be merely one of those regrettable circumstances, due to two branches of science being mutually unaware of what names the other branch was using.

Then again, by pure "chance," a curious commonality links these two conditions: in severe instances of *both* these types of dissociation, the person observes himself as if from outside his own body: hence, the name "dissociation" being selected for both these conditions. Even so, these two conditions are utterly different.

Or so the literature would have you think! Happily, by using channel diagnostics, we see that these two "utterly different" conditions actually manifest the same, highly specific types of alterations to the flow of channel Qi. Whether the condition is "mental" or "physical," the channel Qi behaves in the same, highly weird manner during *both* these types of dissociation.

By observing the flow of channel Qi, we can see that both types of dissociation, the mental (psychological) and the physical (animal-behavior type), are not only closely related with regard to the awareness being located outside of the body – the channel behaviors that ensue in both types are very similar as well.

Even so, there are two major differences between these two types of dissociation: how much of the body is involved, and how long the experience lingers.

---

has genuinely dissociated from a negative experience, he may not have any idea that he has done so, and he might have no memory whatsoever of the event, or no idea that the event caused him pain.

To help understand how "invisible" a dissociation can be, consider that multiple personality disorder, a mental condition in which a person's various personalities might not even know how their other personalities behave or what they have done, has recently been renamed "dissociative identity disorder."

The channel Qi alterations that occur during a purely physical response to loss of blood or to puncture of the skin are body-wide, and they *cease* as soon as the crisis has passed. Either the person recovers, or he dies. In either case, the dissociation-type channel Qi pattern usually only lasts a short while – a few minutes, a few hours, or a few days.

Oppositely, the psychological dissociation that occurs in response to a mental decision, a decision in favor of denial, a decision that "this horrible event is not happening," *may* only affect the specific body part that was injured. *Or*, if the person blocks the pain by dissociation from his heart, the dissociation may affect the whole body. If the dissociation remains untreated, it *might* come and go in response to fear-triggers, and it may last a lifetime. Or it may be constant, lasting for a lifetime. Or it can be treated, by forcing the mind to eventually confront the pain and process the pain.

In either case, pre-death or psychological, the channel Qi flows in the same way: the unique patterns that only occur during dissociation. If the dissociation is body-wide, the channel Qi aberrations can occur body-wide. If the dissociation is in relation to specific body parts, the channel Qi aberrations characteristic of dissociation might only occur in the specific body parts from which a person has become dissociated.

The following case study is an example of a *psychological* dissociation that only affected half the person's body. The dissociation had been dormant for more than three decades. It was triggered by a specific event that recalled the original pain.

Case Study # 10

Numb from the waist down

My patient, age thirty-four, called my office in a panic. I'd treated her several years earlier for an ankle injury, and then for an arm injury. We'd come to know each other pretty well before she'd moved out of town to work on her doctoral degree out-of-state. She called me because she'd been utterly numb, from the waist down, for the last forty-eight hours.

I asked her what she'd been doing the last few days, or maybe even the last week.

She explained that, for the first time in her life, she had fallen in love with a man. She had been a lesbian all her life. She had broken up with her long-term partner more than a year earlier. Now, in her late thirties, she was considering entering into what she hoped might be a satisfying, heterosexual relationship. But the day after she kissed him for the first time, she woke up in the morning, numb from the waist down.

I asked her specifically about any negative associations she had with regard to male sexuality. She had no memory of anything negative, but after several minutes she recalled one seemingly mild, almost cute, situation. When she was nearly four years old, her mother had discovered her lifting her skirt and "showing my privates to the little neighborhood boys. My mother grabbed me and brought me into the house. She told me that I had made the Holy Mother cry. I *loved* the Holy Mother. I was *devastated*. But that was years ago. Now, I think it's funny."

Over the phone, we agreed that this situation *might* be at the root of her sudden numbness. I treated her over the phone. I used a re-associating technique.

She had to allow herself to imagine how she had *physically* felt at the time she was so devastated. As she started to comply, she was surprised at how much *physical* pain she felt when she allowed herself to recreate the "You made the Holy Mother cry" episode. Her stomach knotted up and her abdomen was tight, almost rigid.

Next, I asked her to generate a second set of physical sensations, based on a feeling of expansion in her chest: the feeling that a person experiences in the presence of anything of great beauty or grace.

Finally, she had to combine the two feelings: the physical sensations of devastation and the feeling of expansion in the chest. The expansion feeling needed to be big enough to completely encompass all parts of the devastation-pain sensations. She needed to feel both of these sensations simultaneously: the pain *and* the chest-expansion feeling (aka love) that started in her chest and which spread out until it surrounded the pain. In this manner, she was forcing her mind to feel the pain, and *deal* with the pain. By doing this, she would not need to remain dissociated from a pain that, at the time, had evidently been "too much to bear."

I talked her through this exercise on the phone, and after about ten minutes of feeling her childhood pain while simultaneously feeling the pain being surrounded and held tightly by waves of loving heart energy, the pain diminished. As the pain diminished, she felt sensation returning to her abdomen, her groin, and then her legs. The numbness was gone. It never returned.

Had I been able to feel her channel Qi while we talked on the phone, I probably would have felt an absence of channel Qi in her lower abdomen and legs due to channel Qi diverting deeply interior. Her Stomach-channel Qi would have been flowing backwards or back-and-forth from her feet up to her torso. I can be fairly certain of this, because this is the channel Qi pattern that occurs when a person is numb in this area.

Her case demonstrated a modified (waist down) version of the body-wide pattern that occurs in a near-death experience, which causes body-wide numbness. It is *also* the pattern that occurs when a person mentally dissociates from a particular body part, so that the particular body part becomes numb.

This case study is an example of purely "psychological" dissociation. No physical injury or near-death trauma had occurred. However, this case study demonstrates the weird similarity of *psycho*logical dissociation-type channel Qi flow and *physio*logical, pre-death dissociation-type channel Qi flow.

The link between these two supposedly "completely separate" types of behavior that "by chance" share the same name can be clearly seen by detecting the identical channel Qi behavior that occurs in both of these conditions.

Dissociation and the Stomach channel

The Stomach channel is the channel most *obviously* effected when a person is in a condition of body-wide dissociation. Even in very mild, mentally-induced dissociation, such as that induced while *remembering* a near-death event or, for some people, *anticipating* an unwanted outcome, the Stomach channel Qi may manifest its "backwards" pattern, also

140

known as its dissociation pattern. The Stomach channel alterations will be the main ones discussed in this chapter.[1]

Practice feeling dissociation channel Qi patterns

To understand what is meant by channel Qi "goes backwards" or "vibrates back and forth," have a friend lie down and relax. Feel his Stomach channel Qi. Go through the steps suggested in the "Laying on the Beach" exercise in the sympathetic-mode chapter (chapter five).

After your friend is comfortably imagining that he is lying on the beach, talk him through the following: "You are still lying on the beach enjoying yourself, feeling the warm air on your toes when, suddenly, a tiger comes out from behind the shrubbery. Before you have a chance to get away, he sinks his teeth into your left shoulder and chest. His teeth penetrate your shoulder and chest. He starts to rip your left arm off."

As your study partner experiences this, feel the channel Qi flow in the leg portion of your partner's Stomach channel. If you aren't sure what you are feeling, just hold your hand in one spot, maybe ST-36. Try to notice which direction, if any, the channel Qi is flowing. It may be hard to describe what the channel Qi is doing. Don't bother. Just notice it.

Depending on the verisimilitude of your partner's imagination, the Stomach channel Qi may be going rapidly back and forth, essentially "standing still." If the person is truly feeling the sensations of his arm being ripped off, the channel Qi may actually begin flowing backwards – from the feet towards the head.

Next, feel the channel Qi in the torso portion of his Stomach channel, both inferior (towards the feet) to ST-19 and superior to ST-16. If the partner is really letting himself experience this potentially mortal injury, the Qi will either be missing (gone deeply interior) or will be running backwards all the way to ST-6, on the back of the jaw, and thence to ST-8. (There may be a seemingly Qi-free zone between ST-16 and ST-19.)

Finally, feel any other channels that strike your fancy. Some of the other channels may be very difficult to feel: they may have shunted very deeply interior. The Stomach and Large Intestine channels, in contrast, will be easy enough to feel, but will not be flowing in the right manner and/or the right direction.

Changes in the Stomach channel's basic path

If backward-flowing Stomach channel Qi gets as far as ST-6, on the jaw's "corner," at the back of the mandible, the channel Qi is shunted up to ST-8, on the side of the forehead.

---

[1] The many possible body-wide channel divergences that might occur during dissociation will not be covered here in exacting detail. Nor will the divergent-type patterns that can cause *localized*, relatively small areas of backwards pattern of Qi flow in the vicinity of injury or other blockage-causing situations. Because injuries and blockages can occur anywhere, so can the localized dissociation-type divergences. Therefore, the *possibilities* for localized areas of channel Qi "disappearing" deeply interior and/or backwards channel Qi flow are nearly infinite.

The *Nei Jing* also does not even *begin* to describe all the possibilities of dissociation-based channel Qi disruptions. Instead, the Nei Jing describes a few of the more common, standardized channel Qi divergences, such as those that occur in the UB channel during body-wide sympathetic mode. Even so, included in the divergence section of the *Nei Jing* are references to conditions that manifest in dissociated mode, such as "the Du channel serves as a reservoir."

ST-8 is something of an electrical capacitor: the channel Qi can build up at ST-8, causing a headache. But if *enough* Qi builds up at ST-8, the channel Qi will surge out of ST-8, and short circuit into the nearby Gallbladder channel, causing a surge in Gallbladder channel Qi.

If the backwards flow is mild, Qi may merely accumulate at ST-6 or ST-8. Tooth or jaw pain at ST-6, or a pressure-type headache at ST-8, may develop, brought on by the localized excess of channel Qi.

This build-up of channel Qi, as opposed to a short-circuit on the forehead into the Gallbladder channel, is most likely to occur if the dissociation is only in response to *thought*, to some a mental trigger, as opposed to a response to serious injury or mortal-wound.

Ideally, the jaw pain or headache from such a build-up will cause the person to lie down, process the mental situation, and resolve it. As soon as the dissociation ceases, the Stomach channel Qi will *immediately* begin to flow in the correct direction: any previous build-up of static at ST-8 will then disperse by flowing back down to ST-6. When the dissociation ceases, any channel Qi at ST-6 will resume running down the neck and into the torso, into the usual pattern of the Stomach channel.

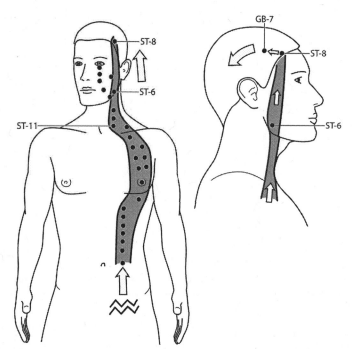

Fig. 8.1 The location for the blockage (the zig-zag lines) in this illustration was selected at random. The blockage might just as easily have been drawn on the neck portion of the Stomach channel or on the foot part of the Stomach channel.

The Stomach channel is supposed to flow from the head down to the foot. In response to dissociation, or in response to a significant blockage along the Stomach channel, the channel Qi runs "backwards," towards the head. When the channel Qi gets to the head, it rises from ST-6, on the chin, to ST-8, at the forehead. From there, it can shunt into the Gallbladder channel. In this illustration, the Gallbladder channel is not shown. Instead, the large arrow on the side of the head demonstrates the direction of the Qi flow in the head portion of the Gallbladder channel. The addition of Stomach channel Qi – the small arrow – to the channel Qi already flowing in the Gallbladder channel increases the overall amount of channel Qi in the Gallbladder's path.

It is easy for the Stomach channel to flow into the Gallbladder channel: the Gallbladder channel is very wide across the forehead, and offers little resistance.

A short circuit

Sometimes, too much channel Qi accumulates at ST-8 to be accommodated at this point. If *enough* channel Qi builds up at ST-8, a person may experience a momentary flash of electrical charge as the channel Qi short-circuits into the vicinity of GB-4.

This flash has been described to me in various ways, by various patients: it's a "zap," "a buzz," and "a tiny spinning inside my head."

This short-circuiting "zap" may occur after a very short period of time of backwards-running channel Qi, if the severity of the injury and the dissociation, and therefore the severity of the build-up of static, is high and of rapid onset.[1]

On the other hand, the zap may occur after several years, or even decades, of channel Qi becoming increasingly stymied by an unhealed injury, scar tissue, or other blockage on the Stomach channel. In the latter case, when the energetic confusion in the vicinity of the blockage becomes, over time, severely altered, *eventually* backwards channel Qi flow offers less resistance than correct channel Qi flow.

For example, an unhealed injury in the foot may, after *decades*, lead to Rebellious Qi in the Stomach channel. In the early years of the Rebellious Qi pattern, a bit of Stomach channel Qi might still be able to trickle past the blockage site. The rest of the Stomach channel Qi may flow backwards, partly up the leg, and then flow laterally, into the Gallbladder channel. But after another decade or so, as the blockage becomes utter, the force of the backwards-flowing channel Qi may become severe enough that Stomach channel Qi flows backward all the way to ST-6, and thence to ST-8.[2]

The leap from ST-8 to GB-4

In terms of life-saving physiology, the design for shunting counterflow channel Qi up to the corner of the forehead is elegant.[3]

---

[1] I had one patient who experienced this localized buzzing on the side of his head every work morning, as he drank his morning coffee and consciously steeled himself (via dissociation) for another day at work.

[2] Blocked plumbing in a house causes the waste water to follow the path of least resistance. Sometimes a mild blockage will cause bubbling noises in the toilet and water moving transversely into other lines until it slowly drains, but a severe blockage might result in raw sewage spewing up from the shower drains. Channel Qi, like water, will flow in the path of least resistance. Water is guided by gravity. Channel Qi is guided by vibratory signals that come from consciousness and thought waves *and* that come from the physical patterns defined by DNA. But with both water and channel Qi, the moving substances can move *backwards* in relation to their guides, if blocked. When this is the case, the stuff that moves, whether liquids or currents of channel Qi, will follow the path of least resistance.

[3] In some British publications, Rebellious channel Qi is referred to as "counterflow" or "retrograde" channel Qi. I prefer the term Rebellious. For thousands of years, the Chinese political system has considered rebellion to be the most dangerous threat to peace and harmony. Using

Consider: if the Rebellious channel Qi of the Stomach were allowed to flow backwards all the way to its origin at ST-1 and Yin Tang, the backwards flowing Qi would flow backwards into the Du channel. Backwards flowing channel Qi in the Du channel can quickly cause loss of consciousness and, if severe enough, death.[1]

To prevent backwards-flowing Qi from touching the Du channel at both Du-26 and at Yin Tang, the re-routing nature of ST-6 shunts any backwards-flowing channel Qi up to the *sides* of the forehead, away from the Du channel.

To review, when Stomach channel Qi is running down the face to the neck, from ST-1 to ST-9, it can pass through ST-6. But if Stomach channel Qi runs *backwards*, *up* the neck, to ST-6, it is re-routed to the sides of the forehead.

In addition to preventing dire, backward flow into the Du channel, this shunt into ST-8, and thence into GB-4, serves an additional purpose. When the Gallbladder channel receives this surge of extra energy from the Stomach channel, this surge serves to sedate the Du channel enough to make the person relax deeply, as if he were *almost* asleep.

This Du sedation via Rebellious Stomach channel Qi increasing the power in the (directionally opposite to the Du) channel Qi in the Gallbladder channel works on the same principle that sedates the Du at 11:00 p.m., when the level of channel Qi in the Gallbladder surges, and induces night-time sleep.

This Rebellious-Qi induced relaxation or somnolence, which can be in motion around-the-clock, so long as the Stomach channel is running vigorously backwards and short-circuiting at the side of the forehead, can be an important factor in healing, following a severe, life-threatening injury.

For example, when a person breaks a leg, resulting Rebellious flow in his Stomach channel Qi will end up at ST-8, and then zap into his Gallbladder channel. This, in turn, will inhibit, somewhat, the Du channel. The inhibition will cause him to be able to rest, or at least be somewhat less active. Between the release of endorphins, triggered when channel Qi flows interiorly along the spinal portions of the UB channel, and the sedation of the Du, he may almost feel somewhat sedated, in spite of the significant injury in his leg. So long as he feels safe, so that he doesn't have to activate an adrenaline override, he may remain in this

---

"Rebellious" to refer to channel Qi running amok suggests how *very* dire this condition can be. Rebellious channel Qi is not just *backwards*, it is a dangerous threat to the harmony of the entire system.

[1] I accidentally produced this loss of consciousness in one of my patients. I was using gold and silver needles to temporarily force a current to flow through the *very* weak patient's lagging Du channel. The two different metals generate a voltage differential, so current automatically will flow between the needles, *from* gold, *to* silver. I thoughtlessly placed the gold needle at the patient's Yin Tang, and the silver needle at Du-14. I had only held the slim metal rods against her skin for a few seconds when her eyes started to roll up into her head, she stopped talking in mid-sentence, and her body went limp. I pulled the needles away, and looked carefully at them. I saw my error: by putting the gold needle at Yin Tang and the silver at Du-14, I'd forced her Du channel to run backwards. She had passed out. I quickly placed the needles in the opposite positions, with the silver at Yin Tang and the gold at Du-14. Within a few seconds, her eyes popped open and her breath quickened. She stared at me, and whispered, "What just happened?"

"sedated" state for as long as necessary. He may feel this way until the break in his leg is healed enough that channel Qi can once again go through – a matter of a few days, or a few weeks, depending on the degree and location of the break.

Following a severe injury, such as a leg-break, *if one is in a safe place*, a person may experience a period of diminished interest in physical activity, a somewhat inhibited appetite, and an increased ability to fall asleep. This "partial sleep" state is created via the partial (one-sided) Du channel inhibition that comes about from the one-sided surge in Gallbladder channel Qi. The Du inhibition is only "half-strength" if the injury only occurred on one side of the body. The channel Qi on the uninjured side of the body may still be running somewhat normally.

Then again, if a person is in danger or is fearful immediately following the leg-break, his body will shift into sympathetic mode. In sympathetic mode, the elevated adrenaline levels will allow him to override the partial-sleep type symptoms of dissociation mode. A person can run for miles on a compound-fractured leg, if he is in mortal fear. Only when he gets to a safe place will his channels cease to flow in the sympathetic pattern. Then, his adrenaline levels will drop. After the adrenaline is neutralized, and his channel Qi switches into dissociated mode, he can succumb to the brain-altering effects of Rebellious channel Qi in the Stomach channel shunting into the GB channel – and rest deeply.

Thanks to the ST-6 shunt, the Du channel does not take a direct hit from backwards flowing Stomach channel Qi. Instead, the Du is merely *influenced* by an increase in posterior-flowing Gallbladder channel Qi – a much weaker force. The elegance of this Du channel protection mechanism never ceases to impress me.

Please, if you ever get the chance to work on someone with strongly Rebellious Stomach channel Qi, take a moment to check out the palpable channel Qi flow running from ST-6 up to ST-8, and into the GB channel.

Other alterations in the Stomach channel during dissociation

In addition to the ST-6 shunt, a shunt also occurs at ST-42. During body-wide dissociation, channel Qi at ST-42 does not travel to the toes. It vibrates back and forth between the top of the foot, at ST-42, and the bottom of the foot, at KI-1.

While the tiger is removing your study partner's arm, ask your study partner to tell you how his foot feels.

Behavior of the other channels during dissociation

Divergences in the other channels, during dissociation, are more variable. Whether or not all the other channels even become involved depends upon the severity and duration of the dissociation.

Consider first the two other channels that flow down to the toes, the Gallbladder and Urinary Bladder channels.

During dissociation, the leg portion of the Bladder channel may run backwards (towards the head), until it arrives at the torso. In the torso, the channel Qi may shunt into the spine, travel up to the midbrain, and be converted into wave energy.

In the case of a dire injury, such as a broken back, the back portion of the Bladder channel might run backwards from the level of the break up to the top of the neck and then flow deep into the midbrain in the vicinity of Du-15. In the midbrain, the channel Qi converts into wave energy, and remains in this state in the "reservoir" that underlies the Du channel. (Technically, the Du channel proper is *not* the reservoir. The reservoir is located *in* the spine and midbrain, which are a bit deeper inside the body than the Du current, which flows just under the skin.)

Also, a pre-death condition or serious injury along the course of the Gallbladder can cause Qi to run Rebelliously in that channel. If the Gallbladder channel runs Rebelliously all the way up to the back of the neck, it then shunts deep into the neck and deep into the midbrain.

The Yin leg channels, Spleen, Kidney, and Liver, should they be influenced by the dissociation situation, will divert into the nearest Yang leg channel, and from there, get into the spine and midbrain.

In the classics this possibility is referred to as "The Yin channel divergences may enter into their Yang counterparts."

During dissociation, the Yang leg channels do not flow backwards from the *toes*. The backward movement begins at the *exit points* of these channels, on the mid-foot. The absence of *any* channel Qi moving in the toes may contribute to the tension and curling under of the toes that is observed in extreme dissociation.

The Yang arm channels, Large Intestine, Small Intestine, and Triple Burner, should they run backwards due to injury blocking their head-ward flow, flow backwards and discharge out the fingers.

The Yin arm channels, Lung, Heart, and Pericardium, should they run backwards, will flow into the chest and thence into the spine and up to the midbrain. In such situations, the absence of Yin arm channel energy in the palm side of the fingers, and/or the backwards-flowing Qi on the dorsal side, may contribute to the rigidity in the fingers that might occur during severe dissociation.

Meanwhile, this increase in channel Qi to the depths of the midbrain *may* keep the most crucial aspects of the organism alive during the crisis.

Far more important than knowing the most common paths of channel Qi during dissociation is knowing how to detect channel Qi. If you can discern movement in channels that suggests missing (diving deeply interior), back-and-forth, or backwards-flowing channel Qi, especially if there is the characteristic *rigidity* in the muscle tone in the areas beneath the missing, backwards or back-and-forth channel Qi, you will at least know to look for something that might be causing a dissociation-inducing blockage.

The blockage might be a physical injury or it might be an emotional dissociation. It might be body-wide or it might be localized. It might be chronic or it might come and go. But if you can feel channel Qi, you will at least have been alerted to the possibility that a dissociation-type pattern may be at the root of the problem.[1]

---

[1] When I say "come and go," all time frames are possible. Mentally-induced conditions may appear only during times of particular stressors, and may last a few minutes, a few days, a few months, or years. Or a few seconds.

Case study # 11

Dissociation following the death of a friend

Female, age 22, with constant pain in right-side ilio-tibial bands. She'd had knee surgery six months earlier to fix "patella shift" in both knees. Patient recalled a bad stumble just prior to the onset of various leg and knee pains. History: five years earlier, had been prone to panic attacks.

Pulse slightly deep in all positions. Tongue: healthy color, thin coat. Voice and energy were strong. Appetite was good, as was sleep. Very positive attitude, and had always been "very healthy."

Diagnosis, at first glance, might appear to be Blood Stagnation, because of the knee and leg pain that might have been triggered by her bad stumble. Then again, her pulse was not wiry, nor was her tongue purple. Her pulses were all deep, but she seemed very vigorous and energetic, with good color in her complexion.

I noticed that Stomach channel Qi was not flowing in her legs below the knees. Assuming the surgical scars were causing this blockage, I needled through the scars, which brought about a temporary correction in Stomach channel Qi flow. But when I tested the length of the right-to-left LI-to-ST channel flow connection by needling at *right*-side LI-4, no corresponding surge in channel Qi in the *left*-side Stomach channel occurred on her leg or foot. I finished the session with gentle (Yin) Tui Na to correct a wrist displacement that I thought might have been contributing to the blockage of right-side LI channel Qi.

She felt less pain immediately following the treatment. The benefit lasted about two days.

The next month she returned. Right knee was very stiff, and felt tight and swollen inside. Right ilio-tibial band pain was severe. Also, left arm tension was worse. (She'd not mentioned this symptom at the first visit.)

I asked questions about the high level of tension in her left arm. She replied that she had been a methamphetamine addict for one year when she was 16 years old. Ever since quitting meth, her arm easily lapsed into strong tension.

I wondered if the use of methamphetamine had caused damage to the Heart and Pericardium channels (a common effect), and wondered if this was causing collateral damage to her whole arm, causing the tension. If this was the case, the lack of correct flow in the LI channel might be contributing to the insufficient channel Qi in the Stomach channels – channel Qi that was insufficient to get past the surgical scars on the knee.

I had a patient whose Stomach channel Qi usually ran backwards. But if I told her a joke or limerick, the Stomach channel *instantly* ran perfectly normally – so long as she was laughing. The instant she finished laughing, the channel Qi would revert to a dissociation pattern. She admitted that she enjoyed being emotionally "turned to stone" because it made her feel safe. Of course, she regretted that it was causing her legs to be rigid, but she couldn't let go of her idea that "something bad might happen if the numbness wasn't there." Only when laughing was she able to temporarily forget about her paranoia, and use her legs somewhat normally.

I needled HT-7, P-6, Ren-17, Ear: center, and after several minutes, left-side LI-4 and right-side ST-36. The patient felt "Little jolts of energy going down my right leg, softening the tension in my knee."

One week later, the patient returned. Her knee and leg had felt better for 1.5 days after the last treatment, but were now worse than before.

Maybe because the surgical scars had been "opened up" by the previous needling, right-side Stomach channel Qi was now clearly running backwards in her leg. I repeated the previous week's treatment, plus performed Yin Tui Na on her right foot, where I'd come across a displaced 1st metatarsal.

Three weeks later, the patient returned. The constant pain in her right foot was much better, but the right I-T band was still painfully tight. The left arm was still very tense, "now and then." Also, her stomach was beginning to be overly sensitive. She felt queasy frequently, and felt frequent bowel urgency.

I examined the channel Qi on her legs more closely, and noticed that there was no Liver channel Qi proximal to LIV-6. There was no palpable channel Qi flowing in the Stomach channel on her lower legs, and there was back-and-forth energy in the ilio-tibial band area.

I needled the same acupoints as on the previous visit and the channel Qi seemed to flow correctly. Then, to get the Liver channel moving, added LU-1, LIV-14, GB-41. With the needles in, the Qi in the Liver channel seemed to run perfectly normally.

One week later, she returned, and her leg pain was worse than ever from ST-31 to ST-36. The foot pain had returned. The stomach and abdominal pain was more severe, and the looming sense of bowel urgency was worsening. The left arm tension and pain were now all the way up to her shoulder. All the channel aberrations had returned.

Obviously, any benefits from the needles were only short-term, and her condition was rapidly worsening.

Also, she had a bladder infection. Again. She told me, for the first time, that she'd had twenty bladder infections in the last four years. (That right there should have tipped me off that some degree of dissociation was going on, but this was the first I'd heard of it. Also, there had been no overt suggestion of bladder problems in her slightly deep pulses.) She was worried because her usual bladder-infection medication didn't seem to be working this time.

I decided to do a new intake, and dig into her history. I asked the date of the first bladder infection and the onset date of her leg pain. She was surprised to realize that they had started at nearly the same time: the bladder infections came first, and two months later the leg pain began.

Constant bladder infections can occur if the channel Qi in the urethra and the bladder itself begins running backwards, carrying bacteria into the bladder from the outside of the body. Ordinarily, the channel Qi swathing the walls of the bladder and urethra runs vigorously down and out, even when no urine is being passed. It is very difficult for a pathogen to travel against the constant downward torrent of channel Qi. Thus, the normal flow of channel Qi in the urethra prevents infection.

Backwards-flowing channel Qi in the bladder is *sometimes* a symptom of dissociation, or a tip-off that something is profoundly wrong with a person's will to live. Based on her twenty bladder infections in four-plus years, I asked, "Do you remember any injury or shock that occurred about five years ago?"

She replied, "No."

Since "No" is a common first response to a line of general questioning, I became specific. I threw out a few of the usual leading questions, pure stabs in the dark – just to get started. "Nothing? No car accident? Death of a friend?"

She stared at me with a strange, blank look on her face. Finally, she said, simply, "Yes."

She hadn't said if it was a car accident, or if it was the death of a friend. So I asked, "Could you tell me about it?"

"My best friend died in a car accident. She'd been my next-door neighbor and best friend my whole life. We were sixteen."

I asked if she could tell me a little more about it, and about how it had affected her.

She said that, strangely enough, it hadn't affected her. She didn't feel anything. She never cried, not even at the funeral. Shortly after that she had started using methamphetamine, but it wasn't really her style, so she stopped after a year. She'd never really thought about her best friend after her death, never even dreamed of her.

I asked her to try to visualize energy running out of her bladder, going down the urethra. She tried it, but it made her feel uneasy. I asked her to continue for a few more moments, and to keep her heart very large and open, surrounding her bladder with loving heart energy (Wei Qi). When she did this, it triggered a *sharp*, sudden onset of her knee pain and ilio-tibial band pain.

I gave her several mental exercises to do right then to help her safely reconnect with and deal with the intense pains she'd felt, and suppressed, following the death of her best friend.

After doing these for nearly an hour, she was able to imagine energy flowing the correct direction in her bladder, and she felt "lighter" in the Stomach channel area of her leg.

She emailed me the next day. She'd had several panic attacks the evening following her treatment. She hadn't had panic attacks in five years. That night, she'd had horrible nightmares; she'd been crying; she'd been hysterical for hours.

I wrote back that she might possibly be beginning to feel the horrible, life-threatening pain of losing her life-long best friend. I asked her to stay in touch with me, to tell her friends and family what she was going through, and to get counseling if she thought it might help. I shared some techniques for helping assuage pain without dissociating from it.

Over the next few weeks she went through agonies of grief and emotional pain.

Her bladder infection cleared up. Her leg pain went away. She can now feel emotion when she thinks about the tragic death of her friend.

Had I continued treating her "fixed, stabbing leg pain" as mere Blood Stagnation, Yin or Yang deficiency, Perversion of Ministerial Heart, or various channel insufficiencies, she very possibly would have continued in the same pattern: feeling a little better for a few hours after each treatment, with the pains then coming on stronger than ever.

As an aside, even in a case like this, where a person is usually highly dissociated, he may eventually learn to feel safe in the acupuncturist's office. As he becomes safe in this somewhat isolated-from-real-life setting, he may "come out of his shell" just a bit. During the moments that he's feeling safe, he may cease dissociating, and feel much less pain and rigidity: his channel Qi may even run perfectly normally while he's in the acupuncturist's office. But there is a good chance that, after letting his guard down in the safety of the office, he'll feel even worse the next day, when he has to clamp down into his dissociations again, after finding himself briefly experiencing unpleasant subconscious thoughts trickling into his mind, subconscious thoughts from which he had been subconsciously trying to stay dissociated.[1]

The diagnosis for this case, in the end, was Shen Disturbance. You might call it "intentional dissociation," or *Intentional* Shen Disturbance (as opposed to the many other forms of Shen disturbance such as Hot Phlegm, Phlegm Misting the Heart, fever, severe dehydration/malnutrition, genetic predisposition, and so on).

Very often, to get lasting progress in this type of Intentional Shen disturbance, the patient must become aware that his *current* pain is linked to his having *chosen* to dissociate from some *other* pain or mortal danger.

Then, the patient must decide if he would rather have his present pain, one that arises from dissociation and backwards-flowing channel Qi – a pain that is probably going to keep worsening – or if he would rather deal with the buried pain from the past.

Until I discovered the underlying cause of this patient's increasing patterns of dissociation, none of my treatments lasted, or provided any real benefit. After I uncovered the friend's death, the only thing I did that provided real benefit was getting *her* to realize that the

---

[1] If a person has given orders to his own subconscious, instructing his mind to feel no pain or to *not* remember something, the subconscious will adhere rigorously to that instruction. If subsequent events arise that threaten to evoke pain or the forbidden memory, including attempts at "healing," the subconscious may respond by creating even more defenses against the perceived interloper. The subconscious is not wise. In some cases, even discussing the "forbidden" subject can lead the subconscious to quickly install fortified dissociation patterns, patterns more severe than before.

This patient had the type of dissociation that is set in motion in response to a *mental command* on the part of the patient. In such cases, the patient himself must either rescind the original instruction or, if he cannot remember the original instruction, he must command his brain to cease taking whatever steps it's using to maintain the dissociation. Attempts by *others* to alter the long-forgotten instructions to the subconscious will *not* alleviate the problem. Attempts to *mask* the deeply rooted self-hypnotic suggestions with new, "positive" hypnotic commands will not be very effective – they will only serve as a thin top-dressing over the previous, deeply ingrained, subconscious instruction.

Treatments will not lastingly get rid of the pain if they are not focused on having the patient *remove* the prior instruction of "Do not feel pain." Instead, such "top dressing" treatments may lead to *very* short-term benefit and, overall, rapidly worsening symptoms of dissociation.

The patient must do this work. There is no needle large enough, no moxa hot enough, no electrodes charged enough, to twist the arm of the subconscious – a subconscious that believes itself to be obediently following the life-saving instructions of the mind. Counseling, acupuncture, and herbs can give support, but the *patient*, ultimately, must destroy the mental habit of dissociation. (See: *Nei Jing*.)

150

bladder pain and the leg pain started at about the same time, and that they both started up a few months after her friend's death.

Once she realized the connection, she did the rest of the work herself. All I had to offer were some techniques for using the heart to assuage physical and emotional pain while staying focused on the pain, thus processing it, rather than hiding from it.

She had chosen to dissociate from her body, rather than deal with the pain. The real "cure" came about when she decided to deal with the pain.

In retrospect, the increasing rigidity in her Stomach channel, causing both the patellar shift and the ilio-tibial band tension, the foot pain, and the backwards flow and/or absent channel Qi flow in her Stomach channel should have made me think of body-wide dissociation from the start.

The inability for channel Qi to surge from the right side Large Intestine channel into the left side Stomach channel – in conjunction with the Stomach channel rigidities – should have made me at least consider body-wide dissociation.

The tension in the arm, relieved *briefly* by needling Heart and Pericardium points in the safety of my office, but returning the next day, should have made me suspect an unmentioned emotional problem that she was refusing to deal with: some degree of dissociation.

All of her symptoms, seen separately, might have been caused by some other excess or deficiency situation. But putting them all together in a tight time frame that linked the twenty bladder infections, the history of panic attacks, and the one brief year of methamphetamine use gave the case study a different hue. Finally putting this all together, I decided to grill her on her history. By this point she'd known me for several months, and there was some degree of trust. Even so, she could think of no trauma in her life that had occurred in the appropriate time frame! It wasn't until I started making lucky guesses that she was able to recall the most violent tragedy of her young life – and the trigger for her ensuing numbness and eventual pain from rigidity.

We are unlikely to see a person in an emergency situation: unconscious and manifesting full-blown, body-wide, pre-death dissociation. But, as demonstrated by this case, we may see patients that are manifesting a few, or many, symptoms that are consistent with some level of dissociation. These symptoms may have their roots in an Intentional Shen disturbance problem that is causing all, or segments, of channel Qi to be moving in the manner of the fourth mode: dissociation.

Although, in this case, the patient was exhibiting Stomach channel patterns characteristic of full-body (blocked heart) dissociation, some patients who have only mentally dissociated from one or two body parts may have only a bit of localized backwards-flowing channel Qi in the vicinity of the highly specific dissociations. This channel Qi might run backwards until it crosses another nearby channel into which it can flow easily. Any path that offers less resistance will be a suitable drain for this localized excess. (Backwards-flowing channel Qi is *always* considered excessive.) A localized case like this might not feature Stomach channel reversal.

Also, some patients manifest localized backwards or back-and-forth flowing channel Qi where the channel is utterly blocked by injury, inflammation, scar tissue, phlegm, and so on. This does *not* signify a mental blockage, necessarily: this constitutes a physical blockage that is causing channel Qi to flow in the path of least resistance – even if "least" means "backwards."

Then again, if the injury, inflammation, phlegm, or whatever fails to heal over a long time, this *failure to heal* may be due to a highly localized mental dissociation that is preventing healing.

A brief discussion of altered self-perception

Outside-the-body self-perception is a significant part of *both* forms of dissociation (psychological and animal behavior). Changes in channel Qi flow show the mechanism for this altered perception.

In both types of dissociation, if the situation is severe enough, some, or even most, channel Qi is shunted deep inside. The Stomach channel runs backwards. Somatic sensory function is inhibited by the release of endorphins and by the turning off, or down, of the heart's function of sensory resonance. As this occurs, whether physically- or mentally-induced, the physical heart and pericardium's role as the receiving/transmitting radio for somatic sensory information is turned off or reduced.

When this happens, the locus of the wave-driven, *sensory* aspect of heart-energetics moves, first into the spine, and then, out of the spine and out of the body, to a location a few inches or a few feet away from the body. Perceptions of where the body is, what it looks like (instead of what it feels like), what it's doing, will then be performed via transmissions that are generated outside the actual body, but which nevertheless register electromagnetically with the brain.[1]

These externally-produced transmissions take the place of the usual heart-to-brain wave transmissions that allow a person to have somatic awareness. Even during emotion-triggered dissociation, somatic awareness may be greatly inhibited. In some cases, the body, and especially the extremities, may even feel cold and/or numb.[2]

---

[1] Self-perception from outside the body is *not* freakishly rare. For example, many people with Parkinson's disease, even in the very early stages where symptoms are minimal, admit they sometimes, or even always, perceive themselves from outside their own body. Sometimes they have done this constantly since early childhood.

For some people who perceive themselves, or some portion of themselves, as being outside the body, attempts to move body awareness back into the physical form can be met with overwhelming fear, disgust, or sheer mental refusal: in a *mild*-mannered battle between the subconscious and the conscious mind, the subconscious will always win.

[2] In all the cases of Reynaud's syndrome (profound inability to restore warmth to the hands and/or feet following exposure to cold, which sometimes lasts for days) that I've seen, the patient tended to *observe* himself, or some of his limbs, hands, or feet, from outside of his own body. Actual sensory awareness in these areas can be missing. I recall one particular patient with Reynaud's. Every week, as I performed Yin Tui Na on her grossly displaced, painless ankle bones, I asked her how her ankle was feeling. Every week, she replied, "How the hell should *I* know?" She honestly had no idea how a person could go about *feeling* his own ankle.

After more than a dozen sessions, she called me at my home number at six in the morning, waking me up. "I can feel my ankle! It hurts like hell! I can feel my ankle!" She then added, inaccurately, "I knew you'd want to know as soon as possible."

152

Case Study #12

The broken arm and the ballerina outfit

Female, age 31, had mild tremor in her left hand while conducting orchestra. She'd recently become the conductor of an important orchestra, and the position was very high-stress. The tremor had started several years earlier, but had been very subtle, and only lasted a few seconds – while she was conducting. Now, it was more noticeable, and lasted longer.

Tongue and pulse were very healthy. Overall health was very good, vibrant.

As I held her left hand to look for any physical cause for her tremor, I noticed a significant lack of channel Qi in her left arm, and the channel Qi in her left, lower-arm Large Intestine channel was running backwards: towards the hand.

I needled points on the Large Intestine, Pericardium, and Heart channels. This seemed to get the channel Qi running correctly.

One week later, she returned. The tremor was unchanged. Her arm presented the same lack of channel Qi that I noticed the week before.

I placed her arm back down on the treatment table, laying it alongside her torso. I asked her to imagine light and feel vitality in her right leg, and then her left leg. She did this easily. I asked her to imagine light and feel vitality in her right arm. Easy. Then, I asked her to do the same in her left arm. She started giggling.

I asked her what was funny. She replied, "I know my left arm is lying by my side, but when I try to imagine it filled with light, I see it bent at the elbow and crossed over my chest. I can't feel it. How can my arm work correctly if I don't even know where it is?"

I needled LI-4 on the left arm. She felt it, and a mild amount of channel Qi started moving through the arm. But her *mental* image of her arm being motionless and crossed over her chest was unaffected by the needle. The needle was evidently moving some current, mechanically, just as it might in a corpse. But it was not in any way effecting her mental *perception* of her arm.

I removed the needle.

I asked her to move her phantom arm, the one crossed over her chest, back into her actual arm. She felt some emotional resistance, but she kept at it. After she got the phantom arm to reside inside her actual arm, she turned to me and said, "I just remembered; I broke this arm when I was four years old."

We agreed that she might have been somewhat dissociated from the arm since that date, but there was no way to know. As soon as she mentally re-associated her imagined arm with her physical arm, the channel Qi began to run perfectly normally. There was no need to insert any needles to keep the channel Qi running, so I didn't.

She came to see me one more time, because she had a story she wanted to share.

After leaving my office at the previous treatment, she'd gone downtown to meet some good friends. She'd been standing on the sidewalk chattering with her friends when one of them suggested a plan for which she felt a mild disinterest.

She felt herself responding with too much vigor, but couldn't refrain from declaring, "If that's what you want to do, you can't be my friend!" She even stamped her foot. She glared at the rest of the women, saying, "And if you agree with *her*, *you* can't be my friends either."

She was appalled at her words and movements even as she was producing them. She immediately apologized, saying, "Sorry! I don't know where that came from. I think it's from stuff I did at my acupucturist's today…"

She told me, "Then the other gals looked at each other, and they looked at me, and they all made excuses to leave.

"I was still feeling a bit alarmed by what seemed like my mouth taking over my brain, when I suddenly realized that what would make everything right was owning a pink ballerina outfit. I walked three blocks to the Dancer's Shoppe, and picked out a pink tutu with a big fluffy skirt. Then, I noticed the price. I didn't want to spend that much. In fact, I wasn't sure why I wanted a ballerina outfit. I don't dance.

"At this point, I realized I was dealing with my inner four year old – the one with the broken arm. So I had a talk with her. I asked if there was anything else that could make her equally happy. She felt that an ice cream sundae would do the job. So I took myself to the ice cream parlor and ate the sundae. And I haven't tremored since, and my left arm feels like it's a part of my body again – even when I'm conducting."

When I've shared this case study with students, I'm sometimes asked why it's pertinent to Asian medicine, since I didn't use needles or herbs to treat her problem. As practitioners of Asian medicine, we possibly should be defined, not as needlers or as herbalists, but as the health practitioners who are the best trained to work with aberrant flow of channel Qi. No other field of medicine has our hard-won knowledge that comes from learning the paths of the channels.

Health problems, including many mental and emotional problems, can be detected by noticing an absence or incorrect flow of channel Qi. Whether we then treat the problem with needles, herbs, or giving instruction in Qi Gong, doesn't matter: when we help a person correct the flow of his channel Qi, we're practicing Asian medicine.

In the above case study, one might say that the effective treatment was a Qi Gong treatment. She had to mentally put her imaginary, non-functioning arm in conjunction with her physical arm. This is certainly a Qi Gong action – and teaching a patient the necessary Qi Gong to correct a channel disorder falls under the heading of Asian medicine.

Many patients do not need needles or herbs. The *Nei Jing* makes the point that, only after the descent into the dark ages, which began around 650 BC (and from which we emerged in approximately 1750 AD), people started losing awareness of their ability to regulate their own physical energy. (In China, this art is referred to as Qi Gong, or Qi Control.) Only after this wisdom was lost did doctors have to start using the crude treatments of herbs and magnetic stones in order to rudely *force* corrections onto patients' channel Qi. ("Stones," in the most ancient times, referred to magnetically charged rocks. Over the centuries, as the understanding of the relationship between magnetism and channel Qi diminished, charged stones were replaced by stone prods, the forerunners of acupuncture needles.) And even with the use of herbs and stones, as the *Nei Jing* points out, if the patient has a mental, emotional, or spiritual problem lurking behind his channel Qi disorder, and doesn't take advantage of the corrections *temporarily* provided by these crude treatments to change his mindset and his consciousness, the illness will not be permanently resolved.

If, by knowing what a person's channels are doing, you can inform the patient how to alter his *own* mindset in order to heal his problem, you are practicing one of the highest forms of medicine.

Physiological changes caused by dissociation-type channel Qi

Short-term muscle changes during dissociation

The tissues directly underlying the flow of Rebellious channel Qi may (or may not) feel hard, tight, or rigid. Going back to the example of the mouse that appears dead in response to being clawed by a cat, the mouse will almost instantly become stone cold. His muscles will be rigid, as if rigor mortis has already set in. When the mouse "comes to," his muscle function immediately reverts to normal.

Long-term muscle changes

When a person has Rebellious Qi running for years, the tissues underlying the flow of Rebellious channel Qi may (or may not) become quite rigid, almost wooden. Many patients with this condition will even describe their legs along the length of the Stomach channel as feeling "like wood." Others, wrongly attributing the steely rigidity of their legs to strength, may be proud of the inflexible, hard, unresponsive muscles in their legs.

If this tissue has been rigid for decades, it may or may not immediately become normal upon reversal of the channel Qi. Instead, the muscles may become extremely limp, flaccid, for several weeks. Then, over the next few weeks, or months, normal ability to contract and relax the muscle may return.

Dissociation and endorphins

When channel Qi flow dives deep within, to the spine, it triggers the release of an enormous amount of endorphins from the spinal nerves, where the nerves emerge near the base of each vertabra. These opiate-like chemicals inhibit the perception of pain. At the same time, endorphin receptors are activated. For this reason, mortal wounds are painless. Also for this reason, self-slashing, also known as cutting, and to some extent acupuncture and tattooing, all of which involve perforation of the skin, release endorphins and activate endorphin receptors. Over-cutting *can* release enough endorphins that a condition similar to opiate overdose may occur: heartbeat and breathing may slow *drastically*. The cutter who was only looking for an endorphin escape may, unintentionally, release enough endorphins to precipitate death.[1]

---

[1] If the cutter can be taken to an emergency room quickly enough, the treatment is naloxone, the same drug used for overdose of opiates.

Tremor and dissociation

Tremor is a normal behavior. It occurs after a person has experienced shock or a severe burst of adrenaline. After the shock is over, as the person begins to realize that everything is OK, he may tremor. Tremoring gets the person's attention. The correct, healthy response to observing oneself tremoring is to quickly assess the physical danger of the situation. If the danger has passed, a person will take a deep breath, and let a "re-adjusting" shudder travel from his head down to the bottom of his spine. This shudder occurs as the brain turns off the elevated UB channel flow of channel Qi that had kicked in during sympathetic mode. After the deep breath and the shudder, the tremoring will cease, and the parasympathetic nervous system can begin to kick in.

For example, if you have ever been swimming in a very cold mountain lake or ocean, you may have experienced a strong shivering or tremoring for a few seconds after you got out of the water. When you started to warm up and realized you were OK, you took a deep breath and shuddered, thus stopping the tremoring.

Tremor is a *normal* transition phase when a person transitions away from dissociation, shock, or severe adrenaline release, and comes back to normal. A person with frequent or constant tremor may have become stuck between post-shock or post-severe sympathetic mode, and a return to normal (predominantly parasympathetic mode).[1]

Shock

In Asian medicine, the medical condition known as "shock" is a form of Yin and Yang Separating. Dissociation is also a form of Yin and Yang Separating: as described earlier, in severe dissociation, a person's self-awareness (Yang) becomes apart from his body (Yin). But shock and dissociation are not *necessarily* related. For example, in some instances, shock is the result of a concussive blow to the head. In some of these cases, breathing *rate* might remain normal, as might heart rate. Qi flow might remain normal, even if somewhat sedated or mildly deepened (slightly away from the surface of the skin). If the Qi flow remains more or less normal, dissociation has not occurred.

---

[1] Many other conditions can also cause tremor. Asian medicine recognizes the role of Heart and Pericardium in tremor, which is related to the fear-based inability to snap back into "normal" mode, thus keeping the heart and pericardium somewhat shut down. Western medicine recognizes that high or low blood sugar, heart disease, and genetics may also cause or contribute to tremor.

Also, *many* western medications, particularly those for asthma, are notorious for causing tremor. To a lesser extent, many of the psychoactive/psychotropic drugs for depression and/or anxiety may also cause tremor or tardive (later onset, even after stopping the meds) tremor, as can some of the anticholinergic drugs – to name just a few.

Chronic tremor is *not* Liver-Wind. Liver-Wind is characterized by motor function thrown into disarray following a sudden, unpredictable onset – like a whoosh of spring wind. This does NOT describe the steady, rhythmic movements of chronic tremor. Liver-Wind treatments, whether acupuncture or herbs, do *not* resolve chronic tremor. Because of my research with Parkinson's disease and related movement disorders, I have worked with hundreds of patients with chronic tremor. *Many* of them had previously worked with acupuncturists who relentlessly treated them for Liver-Wind, to no avail. I have *never* heard of a patient who received lasting (more than a few days, or at most a week) benefit for chronic tremor in response to Liver-Wind treatments.

However, in *some* cases of shock, a person may experience an after-effect of nausea, brought about by reversal in Stomach channel Qi flow: a dissociation pattern. He may also experience poor temperature regulation, another post-dissociation characteristic.

Whether or not a given episode of shock causes dissociation can be determined by the degree to which channel Qi flow has taken on the characteristics of dissociation during or after the episode.

Anesthesia

The condition produced by complete chemical anesthesia is *not* similar to sleep. It is more similar to dissociation. Chemical anesthesia causes powerful reversal of Stomach channel Qi: aspiration of vomit is one of the risks of chemical anesthesia. During complete chemical anesthesia, the body can become very cold, especially the extremities. Also, some people experience alert consciousness during anesthesia, but they perceive events as if the center of awareness is located *outside* of the body. For example, they may observe their own body, and everything else in the room, from a vantage point near the ceiling.

More dissociation-related alterations in channel Qi flow

The zap on the side of the head

Some of my patients who had experienced a strong, one-time "zap" from ST-8 to GB-4 (or GB-5, or GB-6) were relieved to learn of the channel Qi "short-circuit" explanation. They had never known what to make of the memorable jolt on one side of the head, and in most cases, had told no one at the time.

One forty year-old patient told me that he'd not only felt such an event, he had also momentarily lost consciousness – a not uncommon side-effect.

At age eighteen, he'd been cheerfully riding on his bicycle along a quiet country lane, and the next thing he knew he was a quarter mile farther down the road, with no memory of the lapsed time and a strange feeling as if something had gotten rewired in his head. In the privacy of his own mind, he'd referred to the episode jokingly as "my abduction by aliens."

When he first read my description of the ST-8 to GB-4 short circuit (in another book), he immediately recalled his "abduction by aliens." He told me that my description of the experience, and the altered feeling inside the head, exactly described his sensations at that time.

His unhealed foot injury at ST-42 (to which I attributed the backwards-flowing Qi in his Stomach channel) had occurred when he was eight years old. When he was eighteen, ten years after the original injury, the increasing blockage from the injury was finally severe enough to cause the channel Qi in his Stomach channel to back up all the way up to his head, and from there, to build up at ST-8 – and then short circuit into the Gallbladder channel. This short circuit caused the "zap."

When he was forty years old, when I met him, he was still manifesting backwards-flowing Qi in his Stomach channel and Stomach channel Qi flowing into his Gallbladder channel, due to his still-unhealed foot injury.

In other words, a chronic problem that developed in midlife, as a result of long-term excess channel Qi in the Gallbladder channel, had been set in motion decades earlier. The first step was the injury – an injury that never healed. The intermediary step, after ten years of increasing channel Qi confusion on the foot, was channel Qi Rebellion. The rebellion was set in motion when the channel blockage from the foot injury became large enough to completely occlude the Stomach channel from passing over the foot.

By the time he was forty, the long-term backwards-flowing channel Qi in his Gallbladder channel was causing channel Qi aberrations similar to those caused by animal behavior-type dissociation.

Even more fascinating, the patient's foot injury had never healed because he had psychologically dissociated from the foot injury at the time it occurred.

In other words, he had *psychologically* dissociated from an injury, with no apparent ill effect – but thirty years later, because of channel flow sequelae from the still-unhealed injury, he was showing symptoms similar to those of chronic, *animal behavior*-type (pre-death or trauma-based) dissociation. The *link* between the two had occurred when the foot trauma had finally become severe enough to trigger the short circuit on the side of the head, from ST-8 to GB-4 (or GB-5, or GB-6).

Another example: the whirling appliances

Another patient in her fifties recalled a "brain-twirling" event when she was seventeen years old. She said, "I had a flash on one side of my head. The room and everything in it whirled around. I grabbed the washing machine as it flew past and clung to it until things settled back down...but *ever* after that, I felt somehow agitated inside my head, unable to truly relax despite daily meditation and introspection."

She'd been five years old when her foot had been slammed in the car door, an injury to which she had not responded in any way, at the time, because her mother beat her violently if she was hurt or in pain.

Her foot had never swelled at the time of the injury. She had never felt any pain from the injury. When she broke her arm, at age seven, she had also felt no pain. Her mother only suspected the broken arm because she was unable to hold her fork correctly that night, at dinner. The arm was X-rayed, the break discovered, and later, after leaving the hospital she'd been punished, as expected, but she never felt any pain.

When I met her, when she was forty-six years old, the bones in her foot were still grossly displaced, but she never had any pain in her foot (or feeling in her foot) despite a vigorous lifestyle.

She had been having increasing (increasing over the last fifteen years) symptoms of chronic animal behavior-type dissociation (increasing rigidity, arms staying bent, difficulty initiating movement, and tremor – symptoms that match the symptoms of Parkinson's disease –). Her inability to feel relaxed, due to the chronic agitation in the head and a chronic sense of being in danger, had been in place ever since the zap on the side of the head: the moment when the room spun around and the washing machine had seemed to be flying past.

Recovering from the Gallbladder short circuit

I learned nearly as much about long-term changes resulting from dissociation-type channel Qi by studying patients' *recovery* symptoms as I did by directly observing the Qi flow aberrations.

If a patient's Stomach channel Qi short-circuits into the Gallbladder channel for only a short period of time, in consequence of an acute injury or shock, the cessation of Stomach channel Qi shorting out into GB-4 may be unremarkable. When the channel Qi resumes its correct flow, the patient may only notice that he feels more like his old self.

If the patient lives for many years with a well-established ST-8 to GB-4 circuit, his reversion to normalcy may be distinct and unsettling. For example, the patients mentioned above had been dealing for many years with the side effects of living with an internal (brain-based) tremor and other symptoms, including an increasing condition of being either asleep or in sympathetic mode, with decreasing access to parasympathetic mode, over the years. They both noticed a *strong* and strange re-orienting sensation when the Stomach channel Qi ceased shorting out into the Gallbladder channel.

In these cases, part of their treatment required addressing their unhealed injuries. When their childhood injuries on the Stomach channel were healed, and the channel Qi ceased to flow Rebelliously, these patients experienced several *long* seconds of a vibrating sensation in their heads, as if the two sides of their heads had been slightly out of alignment, and were vibrating back into a position of alignment. When the vibration ceased, they felt enormous waves of internal peace – a peace that had eluded them for decades.

The commonality of this recovery experience makes me suspect that long-term increase in asymmetrical Gallbladder channel Qi (only one side of the head) causes the left and right hemispheres of the brain to eventually become somewhat out of sync. In all of the cases of this type that I treated, only one side of the Stomach channel was running strongly backwards – the side on which the injury was located.[1]

Clinical considerations

Needling into backwards-flowing channel Qi: don't do it

If Stomach channel Qi is running backwards, anything that stimulates the flow of Stomach channel Qi, such as a needle or moxa, *or* a magnet that encourages flow in the backwards direction, will very likely increase, at least temporarily, the energy of the backward flow.

---

[1] Parallel (left- and right-side) currents of channel Qi do exert an influence over each other. Therefore, if a left-side channel is running strangely, the right-side of the same channel will reflect this, or "echo" it, to a mild extent. Patients with strongly aberrant Qi flow may seem to have the "wrong" pattern on both sides of the body. It is usually very easy to tell which side is strongly incorrect, and which side is mildly imitating the error. This resonant quality of parallel electrical currents can be beneficial: not only will a healthy current be somewhat influenced by an aberrant one, but the aberrant one may be able to maintain some mild degree of normalcy, despite blockages, due to the influence of the nearby healthy current. In this way, if there *is* an aberration, both channels are only half-altered.

For example, if Qi is flowing backwards from ST-42 to the head, needling the person at ST-36 will probably worsen the situation by stimulating *more* backwards flow of channel Qi at ST-36.

Needling a point under these circumstances is also likely to be very painful. Needling into Rebellious Qi is nearly always painful in a weird, sometimes body-wide, deeply disturbing manner. Many people who have always had a profoundly bad response to needles of any sort turn out to have also had a long-standing backwards-flowing channel situation.

When an inserted needle causes a jarring response or a stunning, electrical shock throughout the patient's body, it is usually because the channel Qi was running backwards at the point of needle insertion. Backwards flowing Qi is always an excess condition. Inserting a needling into the midst of the excess pattern always serves to "tonify" the excess. Never tonify an excess condition.

So-called "sedating" techniques are to be used in a manner that will draw off the excess into some other area. The needle insertion *must* occur in an area where the channel Qi is running correctly. It is the *re-routing* of the channel Qi that constitutes "sedation" in these cases, and not any particular method of insertion or stimulation technique. Do not perform any style of needling into channel Qi that is actively flowing backwards. It will only worsen the situation, and inflict unnecessary pain on the patient.

If a person has an accumulation of channel Qi at ST-8, needling or applying moxa at ST-8 will *not* be helpful. If anything, the treatment will attract *more* channel Qi to ST-8, and is likely to trigger the short circuit into the Gallbladder channel, if it isn't already occurring. This method of treatment is contraindicated, as it is considered "tonifying an excess condition."[1]

As noted already, we are not likely to see a patient in clinic who has just received a mortal injury or who is preparing for immanent death. Instead, we are likely to see patients in whom this channel Qi pattern has developed in response to unhealed injury, including scar tissue, phlegm blockages, or short-term or long-term mental/emotional dissociation. Treatment in these cases must address removing the blockage.

If the underlying cause of the problem is mental/emotional, the job of the acupuncturist or herbalist is to help the patient alter whatever mental state is triggering the dissociation. Treating Heart and Pericardium points, Yin Tang, or Ren-17 can be supportive, along with anything that will help the patient breathe more deeply and relax, while the patient works on getting his consciousness back into the blocked area.

---

[1] So-called "sedation" techniques do *not* reduce the amount of channel Qi flow. Nearly everything you learn in your books is wrong on this subject, the result of centuries of blind theory. All needles function in the same way, no matter how they are inserted, removed, or manipulated: they all serve as *attractors* for electrical charge. A needle can only sedate an excess situation if it is inserted into a location that has *deficient* channel Qi, and inserted in such a manner so that the very *tip* of the needle taps into the area where channel Qi is excessive. In this manner, the needle serves to draw off the excessive channel Qi by allowing the current to flow along the sides of the needle, letting it flow into an area of deficiency.

Short- and long-term dissociation

A short-term psychological dissociation may be triggered by a situation in which a person *feels* as if he is going to die or wants to die. For example, very recent death of one's child or the recent death of a very-long-term spouse can induce such strong disarray in the heart that the person may feel as if he is preparing for death himself. In such a case, the person may find himself accumulating channel Qi at ST-8, and feeling headache pressure at this point. Or he may even feel the lethargy or drowsiness induced when channel Qi shunts from ST-8 into GB-4.

In many of these cases, the dissociation may slowly ebb, over a period of months or years.

On the other hand, some patients gradually, over years, develop long-term, *psychologically*-induced dissociation. These cases are of two types: body-wide dissociation because the person has taught himself to habitually cope with stress by emotionally "playing dead," or localized areas of dissociation in the vicinity of unhealed injury, phlegm blockage, negative memories, and so on.

In the first type, which is a mental trick of making oneself "emotionally dead" when dealing with unnerving or unpleasant situations, the dissociation-type channel Qi pattern may be body-wide. The sensations of physical restriction and movement inhibition or muscle rigidity can come and go as quickly as the fleeting *thought* of *someday* being in a potentially stressful situation. The come-and-go nature of these symptoms, which correspond to the come-and-go mental processes of the patient, confirm that the problem, no matter how intense or painful, is *purely* a Qi problem – not a Blood Stagnation problem.

In these cases, the patient has to retrain his mind to not rely on dissociation for dealing with things he doesn't like. While physical treatment may help the patient a little by holding open an energetic door via stimulating the heart-mind reconnecting energy patterns at Yin Tang or Ren-17, the patient must "go through" that door by himself. He must *change* his pathological modus operandi. Otherwise, all the acupuncture, counseling, or other treatments in the world will never yield more than temporary help.

In the second type, which does not come and go, and which is caused by unhealed injury, scar tissue, congealed phlegm, and so on, psychological-type dissociation may *also* be at work. However, this is a localized dissociation, and may be turned off by needling through the blockage *or* simply drawing the patient's attention to the area.

These localized dissociations occur when the patient has mentally compartmentalized the injured area away from normal consciousness. By so doing, the patient has created a situation in which an injury has long been *unable* to heal. The patient has told his mind to dissociate from the body part where the injury resides: he has essentially made the injury non-existent to his mind: the body cannot heal that which it does not *know* about.

The presence of the blockage and the chaotic energetics that build up in the vicinity of a relatively small, localized, unhealed injury *might*, over the long-term, create, eventually, a distorted flow of channel Qi. This distorted, and sometimes even backwards, flow, by following the path of least resistance, will sometimes merely flow into another channel. However, sometimes, when an unhealed injury blocks a significant point on a channel, such as an exit point, the path of least resistance must be a backwards flow of channel Qi. Then, the brain may respond to this backwards flow as if dissociation is occurring: as if a life-threatening injury is ongoing.

Due to long-term injury, a pattern of aberrant channel Qi flow can slowly be set in motion, in some segments of the body, that is indistinguishable from the flow of channel Qi that occurs during times of severe blood loss or mortal injury.[1]

Case Study #13

Foot dragging with come and go channel Qi flow, and singing

Male, age 48. Increasing foot dragging of the right foot, poor coordination in his legs.

History included a multitude of foot injuries beginning in childhood. His right foot was slashed open by a sea shell while his parents were engaged in a hellish fight at the beach. Although he recalled, intellectually, that his parents' fight combined with the foot agony had been the greatest pain of his life, he had no memory of what the pain felt like. A few years later, the top of his foot was smashed by a softball pitch. The next year, a rusty nail had gone through his foot. The rusty nail incident was fearful to look at, but he had experienced no pain during the injury.

Examination of the foot revealed multiple scars. For most of the scars, as I pointed them out, he had no memory of having received them, *nor did he know that the scars were there*. It was as if they had been invisible.

When asked to close his eyes and imagine his right foot, he was unable to do so.

Qi was running backwards from ST-42, in the center of his right foot, up to ST-6, on the back of the jaw.

I treated the foot injuries/bone displacements with Yin Tui Na. Then I needled through the various scars, allowing channel Qi to resume flowing through the various channels of the leg that were affected. However, even after the injuries began to heal and the channel Qi was able to flow correctly, his channel Qi *sometimes* reverted into a back and forth pattern characteristic of dissociation.

---

[1] Because these situations are not overtly discussed much in the "classical" literature, students may think that cases of body-wide and localized dissociation are rare. They are not. For example, statistics show that by age 70, 4% of the U.S. population has beginning symptoms of Parkinson's disease. This disease is characterized by Rebellious flow in the leg portion of the Stomach channel. Some people with Parkinson's frankly admit to having used dissociation from the physical body since childhood, as a mechanism for avoiding physical or emotional pain – and at some point, have forgotten how to re-associate. Other people with Parkinson's have an unhealed childhood foot injury from which they have *locally* dissociated.

Many other, milder, forms of pathology can be traced to Rebellious Qi patterns that were set in motion from some type of dissociation. The *Nei-Jing*'s way of addressing this subject is to repeat, again and again, that people must stay in contact with wisdom and truth (heart), or else they cannot be successfully treated. This is a reference to the detachment from heart and truth that occurs when a person pretends, consciously or subconsciously, that he doesn't feel all or a part of his body.

I have met many people who are proud of their ability to dissociate or to become numb to pain. Many even insist that dissociation from the body is the way to attain spiritual transcendence. This is incorrect. Transcendence occurs when pain is looked squarely in the eye and transformed into its energetic components, thus dismantling the pain, and allowing its energy to return to its source. *Hiding* from pain, lying to oneself about having pain, and *suppressing* the responses of the body is *not* the way to go deep within, to discover the source of the body's energy, and to learn how to convert energy, even terrible, disruptive energy, back to it's origin: pure love.

If he was deeply relaxed, the channel Qi would flow correctly. But if he roused himself to the level of consciousness needed to talk or move, the Qi in the leg portion of his Stomach channel ran back-and-forth. He was still unable to imagine himself having a foot.

When asked to sing a childhood song for me, his Stomach channel Qi flowed correctly all the way down to his foot, and over into SP-3, even while he was completely alert. Singing is a job that requires using the melody line-recognition area, a brain area located in the frontal lobe, immediately adjacent to the frontal midline, an area that connects both to the *heart* and to the music memory area in the deeper part of the brain,

By singing, and thus accessing the heart and forcing the heart to employ the *pre-injury* parasympathetic mode energetic pattern that his brain associated with the childhood song, the body's channel Qi could temporarily resume flowing in parasympathetic mode – as it had presumably done, prior to his first foot injury. *He was even able to have somatic awareness of his foot so long as he was singing.* As soon as he stopped singing and refocused on his foot, his Stomach channel Qi slipped back into back-and-forth, and he ceased having somatic awareness of his foot.

In terms of cognition of his foot, he could not be in parasympathetic mode unless he tricked his heart by singing. As soon as he stopped singing and was asked to think about his foot, he dissociated from his foot.

Although needles were inserted into his foot, and various pericardium and heart points were accessed, he was not able to regain somatic awareness of his foot without singing songs from his *childhood* – songs that preceded the first foot injury. When asked to mentally work on re-associating with his foot, he refused. He insisted that the foot problem, if not treatable with regular medicine, must be a punishment from God, and he was willing to accept God's judgment. He also admitted a greater fear: if he re-associated with his foot, he would be unable to escape from the pain of his parents' bitter argument.

It is worth noting that patients who have adopted a mental posture of dissociation from some body part are often highly reluctant to perform the mental work necessary to command their brains to re-associate with the dissociated body part. They can be very emphatic about the logic behind their reluctance: they feel, correctly, that resuming a sensory relationship with that particular body part will force them to experience a pain that's been put "on hold." Sometimes, they fear that re-associating with the injured body part will cause pain in some other part of the body, such as the heart – an emotional pain.

Even if the long-term effects of the dissociation-induced pains are worse than the original pain, they may still refuse to mentally address the unhealed mental aspects of the injury. For example, in this case, the patient could barely walk, unless he was singing – something that he particularly disliked doing (because it caused him to be aware of his foot). The patient ended up getting disability because he could no longer walk – and he refused to consider any sort of psychological mental retraining that might allow him to re-associate with his foot, heal from the original pain, and move on.

He was willing to experience various acupuncture treatments for Calming Spirit and so forth, and spent many happy hours in counseling, but no matter how peaceful he became during these treatments or how much he talked about his past pain, he was not interested in anything that would require him to actually feel or in any way deal with his foot situation. He even refused to consider the idea of offering up the problem to a higher power, because this would cause him to "lose an important part" of himself.[1]

An Asian medicine diagnosis of this case would begin with Blood Stagnation in the foot at ST-42. After correction of the Blood Stagnation problem, the diagnosis would have to change to one of Intentional Shen disturbance. His refusal to re-associate with his foot was a mental preference for disability rather than dealing with what would have been a short-term, process-able pain.

The above case study is not atypical of cases that involve dissociation from some body part: the patient may be highly reluctant to re-associate with that body part, even if the acupuncturist is able to restore the channel Qi's *physical* ability to flow. Even with the physical obstruction gone, an acupuncturist or herbalist cannot and should not try to force change upon a mind that has *decided* to maintain a particular stance.

Until the mental/emotional situation is addressed, either by dealing with it or surrendering it to a higher power, it will not be corrected.[2]

In summary, dissociation symptoms can range from localized (just a limb, organ, or a particular muscle) to body-wide. The symptoms can be mild or severe. They can be induced by physical blockage of a channel *or* mental denial of some area, with a concomitant absence of channel Qi or a perversion of channel Qi (back-and-forth or backwards), in that area.

In cases where channel Qi can be restored by needling, but returns to the backwards or missing mode a few minutes or days after the treatment is over, either an undetected physical blockage is still in place *or* mind-induced dissociation may be playing a part. If Intentional Shen disorder is causing dissociation from the whole body or some body part, the problem is *best* treated by teaching the patient to be actively involved in rescinding those previous instructions to his subconscious that called for dissociation.

---

[1] This person was not Shen disturbed, in the classic sense, although it might be easy to jump to that conclusion. As any experienced doctor will attest, many, if not *most,* people would rather die or suffer pain than change.

Whether the issue is weight, drugs, cigarettes, or negative behavioral patterns, most humans would rather suffer than change or "give away" their habits and sense of uniqueness. Even patients who come to us because they've decided to change their lives are very often reluctant to change the self-identity factors that are most significantly contributing to their problems.

[2] Sri Sri Daya Mata, highest disciple of Paramahansa Yogananda, was told by a student in satsanga (spiritual seminar), "Everyone says that we're never given more problems than we can *deal* with. But that's not true: I've known people who fell apart from their difficulties."

Daya Mata replied, "That's because they *didn't* deal with them."

Summary of the last four chapters

Channel Qi flow patterns can shift significantly away from the healthy, *parasympathetic-mode* pathways – the basic, main routes of the primary channels that we learn (more or less accurately) in school.

When, due to fear or negative thoughts, a person shifts out of parasympathetic mode and into sympathetic (flight, fight, or freeze) mode, his channel Qi flow patterns become dramatically altered, diverging into specific, sympathetic-mode flow patterns that increase channel Qi flow to the heart, lungs, and adrenal glands.

In sleep, many of the channels barely flow at all, and the most powerful channel of all, the Du, is inhibited.

In response to dissociation, channel Qi ceases to flow normally and, instead, moves back and forth, backwards, or dives deeply interiorly.

"Pain" can ensue if these non-parasympathetic patterns continue when they are no longer called for.

A medical practitioner *can* recognize if any of the non-parasympathetic patterns are inappropriately present. He can do this using either intuition *or* he can do it by directly feeling the flow of channel Qi.

Then, unless the patient has created mental instructions commanding himself to hold on to the incorrect pattern, the practitioner can use his channel Qi-shifting skills of needling, moxa, magnets, herbs, and so on, to temporarily suggest how corrections in channel Qi flow might feel to the patient. It is up to the patient whether or not the suggestion will be accepted and maintained.

This is the essence of acupuncture.

"Meridians are most fundamental not only to determining life and death, not only to treating all diseases, but they are also most fundamental to redressing the balance between deficiency and excess. Hence, it is very important to have a mastery of meridians."[1]

Chapter nine

Applications of channel Qi diagnostics

Excess or deficient are the two possibilities for channel Qi.

Channel Qi itself doesn't get hot or cold, or Yin or Yang. As for the Five Elements, the Five Elemental forms of channel Qi have nothing to do with whether or not, and where, channel Qi is flowing.

With channel Qi pathologies, it all comes down to excess or deficient.

If channel Qi in some location is blocked, stagnant, attacking, or flowing into some schema that doesn't fit parasympathetic mode, it's a problem of excess – *at that particular location.*

If channel Qi is *not* present in a place where it's supposed to be, or is running weakly, then the channel Qi is deficient – *at that particular location.*

In nearly all cases (except for utter starvation, profound depression, or loss of will to live), deficient channel Qi in one location is caused by excess channel Qi in another location. This is to say, channel Qi is missing somewhere because it's blocked or being shunted somewhere else.

Selection of acupoints for treatment will depend on whether you are focusing the treatment at the excess location or at the deficient location, or both.

Defining symptoms as excess or deficient: school days

We start a course of study in Asian medicine with the real basics: if the person is wearing lots of clothes on a warm day, he's probably cold (deficient). If he's red in the face and eyes, he's probably hot (excess). If his voice is too loud or too belligerent, he's blocked up somewhere (excess). If he's hunched over and whispering, he's weak (deficient).

As a student, I puzzled over the above platitudes about clothing and loud voice, and so on, and carefully memorized them. I wrote in my class notes, "A person who dresses warmly is probably cold," as if this painfully obvious conclusion held some magic key that would be revealed later.

---

[1] Ling Shu, chapter 10-1, from *A Complete Translation of Nei-Jing and Nan-Jing,* translated by Henry C. Lu, PhD. International College of Traditional Chinese Medicine of Vancouver, 2004.

It turns out, it didn't.

The main reason for reviewing these *self-evident* conditions was to teach us how to transform everyday ideas such as hot and cold, and the somewhat more obscure ideas such as Yin and Yang, into two medical terms: excess and deficient.

Without Asian medical training, we might not automatically apply the words excess or deficient to a person who is physically hot or cold, emotionally fired up or inhibited.

But these two words, excess and deficient, are the essence of a medical theory in which illness occurs because some areas are getting too much channel Qi and some areas are not getting enough.[1]

---

[1] Many students do not understand that the basic principles of Asian medicine are extremely simple, as simple as the common English expression, "Feed a cold and starve a fever." So many of the first year "diagnostic principles" are based on conditions that should be obvious, conditions that should be apparent to everyone.

I'm always amazed when students tell me, with a straight face, as if he has deduced something deep and mysterious, "The patient is wearing several layers of clothing even though it's a warm day, so I suspect a diagnosis of cold!"

Well, of course! You shouldn't need to take a medical class to recognize that!

As an aside, a *very* few medical students are so academic and so out of touch with human behavior that they *do* need to be taught, in class, to look out for these most obvious signs and symptoms. But a student who needs to be taught the obvious, a student who needs to be told, "*If* a person wears a jacket when it's hot, it means he's cold," a student like this must ask himself if he truly has the knack of observation, or an aptitude for medicine.

For example, a panicked clinic student rushed into the conference room to tell me, "My new patient is so deficient, I'm afraid she's going to die! I don't know what to do!" I asked a few questions. The patient was 28 years old, female, and "she can barely get out of bed in the morning." The student was already planning a Super-Tonic herb formula, but was afraid to needle the patient for fear of sending her into an immediate decline, possibly death.

I hurried to the patient's room. Awaiting me was a vigorous, rosy-cheeked woman who looked like an athlete. I quickly learned from her that she was a dance major at the university, and the night before, she'd worked out so vigorously with some new movements that, this morning, she laughingly told me, she was so stiff she could "hardly get out of bed."

My clinic student had been taught in her first year diagnostics class that, in cases of extreme deficiency, a person might not even be able to get out of bed. Therefore, when the patient said she could "hardly get out of bed," my student had flown into a panic. Meanwhile, the robust, jolly patient had only come in for a preventive tune-up because lots of her fellow students had been getting the flu.

I excused myself and went looking for my student. I found her in the herb room, throwing tonics together. When I suggested to my student that she had over-reacted, and that her patient was perfectly healthy, my student became angry with my stupidity: "She's only 28, and can barely get herself out of bed!"

After explaining matters more fully to the student, who was at first hesitant to believe me, and then disappointed, I had to wonder if this student had even the *basic* observational skills necessary to be a good doctor.

After first writing up this example (in an earlier edition), I was told by a student that the above anecdote made her fearful of forming an incorrect diagnosis, and therefore I should not include this example. So, let me clarify: I'm not trying to create fear. I only included this example to remind students to keep their eyes open to the obvious. Medical instructions from the *Nei Jing*, written up in the dark ages when, evidently, some people weren't even able to recognize when a patient was cold or weak, should not be held, in modern times, as mystical gospel.

168

Back to the point, with channel Qi diagnosis, it all boils down to excess or deficient.

Diagnosing a patient

When a patient first enters the room and begins talking, we use basic observations such as those we learned in first semester in order to immediately determine if the patient's immediate symptoms are more related to conditions of excess or conditions of deficiency.

Next, after taking in these basic observations, we ask for symptoms and a few details, such as the date of onset and whether the symptoms come and go. For many, if not most, practitioners of Asian medicine, the interview, not tongue or pulse, is going to be the primary source of diagnostic information.

After the question and answer session, the pulse is felt, the tongue is observed.

After assessing all this information, a practitioner with a year or two of medical school under his belt has a *pretty* good idea of what body parts and/or channels are most *likely* affected.

This is the point at which the channel Qi should be felt. Unless something very strange is going on, feeling the channel Qi flow in the most likely area should only take a few seconds.

The practitioner can save time by only detecting the flow of channel Qi in these most *likely* areas. There is no need to spend time feeling for channel Qi flow in *all* the channels if the symptoms give a pretty good idea of where to start looking.

For example, if the patient is complaining of knee pain, we might start off by detecting the flow of channel Qi in the vicinity of his knees. We probably *won't* start off by checking the flow of channel Qi in the Pericardium channel.

Of course, there's always the possibility that we'll end up checking out the Pericardium, as in the case study in the previous chapter, demonstrating dissociation, in which leg pain was being caused by emotional damage.

Still, we start by examining the areas that are the most *likely* suspects. As the old saying goes, "If you're hanging around the corral and you hear hoofbeats, you should first think, "Horses!" not "Zebras!"

After noticing what the channel Qi is actually doing, and finding the place where the channel Qi is running wrong, in a manner that might account for the symptoms, a practitioner can then determine a precise treatment plan – one that will rectify the channel Qi aberration that he's found.

For simple problems, the six *most likely* findings will be that channel Qi in some particular location is either:
1) flowing weakly
2) congested (running slowly and heavily in one area, causing an area downstream from the congestion to be weak)

Use some common sense. The real purpose for all those basic intake instructions (looking, smelling, touching, etc.) is learning how to translate *blatantly obvious* symptomology into the technical terms "excess" or "deficiency."

3) blocked so that the channel Qi seems to disappear
4) stuck in some wrong mode (stuck in a divergent pattern)
5) flowing into a wrong channel (attacking)

or

6) flowing backwards, also known as flowing Rebelliously, or Counterflow.

If you find any of the above aberrations, you can select some appropriate locations for needles that will rectify the specific channel irregularity.

The following section considers the above six conditions, one at a time, and explains the needling strategy appropriate for that condition.

Selecting acupoints

All needles work in the same way: they attract channel Qi to themselves.

1) Channel Qi is flowing weakly.

Where channel Qi is running weakly, needles can attract channel Qi into the area that's weak, and thus increase the flow of channel Qi. Of course, if the flow is weak in one place, it's probably excessive somewhere else, but the area of excess might not technically matter, so long as the channel Qi is actually flowing, albeit weakly, along the correct course of the channel.

For example, say a patient's appetite is still a bit poor after having food poisoning two weeks ago *and* you can feel that the Stomach channel is running weakly. By simply needling one, or a few, of the main points that stimulate the Yang Ming channels, this patient's Stomach channel may become reinvigorated.

For example, needles inserted into ST-36 and LI-4, two "high energy" points of the Yang Ming system, may provide enough stimulation to the Stomach channel that it picks up in tempo and vigor, flushing out any residual "wobbles (bits of stagnation, aka excess) in the Qi flow, that might be left over from the illness.

Explanation for the acupoint selection:

In this very simple scenario, we don't know where the channel Qi is stuck, or "excessive." Maybe it's the Liver channel, maybe it's in the Du. It might not matter. Most likely, the channel Qi got driven out of whack during the illness, and never slipped back into the correct flow pattern. But we do know that the patient no longer has the food poisoning – so if we can get channel Qi back into the Stomach channel with a quick stimulation of the Stomach channel, we will have done our job. The stuck place may well self-correct once the Stomach channel Qi is flowing again.

A needle at LI-4 will temporarily pull a little extra Lung channel Qi into the LI channel, drawing on channel Qi that would ordinarily be flowing towards the tips of the thumb and index finger. The temporarily increased channel Qi in the LI channel will then flow in its path of least resistance up to Yin Tang, and then into the Stomach channel.

Meanwhile, the needle at ST-36 will serve two purposes. It will temporarily attract channel Qi to itself – channel Qi that possibly should have been in the Stomach channel, but which was going somewhere else (maybe diverting into the heart, or something else uncalled for) – *and* it can ensure that the sudden increase of channel Qi coming into the Stomach channel from the Large Intestine channel doesn't overflow the banks of the sluggish Stomach channel. We don't want the sudden flood from the Large Intestine channel to spill over into some channel other than the Stomach, for example, or into the heart via the Stomach channel's sympathetic mode divergence.

Having a little lightening rod (an acupuncture needle) at ST-36 helps insure that the new surge of channel Qi into the Stomach channel from LI-4 will flow *straight* down the Stomach channel all the way to the leg. For this reason, ST-36 will have been inserted before LI-4, so that when the temporary increase from the LI channel starts to move, it will have an attractor already in place at ST-36.

In a healthy person, channel Qi flows from LI-4 to ST-42 in approximately three seconds. You can't insert needles quickly enough to beat the flow of channel Qi. It's best to insert first those needles that will serve as guides to incoming channel Qi.

With a simple channel Qi weakness, as described in this case, a simple treatment that temporarily increases the flow of channel Qi in whatever channel was deficient may well be adequate. After the treatment, if there are no significant obstructions, the channel Qi will continue to flow in an improved manner in the Stomach channel.

If you don't worry about channel Qi, and just use "point prescriptions"

In a simple, straightforward case like this, even if you *don't* know what the channel Qi is doing, you will probably have very good luck just falling back on the generic point prescriptions for weak Stomach. We learn in school that we can just needle ST-36 for a weak stomach, because this point makes energy course more vigorously through the stomach channel.

2) Channel Qi moving slowly because it is congested

If channel Qi is moving slowly because it is congested (not running straight and true), a needle can be inserted *downstream* from the area that is congested. The needle acts like a lightening rod, attracting channel Qi to itself. In this manner, it drains channel Qi out of the congested area by offering a straight and low-resistance route for the channel Qi to flow. The hope is, once the Qi becomes straightened out, it will stay that way.

For example, say the patient has been fighting a lung-flu bug for a few days, and now he's in the fever stage. The channel Qi in his lower arms is congested – moving in a confused pattern. This congestion in the lower arm is slowing the flow of channel Qi in his Large Intestine channel from LI-4 to LI-10, causing LI-11, at the elbow, to be sore (sensitive from lack of channel Qi: no go through = pain). We usually say that this is an excessive condition at LI-11, because of the overall fever, and the pain at that location.

But in fact, the pain is caused because of an excess *prior* to LI-11. The stagnation in the lower arm, *prior to LI-11*, is causing the no-go-through pain at the elbow.

A needle inserted at painful LI-11 will attract to itself the Large Intestine channel Qi that is wandering around in the lower arm, confused by the pathogen.

This attraction will get the channel Qi moving more briskly into the elbow area. The force of the sudden electrical attraction may break up the illness-induced pattern of confused, congested channel Qi in the lower arm. If the attraction of the needle is stronger than the influence of the bug, the needle will win: the channel Qi will flow towards the needle.

Analogy

When debris from a storm creates a dam across a river, the water builds up behind the dam. The confused channel Qi in the lower arm is like the water building up. If a hole is made in the dam, water will flow into its correct path. As the water speeds through the hole, it may very well carry some of the debris along with it. Getting the water moving may serve to get rid of the dam.

A needle inserted at a deficient LI-11 attracts lots of channel Qi to the needle: the same as a hole in a dam. As a surge of channel Qi starts moving through the elbow area, more and more of the channel Qi is able to flow into the upper arm part of the LI channel. The channel Qi movement induced by the needle may even break up the dam (drain the excess, correct the flow pattern).

Explanation for the acupoint selection

We felt the flow of channel Qi: the flow was sluggish in the lower arm portion of the LI channel, and was sluggish or missing in the upper arm portion of the LI channel. We inserted the needle at LI-11 to "drain the excess."

Although we say that the needle at LI-11 "sedated" the excess, the overall amount of channel Qi in the patient's body was *not* "sedated" or "reduced." Rather, the excess just prior to LI-11 was induced to get moving, thus reducing the blocked portion of the overall situation.

Needles don't tonify or sedate "points." Needles tonify or sedate the *flow* of channel Qi.

Any acupoint that is known for helping "sedate an excess," such as LI-11, is an acupoint that is located *just past* a place where channel Qi *tends* to get stagnant or congested in specific pathological conditions.

In the above case, *if* the channel Qi congestion had been in the *upper* arm (a less common occurance), needling LI-11 would *not* have helped. Needling LI-11 may have actually done harm to the patient if the congestion was in the upper arm.

For that matter, if the congestion was in the upper arm, needling the elbow would have attracted more channel Qi into LI-11, which would then *try* to move into the already congested upper arm. The upper arm, if congested, would be an area of fullness, of excess. By needling at LI-11, we would have been tonifying (attracting channel Qi into) an area of excess.

We shouldn't do such a thing. We are warned in first semester never to tonify an excess condition.

Then again, if we had felt slow movement, or had felt channel Qi congestion, in the upper arm portion of the LI channel, and also felt a *lack* of channel Qi in the shoulder area of the LI channel, we could needle LI-15, at the shoulder.

172

In school, we learn that, if a person is just coming down with an illness, and the channel Qi is starting to run poorly, weakly, from the Lung channel to the Large Intestine channel, needling LI-4 can be helpful. We are also taught, formulaically, if a person is feverish, we do *not* needle LI-4, we needle LI-11.

In the patois of Asian medicine, we say that the first instance is deficiency, and LI-4 is often a useful place to "tonify." The second instance, fever, is excess, and we "sedate," or "drain."

In fact, what we've done in both cases is *move* the channel Qi. If there isn't enough channel Qi, we insert the needle at the beginning of the area that is weak. This draws channel Qi into the area. If there is too much (congealed or stagnant) channel Qi, we position the needle at the *end* of the congealed area: at the area where the channel Qi *starts* to become insufficient.

In either case, we haven't actually increased or decreased the overall amount of a person's channel Qi. All we've done, with the needles, is move things around a bit. Unless we set out to draw a significant amount of blood, we aren't actually getting rid of channel Qi when we sedate: we are just pulling some stuck channel Qi *out* of the area in which it's become stuck, in the hope of increasing the channel Qi flow in the area where it's become deficient.

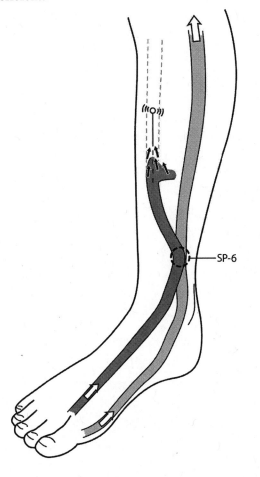

It is always easier to *pull* channel Qi back into its correct path than to try to *push* channel Qi into a straight path. In the case of congestion, the needle is most helpful if it's inserted at the downstream end of the congestion, where the channel Qi flow has started to become deficient.

Fig. 9.1 *Pulling* the channel Qi back into its correct path, and breaking up the blockage that was making the Liver channel (the darker channel) attack the Spleen channel (the lighter channel). The tiny black arrows show channel Qi being attracted to the needle.

Draining a puddle

You may already know this

principle, in which case, this next bit is redundant. Just skim, or move to the next section. But if you're new to the idea of pulling the channel Qi along, as opposed to trying to push it into the right place, consider the parallel of *neatly* draining a puddle. To do a *neat* job, you create a little drainage ditch running downhill, away from the puddle: a path of lowered resistance.

You do not add *more* water to the puddle in the hopes that the borders of the puddle will somehow become overwhelmed and crumble, so that the built up water will then wash away. This might work, but it will be a messy job.

The needle is the drainage ditch. It offers a path of lowered resistance. Whether we are trying to get more channel Qi into a deficient area or pull channel Qi away from an excess area, the needle always works the same way: it attracts channel Qi to itself.

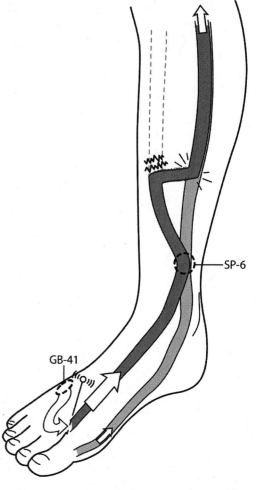

Fig. 9.2 Attempting to **push** the channel Qi.

The needle in this picture has been inserted at LIV-3 (near the big toe) in an attempt to push channel Qi up the channel towards the blockage, and straighten the blockage out. The needle is attracting channel Qi from GB-41, the exit point of the Gallbladder channel, as well as any Liver channel Qi that might be in the toes.

However, the desired outcome, straightening out the blockage, is rarely attained: because of the blockage higher up in the Liver channel, the odds are good that any Liver channel Qi that *is* attracted, via the needle, will still hit the Liver channel blockage and attacking the Spleen channel.

Not only that, the patient may experience pain in the leg, either at the site of the blockage, or at the needling site, because of the increased amount of channel Qi being stymied at the blockage.

Note the larger-than-usual arrow in the Liver channel. This larger arrow represents the additional Liver channel Qi that is being drawn into the channel because of the needle. The smaller-than-usual arrow in the Spleen channel, near the toes, represents the decreased amount of Spleen channel Qi that is able to flow, because of the attack on the Spleen channel, farther up the leg.

174

In school, in the first semester, we are repeatedly reminded to never tonify an excess condition. From an acupuncture standpoint, this means never insert a needle that will bring more channel Qi into an area that is already congested. *If* you needle in such a way as to increase the flow of Qi into an area of congestion, blockage or any form of excess, the patient will probably feel pain, and your needling will only work, if it works at all, because of the defibrillation principle – a principle based on randomized shock. Randomized shock is hardly the most elegant way to treat a highly specific electrical problem.

3) Channel Qi blocked by an obstruction

If the channel Qi is blocked by an obstruction, such as injury (broken, twisted, displaced or torn tissues), severe inflammation, scar tissue, or emotional dissociation from some body part, the obstruction should be treated before needling is attempted.

For an obvious example, if the patient has a compound fracture (broken bone sticking through the skin), the bone needs to be reset before needling is performed in the area.

If tissues are displaced, twisted, or torn, then some amount of physical resetting is usually called for before the needles are inserted. Despite hopeful insistence on the part of many acupuncture students, inserting acupuncture needles will *not* untwist a twisted ankle. Needling will *not* cause displaced bones to snap back into place. Needles will *not* remove splinters or pieces of broken glass. Needles will *not* perforate scar tissue unless inserted directly into-and-through the scar tissue. Needles will *not* necessarily cause a person to suddenly recover emotional equanimity in an area from which a person has dissociated.

If a physical or emotional obstruction is present, the obstruction must first be addressed and, hopefully, removed.

Whether the channel Qi diverts around the obstruction while staying close to the surface of the skin, or dives deeply interior and re-emerges somewhere downstream from the obstruction, or shunts into another channel altogether, the excess/deficiency locations are the same: the area upstream from the blockage is excess. The blockage causes the channel Qi to puddle up behind the obstruction and become excessive. Oppositely, downstream from the blockage, the length of the channel that has no detectable channel Qi (a distance that can range from a fraction of an inch to several feet) is the deficient part.

For broken bones or twisted or torn tissues, some form of Tui Na may restore the displaced tissues to their correct location.

For example, with a dislocated shoulder, Yang (overtly physical) Tui Na is appropriate.

With more subtle injuries, or old, forgotten, or now-painless injuries, Yin (subtle) Tui Na may be more appropriate.

In really nasty cases, such as a compound fracture, a bit of Yang Tui Na may be necessary to pull the ends of the bone apart so that they can be fitted back together: after this, Yin Tui Na may be necessary to give *all* the various injured tissues in the area the support they need to move back to their correct positions, and to allow the bone to settle into the most perfect resetting.

This subject, giving hands-on support to physical injury or fear, is *so* obvious that it is not even addressed in the Nei Jing. Sadly, because it is not addressed in the most ancient classics, this subject is often ignored in schools of Asian medicine. Many westerners think of Asian medicine as nothin' but needles, or limited to acupuncture, moxa, cupping, magnets, lasers, and herbs. Even some Asian medical students fall into this limited type of thinking.

When I was in school, a few of my fellow students were determined that needles, and needles alone, should be able to cure anything. I remember watching, and flinching, as my fellow students needled vigorously into a patient's ankle that was clearly twisted, sending the patient into paroxysms of pain. I also recall students who were fairly clumsy in their physical handling of patients, insisting that the Tui Na and shiatsu classes were "a complete waste of time."

These students were forgetting that *basic human nature* tells us, in such cases, to hold and support a torn or twisted area, to give comfort to the injured tissues. This is the essence of Yin Tui Na. In the security of being held – a most basic human form of support – the injured tissues are able to relax their micro-muscle tension and large muscle displacement. When this relaxation occurs, the displaced tissues may quickly drift back or snap back into their correct locations – with no forceful, intentional directing of movement on the part of the practitioner.

The only "force" in Yin Tui Na is firm, *generalized* support, provided by snugly holding one's hands over as much of the injured area as possible. If you think of Yin Tui Na as a way to turn your hands into a human Ace bandage (elasticized wrapping), you've got the right idea.

But human hands are far better, more perfectly supportive, than mere bandaging. An injury will sometimes respond very quickly to human support, and put its broken bits, displaced parts, and twisted thingees back into place all by itself.

In most cases, unless there is something as overt as a compound fracture or displaced shoulder or hip, there is no way the practitioner can possibly know exactly what hard and soft tissues need to go where. There is no way to manually force these types of post-injury corrections. By using Yin Tui Na, the body gets the support it needs so that it can fix these things by itself.

Then again, with something as overt as a displaced head of femur, or dislocated shoulder, Yang-type, which is to say, overt, even vigorous, Tui Na might be needed to muscle the bone back into place.

Only after all the tissues are back where they are supposed to be can needling be used to painlessly move channel Qi back through the injured area, speeding the healing.

I often remind students of the above principle by asking them, "When putting up a house, what do you install first, the framing or the electrical system?"

If a person has displaced tissues, his "framing" needs to be repaired before his electrical system (channel Qi) is strung back up.

Next on the partial list of possible obstructions is severe inflammation. If an area is grossly red and inflamed, whether from infection, injury, or rash, applying a cooling cloth might be helpful. After even just a few minutes of cooling, the needling can begin – and it will be less painful, more helpful.

An alternative to cooling the area is needling the opposite side of the body. For example, if a person's right knee is painful, red, and swollen, so that channel Qi is not getting through the knee, the odds are very high that the person's *left* knee, though undamaged, will,

176

because of resonance, be manifesting a mirrored channel Qi aberration. By fixing the channel Qi flow on the left, undamaged knee, the channel Qi of the right knee may very well be altered enough to provide significant relief and accelerate the healing.

Next, the channel Qi might be obstructed by scar tissue. Scar tissue is electrically non-conductive, like rubber. If the scar tissue is thick enough (visible to the naked eye), channel Qi will probably not be able to pass through it. The subsequent diversion may be significant enough to cause health problems. A later chapter gives suggestions on treating scar tissue.

Finally, if the obstruction is psychological, the patient will need to work on his attitude towards the injured area. A quick test for dissociation is asking the patient to imagine light in the exact part of his body where the channel Qi is blocked.

If he cannot imagine light in the area where channel Qi is blocked or running incorrectly, or if the area in question is dimmer or darker than the same body part on the opposite side of his body, be aware that the "darkness" he sees is coming from his mind – not his body part. If he is unable to *change* his mind so that he can imagine light in the area, you still might be able to help him, if you have training in psychological counseling for dissociation. If not, the patient may benefit from professional counseling.

You might *try* needling into the area, to see if the needle's attraction of channel Qi into the area is able to bring light into his mind's image of the area. You might also want to check what happens with the patient's Heart and Pericardium channels while he does this imagery work. If these channels weaken or divert while the person tries to focus on the injured area, then these channels may want needling, as well.

Sometimes, a bit of Yin Tui Na will enable a patient to imagine light in an otherwise "dark" zone.

If the needling of the obstructed area and/or needling the Heart or Pericardium channels at points of weakness *does* bring light to the area, great. Proceed as you would with any other channel problem: tonify to bring channel Qi into the area or drain excess out of the area, as needed.

Then again, a mere needle may not be able to override a Shen disturbance. No needle in the world is big enough to override the convictions of a terrified mind.

Acupoint selection

Moving on to the subject of selecting acupoints for the above situations: in many, if not most, cases, removal of the obstruction will allow channel Qi to *immediately* flow in its correct pattern. Often, no needling is necessary.

However, if, after correcting a physical or emotional obstruction, channel Qi is reluctant to resume running in its correct path, the point selection should follow the thinking already discussed: needle into the area where channel Qi is deficient, as close as possible to the location where it had previously been blocked. Thus, you can gently attract channel Qi back into its correct path, and out of the area where it had become congested or backed up.

For example, if the ulna was broken near the wrist and channel Qi fails to resume flowing in the Small Intestine channel even after Yin Tui Na restores all the tissues to their correct place (a remote contingency – usually the channel Qi is happy to flow, once its way has been made clear of obstruction), a needle at SI-19 (to serve as an attractor) and a needle at SI-7 (just past the point of fracture, where the channel Qi has become deficient) should be enough to restart the flow of channel Qi in the area.

Practical measures

Even if channel Qi resumes flow by itself, a person who has made an appointment with an acupuncturist may feel more confident about his ability to heal if he gets needled in one or two locations. Also, misunderstandings as to the nature of our medicine lead some insurance companies to only reimburse if needles are inserted – whether or not correct Qi flow has been restored.

Until such time in the distant future when patients get insurance coverage on the basis of Qi flow restoration, go ahead and needle the patient in whatever areas will accentuate the good work that you have already done – even if the Tui Na, the cool compress, or the counseling have restored the flow of channel Qi without the use of needles.

4) Channel Qi stuck in some divergent pathway

If channel Qi is stuck in some divergent pathway, the location where the channel Qi diverts from the primary channel is the location of the "excess," and the amount of channel Qi that stays in a divergent channel when it is no longer needed there is also an excess.

To treat this condition, insert a needle in the portion of the original path downstream from the divergence: the part of the path that is now deficient. You can place the needle as close as possible to the location of the divergence, which might happen to be an "a shi" location (a spot that doesn't have the status of an official acupoint), or you might go a bit further down the channel, selecting the first named acupoint after the diversion.

Acupoint selection

For example, if a person's Stomach channel Qi is stuck in the pattern of diverting at ST-13 into the heart (sympathetic mode), you might want to insert a needle into ST-14 or ST-15 or even ST-19. (See Fig. 6.1.) Once channel Qi is flowing through the upper-torso portion of the Stomach channel, you may wish to add a needle or two into the toe points of the Stomach channel, to fortify the parasympathetic position.

Next, because the stuck pattern was one of sympathetic mode, you might check to see what the Ren channel is doing. If the body has become stuck in sympathetic mode, the Ren channel at Ren-12 might still be shunting channel Qi into the Stomach channel – its modus operandi during sympathetic mode. If so, this shunt will be creating a mild deficiency in the Ren downstream from Ren-12. If so, needling Ren-14, -15, -16, or –17, which are the nearest to the deficient areas, will attract channel Qi away from the Ren-12-to-Stomach-channel shunt and back into the Ren proper.

You'll be able to quickly tell if the Ren needs work by detecting what the easy-to-feel Ren channel is doing.

On the other hand, you might want to bring your patient's attention to the situation, show him the location of the problem, and have him mentally move the energy back to the surface of the skin in the vicinity of the sympathetic divergence at ST-13.

If, after he does this, the channel Qi flows correctly, the problem is solved – and the patient can treat himself in the future.

Don't worry about losing a prospective long-term client's money by teaching him how to treat himself – a patient who learns from you is a patient who will be quick to think of you during his next health problem, and quick to refer you to his friends.

Then again, a channel might be stuck in a sympathetic divergence because the person is still fearful or stressed. If you only treat the channel Qi with needles and the person remains fearful, you have only given very short-term relief. This patient needs to understand the degree to which fear or stress is keeping him sick. He must either learn new coping skills, or find a way to remove himself from a stressful situation – or get used to being in pain. In such cases, the benefit of acupuncture may be only palliative, and short-lived. On the other hand, spending even a few moments in parasympathetic mode after having been stuck in fear-mode may provide a window of light for the patient, inspiring him to get to work on his fears or stresses. Even if the benefit is only short-term, providing comfort is worthwhile.

Or the person may be stuck in a sleep-mode divergence because of a blow to the Gallbladder channel on the head, or maybe something that's causing the Stomach channel Qi to run rebelliously into the Gallbladder channel. In cases like this, you will need to treat the injury. Tui Na might be the appropriate way to approach an unhealed injury that is keeping someone's channel Qi stuck in a non-parasympathetic mode.

Than again, in cases of dissociation-type channel Qi divergences (for which you can use the "can you imagine light in the area with incorrect channel Qi?" test), the divergence is appropriate – so long as the dissociation is present.

Until the dissociation ceases, the channel Qi *should* flow in this protective, life-inhibiting mode. You will not be able to over-ride this flow pattern with a needle, in a lasting way, if the person remains dissociated.

The person may need counseling, or time, to help process whatever he's dissociated from. Then again, gentle needling in the areas that are profoundly deficient (particularly the toes and fingertips) *may* help get channel Qi moving again. Whether it continues in the restored, healthy pattern will depend on whether the person ceases his dissociation.

As an aside, the natural way to get out of the dissociated mode, the method preferred by animals, is nuzzling, licking, or snuggling with the shocked or severely injured patient. Primates, including humans, can hold the dissociated patient closely to a supportive heart, thus comforting the patient until his own heart resumes parasympathetic resonance.

In the acupuncture office, we cannot perform these most basic and natural actions. However, if a patient is told that, in nature, this is the sort of treatment he would get, he might be able, on his own, to find a friend, family member, or spiritual guide (even a disembodied one) who can physically comfort him; talk therapy is usually ineffective in treating dissociation. While being thus supported, he can work on turning his heart back on with regard to the physical or emotional pain, until he can once again imagine light through his whole body.

In the above situations, in which tissue displacement from injury, scar tissue, fear, stress, or dissociation is causing the channel Qi to remain stuck in a divergent pattern, rectification or removal of the displacement, scar, fear, stress, injury, or dissociation will usually allow spontaneous reversion of the channel Qi into the correct path: no needling will be necessary.

Of course, the patient probably came for needles or moxa, so you might want to insert a few needles, use moxa, apply cups, or do something, anything, technical, in areas where they will cause the least disruption to the area that is now starting to heal.

5) Channel Qi attacking

If channel Qi is attacking, flowing out of its correct path and into a wrong channel, the needling will follow the same idea as in situation #4, above: insert a needle into the (now) deficient part of the channel which is doing the attacking. Insert the needle fairly close to the place just past where the channel Qi diverted.

If the diversion occurred in response to some illness or injury that has long since healed, and is now occurring only from habit, a few needles downstream from the divergence will suffice to bring the channel Qi back into its own bed. An additional needle or two to attract the channel Qi to flow the length of the channel may also be helpful.

However, if the divergence is being caused because of some physical or emotional obstruction, that obstruction must first be removed.

After removal of the obstruction, the channel Qi may automatically resume its correct flow pattern. If not, a few needles into the (now) deficient part of the channel, just downstream from the location of the divergence, should bring the errant channel Qi back into its correct path.

Acupoint selection

For example, if Liver channel Qi just before (inferior to) LIV-14 is attacking the Stomach channel, and the initiating illness or stress has passed, needling LU-1 (as an attractor point) and LIV-14 (the point downstream on the Liver channel closest to the point where the Liver channel Qi is going astray) may induce the Liver channel Qi to snap back into place.

Of course, if the person continues submitting himself to stressors, or if he allows himself to indulge in any of the seven pernicious emotions (self-pity, jealousy, resentment, etc.), his Liver channel may soon resume its attacking ways.

6) Channel Qi flowing backwards

Backwards flowing channel Qi is an excess condition. A needle inserted into backward flowing channel Qi will attract energy to itself. The source of the attracted energy will be the backward flowing channel Qi. For example, if channel Qi is running from ST-42 to ST-31, a needle inserted at ST-36 will attract channel Qi from ST-42. The overall effect is an increase in the amount of backwards flowing channel Qi.

Needling into a backwards flow of channel Qi constitutes tonifying an excess condition. Therefore, we never needle into channel Qi that is flowing backwards. Also, it can

180

be painful for the patient, and cause a sensation throughout the patient's body as if he'd stuck his finger in a low voltage electric socket. Don't do it.

If channel Qi is running backwards, it's either because an unhealed injury is so thoroughly blocking the path of channel Qi that the path of least resistance moves the channel Qi in the opposite direction from usual *or* because the person is either partially, or all, in dissociated mode.

In body-wide dissociation, the Stomach channel Qi runs backwards, or back-and-forth (an excess condition that is a brother to backwards). The other channels may also be running back-and-forth, or impossible to feel.

I hesitate to say "impossible to feel," because I fear that some student with poor Qi-detection skills, when he can't feel channel Qi in his patients, will decide that all his patients must necessarily be dissociated. Keep in mind that dissociation is a fairly rare condition, a condition more associated with shock and immediate trauma – a condition that is more likely to be seen in the emergency room than in the clinic. Still, these situations *can* manifest as chronic conditions, and a health practitioner will be well-advised to keep an eye out for them. As an aside, based on my limited experience, it seems that people who are highly cerebral, analytical, and self-controlled are *more* likely to have created intentional, even if now subconscious, dissociations than people who are less cerebral and more impulsive.

Acupoint selection

If the channel Qi is running backwards and you suspect injury, rather than dissociation, let your hand track the backwards-running channel Qi to the point where it starts. That will probably be the site of the unhealed injury that's causing the blockage.

Treat the injury using Tui Na or whatever gentle form of treatment is able to coax the body to consider healing the injury. After the injury has healed, or in some cases, even started to heal, the channel Qi flow may automatically resume flowing in the correct direction. In many cases, no needling will be necessary. If it does not automatically flow correctly, a few needles just downstream from the now-healed or healing injury should be enough to get channel Qi once again flowing through, and past, the injury spot.

If the blockage is caused by scar tissue, you may need to needle the scar. As with the above, once the blockage is broken down enough so that channel Qi can get through, it will probably flow correctly with no further assistance from you.

If the problem is one of accidentally being stuck in dissociation, you might want to consider needling Heart and/or Pericardium channel acupoints, or Du and/or Ren points for Heart and Pericardium, or Yin Tang. If this works, the backwards flow of Qi should cease almost immediately, and normal channel Qi should start to flow. If these heart and pericardium calming points do not work, you may need to talk with the patient about working on letting go of shock or fear so that he can literally reconnect the dissociated body parts, or all of his body, with his heart.

Much has been written elsewhere on this subject, and this type of counseling is too involved to be discussed here.

If the heart and pericardium stimulating points do *not* work, and a patient's channel Qi continues to run in a dissociated path, and you are convinced that the problem is *not* a physical blockage but is an emotional one, you still might try needling some of the points on the fingertips and toe tips. These points can sometimes bring a person back into parasympathetic mode, at least temporarily.

You *might* opt to bring the patient's attention to the fact that channel Qi is running as if he has dissociated from his entire body, or from the body part in question. Ask the patient to try to visualize light in the area in question. If he cannot do it, he is harboring an emotional problem that will *not* be lifted with mere needles. On the other hand, if the patient can visualize light throughout the area in question, have him do so, and insert some gentle needles in the ends of the effected channels – just past the exit point.

For example, if the backwards Qi flow was in the leg portion of the Stomach channel, but the person *is* able to imagine his leg filling with light, and even notices a warming or decrease in numbness in his leg as he does so, insert a needle into ST-43 or 44, just past the channel's exit point at ST-42. Needling just past the exit point ensures that you are 1) not needling into an area with backwards flow of channel Qi and 2) stimulating a shift back to parasympathetic mode.

However, if these points do not help the patient to create and/or *sustain* a mental image of light within his own leg, or if they work only briefly (just while they are inserted, or last only a short time after they are removed), the patient may have some emotional work ahead of him.

Some patients are able to slide back and forth between healthy and unhealthy neural modes, depending on situation. It's always VERY important to ask the patient if his problem comes and goes, and if so, what the triggers are.

For example, if a person gets pain or numbness from dissociation while in a stressful situation (instead of using sympathetic mode, which would be healthier), even though he feels perfectly OK while he's at home in the evening, or feels fine in the acupuncture clinic, or feels fine so long as you are in the act of treating his Heart and Pericardium points, you aren't going to be able to get meaningful results with acupuncture.

Instead, this person needs to learn how to stay connected with his body and heart, *when he is stressed*. Counseling and retraining exercises can help. Needles will not.

Many students have a difficult time understanding this. Consider – if your patient likes coming in for treatment because the treatment calms him, and he's able to be calm in other situations as well, but he continues to have various health problems when stress gets to him, those health problems are not coming from a standing displacement of channel Qi. Those problems are arising anew, every time, because the patient has learned to create distressed channel Qi flow patterns whenever he feels stressed. There is no way that an acupuncture needle, inserted during calm times, is going to change the mental habit of reverting to a distressed channel Qi flow during times of stress.

The real problem here is a mental *habit* that the patient uses during times of stress. Temporary amelioration of stress, via acupuncture in a calm setting, will NOT change the ingrained mental habit.

For example, acupuncture *can* be extremely helpful for restoring equanimity to a person who is stuck in dissociated mode or in shock because of a recent earthquake. Acupuncture will *not* be helpful in changing the stress-related mental, and, therefore, channel Qi behaviors of a person who has taught himself to dissociate from his body while enduring regular battering by a violent spouse. In the latter case, the person might be able to feel calm, and feel a reduction in dissociation-related health symptoms, during his treatment, but as soon as he returns to the ongoing abuses, he will revert back into warped channel Qi mode, due to mental habit.

The *Nei Jing* makes this point over and over and over. We can only provide lasting, meaningful assistance in those instances where the patient's mental equilibrium is already well-regulated by wisdom, inner peace, and a lifestyle in harmony with universal law. Our job is to assist those who, despite their striving for correct mental and spiritual attunement with the universe, have nevertheless found themselves in a situation in which they need a bit of guidance to correct for a channel Qi situation that they have gotten themselves into: one that is too complex or too obscure to deal with on one's own.

In such a case, the acupuncturist can step in and point the way. The acupuncturist is supposed to help track down the site of the problem: diagnosis. Then, he can work with the patient to figure out why the channel Qi has become aberrant: root cause. After that, working together, the doctor using needles to direct the channel Qi, the patient using his mind to correct any errors in awareness of the problem area, they can get the channel Qi to flow correctly. After that, it is the job of the patient to recognize the sensations of correctly flowing channel Qi and the heart-based sensations associated with having the channel Qi flow correctly.

If the problem has been triggered by one of the seven pernicious emotions, it is also the job of the *patient* to retrain his mind so that he is no longer susceptible to these ego-temptations. You can give him suggestions about retraining his mind, but the patient must do the actual work.[1]

---

[1] Acupuncture and herbs do *not* treat body, mind, and spirit. Acupuncture treats the *body*, via channel Qi. Herbs treat the *body* via altering the flow of channel Qi, by chemistry, or both. Mental attunement with the heart treats illness of the mind (wrong thinking), Soul attunement treats spiritual ignorance (delusion that one is apart from the universe). The earliest use of the phrase "healing of body, mind, and soul" that I can find, a phrase so frequently and incorrectly connected to acupuncture needles (of all things), was first presented in English in 1925 as the subtitle of a yoga journal: *East-West Magazine: devoted to healing of body, mind, and soul*. The point of the articles in the journal (now titled *Self-Realization: devoted to healing body, mind, and soul*) is, if a person lives correctly and works regularly at spiritual attunement, he can attain soul-realization. *Then*, when he has spiritual health, his other health problems, be they mental or physical, will easily be dealt with. This is in keeping with the teachings of the *Nei Jing*.

Acupuncture and herbs do *not* treat the mind. For clarity here, the word "attitude" might be better than the word "mind." Our medicine *cannot* change a person's attitudes, his emotional choices. The original meaning of "mind" in the phrase "healing of body, mind, and spirit," has to do with attitude. When attitude is aligned with universal love, the ensuing thoughts of the mind reflect wisdom. Oppositely, when attitude is aligned with ego, it is subject to a thousand mental errors.

As an aside, when a person says, "Of course I am justified in being mentally negative, because I was scared/hurt when I was a child," this person is expressing an attitude of self-pity. Any channel Qi problems associated with his habits of mental resentment will not respond lastingly to acupuncture so long as that resentment is able to recreate the illness pattern. If the patient wants to cling to the ego-based, negative attitude, we cannot lastingly, effectively treat this person's health problems with needles.

This is not to say that mentally-induced pain and suffering is insignificant, or that the person should just "get over himself." Not at all. All "normal" humans suffer, to some degree, from wrong mental attitudes. (Continued on the next page.)

Summary

In summary, nearly every physical health problem can be tracked down to the channel Qi aberration that is inhibiting the channel Qi from "going through." In nearly every case, the channel Qi is being blocked and building up (becoming excessive) in some area, and subsequently is deficient somewhere downstream.

By needling into the deficient area, drawing channel Qi away from the blocked area, balanced channel Qi flow can be restored.

In cases where physical obstruction or emotional blockage is contributing to the inhibition of correct channel Qi flow, the practitioner may wish to first work on removing the physical or emotional blockage.

If the patient is keen on getting needles and doesn't want to have you "waste time" removing the blockages or stagnation with cupping, Tui Na, counseling, or other appropriate modalities, you still might want to spend just five or ten minutes on physically removing the blockage or on counseling, and then needle into the area that is deficient. If the acupuncture is performed while some portion of the blockage is still in place, the patient may need more treatments than he would if you were allowed to just focus on the blockage. Still, if this is the patient's preference then, by all means, comply with the patient. Better a slow recovery than a non-recovery because the patient, thinking you don't use enough needles, doesn't return.

Mentally-induced suffering is a form of sickness deserving of the highest compassion. Significant effort may be required to overcome it. However, this work cannot be done with acupuncture needles and herbs alone.

Our medicine can prod a person to bestir himself out of an emotional sulk, if he has slid into one inadvertently. But if a patient is *choosing* to align himself with ego-based mental processes, however unwittingly, there is nothing we can do about it *with needles and herbs*.

If, in our capacity as counselors, we have the ability to pinpoint the negative emotions that are contributing to the illness, we can alert the patient to them.

I've been impressed by the large number of patients who have resolutely changed their negative attitudes when their wrong thinking has been pointed out to them, or when they've been shown how their clinging to emotionalism is causing their physical pain. So we can provide help in many of these cases. But not with an acupuncture needle.

Of course, there are *some* mental illnesses that are *not* caused by wrong attitude, which is to say, *not* caused by the seven ego-based emotions. These mental illnesses are sometimes the sequelae of illness patterns or injury: External Influences. For example, many pathogens exert a negative effect over the mind. When we're feverish, the mind is easily addled. In Asian medicine terminology, mind-altering illnesses can result from Excess Sun-Heat (sunstroke), or Damp Heat from an External illness (pathogen) being retained in the Gallbladder (which then Mists the Heart and Disturbs the Shen), Blood Stagnation disrupting the Shen (stroke from clot or internal bleeding) or from a blow to the head, to name just a few. Still other mental disorders have a genetic component.

In cases where the mental problem is actually a physical problem stemming from one of the External Influences, we can use acupuncture and herbs to help clear the body of the results of pathogen, injury, or external excess. If a patient's mental processes have become clouded by illness or injury, our medicine *can* help treat these body-based problems, and thus help restore mental clarity.

184

"Those who practice acupuncture therapy simply by trial and error irrespective of the established laws will suffer premature death as a punishment by heaven."[1]

Chapter ten

Real-life case study examples

The preceding chapter only gave simple treatment examples for the six basic aberrant channel Qi situations. In actual practice, cases can be a bit more complicated. But no matter how complex a case, the principles of the preceding chapter still hold.

This chapter features case studies that demonstrate each of the six situations described in the previous chapter – and the importance of tracking the paths of the channel Qi. The first five case studies were taken from patients in my private practice during the course of one week: the week that I was writing up this chapter. The sixth case study, the one demonstrating Rebellious channel Qi, comes from a previous week, but still serves as a great example.

1) Deficiency in a channel

Case Study #14

Snakebite

Female, 62 years old. Bitten on her left hand at LI-4 by a rattlesnake six months earlier. She had been taken to the emergency room and treated with eight units of sheep-derived antivenin. By the time she got to the hospital, her left arm was already badly swollen and numb from the hand to the shoulder. The swelling never got further than the shoulder.

Six months later she came to see me because her left arm still didn't feel "right," wasn't as strong as it should be, and she felt "unbalanced" in her body ever since the event.

Her pulse on the left side was strangely wiry and excess in all positions, riding above the skin like a hard garden hose through which hydrolic pumps were gushing torrents of fluid, in spurts. As soon as I felt her pulses on the left side, I said out loud, "Wow, that's different," at which point her pulses immediately became deep and almost impossible to feel. I laughed and told the patient what had happened to her pulses in response to my remark. Immediately, her pulses presented in a pleasant, perfectly harmonized movement. Oh well; so much for relying on her pulses.

---

[1] Ling Shu, chapter 9-1 (last sentence of paragraph), from *A Complete Translation of Nei-Jing and Nan-Jing* translated by Henry C. Lu, PhD; International College of Traditional Chinese Medicine of Vancouver, 2004; p. 405.

"Punishment by heaven" is a reference to the universal karmic laws of cause and effect.

Her tongue was healthy.

Almost no Qi was flowing in her left-side Large Intestine channel, from her hand to her face.

I was planning to needle LI-4 but, before I did, I wanted to create a situation that would guarantee that any channel Qi pulled into the LI-4 area by my needle would immediately be drawn up the LI channel, to the face, instead of getting confused in the snake-bite area of the hand.

So I started the treatment by needling Yin Tang, the terminus of the Large Intestine channel. I was ignoring the snake-bite area on the hand.

Next, although the problem was in her *left* hand, I inserted a needle into LI-20 on the *right* side of her face. – the Large Intestine channel crosses over the upper and lower lips, and ends up on the opposite side of the body before it gets up to the forehead, at Yin Tang. The channel Qi on right-side LI-20 comes from the *left* arm. I was still ignoring the snake-bite area on the hand.

Next, I inserted LI-15 on the *left* (snake-bite side), followed by LI-11 on the left.

Channel Qi was still not flowing in her Large Intestine channel, because it was still blocked on the hand, down at LI-4. But I could now be certain that when I needled LI-4 and brought a surge of channel Qi into the Large Intestine channel, that channel Qi would also be influenced by the collection of Large Intestine points that were already in place. Those already-inserted needles would act like lighting rods – attracting the channel Qi to themselves. When that Large Intestine channel Qi did start to flow, it was certainly going to be attracted to stay in the LI path!

Finally, after all the "lightening rods," or "guide" needles were in place, I needled her left-side LI-4 and LU-7.

Channel Qi surged into her hand at LI-4.

The guide needles worked. I felt the channel Qi as it quickly made its way up her arm, the side of her neck, and into her face. As it got to her face, her face visibly let go of its subtle grimace. She exclaimed, "Oh! I feel so much better! My head feels balanced!" She explained again, "I'd been feeling so unbalanced in my head and upper body, ever since the snake bite."

I left the needles in for forty minutes. When I took them out, she sat up quickly, marveling at how different she felt and waving her arms up and down, back and forth.

This simple type of problem, in which a person has had a disruptive event or injury at a specific location, after which the channel Qi remains aberrant even though the original cause for the blockage is gone, often calls for local (at the location of the problem) needling, and "just acupuncture and nothin' but acupuncture."

No Tui Na, counseling, moxa, cupping, or herbs were necessary. Her *overall* energy levels were not deficient. She just had a deficiency of channel Qi in one channel. She did return one time for a follow-up treatment. She felt that her channel Qi was flowing almost normally, but she wanted the assurance of another acupuncture treatment, the same as the first. Following the second treatment, she called my office to tell me how different she felt since starting the treatments: how great she felt.

Discussion

Even without thinking about channel Qi, even a beginning student would probably have treated this person appropriately. Just using the idea of "local acupuncture," in which a needle is inserted into the problem area, would have been fine. In this case, "local acupuncture" theory would have called for a needle to be inserted into LI-4, the area of snakebite. Such a treatment might well have gotten the same result.

Then again, someone trying to get fancy, using points such as SP-9 or LI-11 to "clear heat and/or toxins" might not have gotten any result – there was nothing wrong with the channel Qi at SP-9, and there was no channel Qi at LI-11 to work with – as demonstrated by the lack of response when I inserted the needle at LI-11.

2) Congestion causing deficiency downstream

Case Study #15

Sequelae of the flu: phlegm in the Ren channel

Male, 57 years old, had recently finished fighting a strong, three-week flu that had caused cough, fever, phlegm in his larynx, facial sinuses, and eyes, plus an assortment of typical flu symptoms. All these symptoms were now gone, but he had a residual asthma-like coughing and chest spasms that seemed to be triggered by a wide range of seemingly random activities, including eating, being exposed to a temperature change, and even in response to saying, "I haven't coughed in a while."

Every morning for over a week he'd expected the asthma to be gone or lessened, because the flu was long gone. But with each passing day, the asthma seemed unchanged.

His pulses, as always, were extremely deep. (In my experience, heavy-boned Norwegians tend to have very deep pulses even if they are in prime condition.) His tongue was very slightly red, as always.

His Lung channel seemed to be flowing just fine, as was his Kidney channel. The usual asthma points were not tender: channel Qi was flowing fine in his spine and along the Hua To Jia Ji area just parallel to the spine, including at Ding Chuan, the Jia Ji asthma point.

His Ren channel, of all things, was not flowing well. The Ren channel felt weak and sluggish downstream (moving towards the throat) from Ren 12, and stayed sluggish all the way to Ren-16 – after which, it disappeared altogether. There seemed to be no channel Qi from Ren-16 to Ren-24.

I inserted a needle at Ren-16, threading it down towards Ren-15. It attracted no channel Qi.

I inserted a needle at Ren-24 – a very "strong point": one with a significantly lowered voltage differential. Still no channel Qi moved through the needles.

I inserted a needle at Ren-15, threading it down towards Ren-14. Nothing.

I inserted a needle at Ren-14, threading it down towards Ren-13.

I inserted a needle at Ren-13, threading it down towards Ren-12.

I decided to stimulate the upper end of the channel, and inserted needles into Ren-19 and -20.

From Ren-19 to Ren-13, was a line of almost-connected needles. But there was no real flow of channel Qi.

It did seem as if I could begin to feel a faint response, a tug, in the needles. But even so, it certainly wasn't good enough. There was no feeling of channel Qi flowing through the area.

Phlegm

Phlegm, in Asian medicine, refers to a disorganized jumble of tissue, fluid and or channel Qi. This jumble is electrically non-conductive. In terms of electrical conductivity, "Phlegm" is similar to a rubber eraser. A rubber eraser is a recognized non-conductor, an item whose molecular make-up is an utter jumble of long, confused strands, nearly impermeable to electrical currents.

In living systems, channel Qi has a very difficult time flowing through the molecular jumbles found in mucus, edema, or scar tissue, and the confused electrical disarray of confused channel Qi and confused thinking (all are various forms of Phlegm).

Because Phlegm is non-conductive, the application of needles is often useless. Hence the common warning, "Phlegm is one of the most difficult problems to treat."

His illness had been characterized, physically, by mucus-y phlegm. It seemed the illness had left some residual "channel Qi phlegm," or you might say "highly confused channel Qi," in its wake.

I needed to find some way to temporarily *force* a linear current through the confused, curly-cued, tangled wad of electrical static in his upper Ren channel.

I did not want to use e-stim in the vicinity of his heart.

Instead, I taped a thick silver needle to his chest at Ren-18, and a thick gold needle on his chest at Ren-14. This would cause the channel Qi to flow from Ren-14 up to the "lightening rod" at Ren-18.

The slender, two-inch wands of gold and silver "needles" are somewhat blunt, shaped like mildy engorged acupuncture needles, and are not intended for insertion *into* the skin.

The voltage differential between gold and silver caused a current to flow over his skin, flowing *from* gold *to* silver, even in the nearby presence of the confused, non-conductive electrical jumble going on just *below* his skin.

Within a few minutes, the steady DC flow from the gold-to-silver was causing some of the patient's channel Qi to align itself with the current created by the metals: from Ren-13 to Ren-19.

The patient said, "That feels weird! In a good way."

After a few more minutes, I could feel that the acupuncture needles were starting to pick up some channel Qi: I could feel a "tug" on the needles when I moved them just the slightest bit.

I left the gold and silver needles in place for 45 minutes. Each time I checked on the patient, he reported, "This feels so weird! It feels really good, as if my chest were coming back to life. Don't take the needles out yet."

When I removed the gold and silver needles, the other needles were vigorously charged with channel Qi.

After I removed all the needles, I could feel the channel Qi correctly flowing through the Ren channel. I instructed the patient to run his hand gently from Ren-14 to Ren-19 ten or twenty times, every morning.

Over the next few days, his asthma-like coughing and chest spasms steadily decreased.

Discussion

Phlegm is notoriously difficult to clear. If the channel Qi is sufficiently obstructed, physical actions such as massage, chemical dispersal via herbs, or electrical restoration may be necessary.

Had this patient been treated with asthma points in the ears, Hua To Jia Ji, or with points that tonify Kidney, he would have received no benefit: channel Qi flow in all those places was just fine. Any treatment that didn't deal with the congestion in the Ren channel would be missing the point – and wouldn't give a result.

If I hadn't wanted to use gold and silver needles, I might have been able to get the same effect by running my hand from Ren-14 to Ren-19 several hundred times, or maybe a thousand times. The static generated by this movement would have had an effect similar to that of the gold and silver needles.

In this case, needles had been inserted into the deficient area. However, that wasn't enough. The congestion was too severe. In a pond analogy, we might say that the pond had become so sludgy that it couldn't flow, even after the dam was broken.

Therefore, treatment had to be applied directly to the area where channel Qi was stagnant: the area of excess.

However, we *never* want to tonify an excess condition. Therefore, all the needles inserted into the area of excess were connected to needles outside of the excess area: the needles inserted into the congested part of the Ren channel were all threaded into place from a starting point downstream from the congested area. If these needles in the congested area (Ren-13 through Ren-16) attracted *any* channel Qi movement, it would instantly be pulled into the downstream area (Ren-19 and Ren-20) – where channel Qi was deficient.

The use of gold and silver needles did not tonify the area. The gold and silver needles created an on-the-skin current that ran in the correct direction. It did not actually attract any additional channel Qi to the congealed mess below the surface.

Just using the point indications that we learn in school, phlegm is notoriously difficult to treat. However, by actively directing channel Qi and helping it flow over or through the congested area and out into the deficient area, we can often treat phlegm very effectively.

By the way, we learn in school that ST-40 is helpful for phlegm. This point does not help with mucus-y phlegm, literal phlegm. The phlegm for which this point is helpful is metaphorical Phlegm misting the Heart: for example, Shen disturbance from Phlegm misting the Heart following an External-Wind disorder whose residual heat has become lodged in the Gallbladder.

3) Blocked so that channel Qi seems to disappear

Case Study #16

Long-term ankle pain and asthma

Male, 27 years old, professional golfer, had right ankle pain and swelling for over a year. He'd used basic anti-inflammatory drugs for six months; they hadn't worked. He'd tried physical therapy for a few months, with no results. His doctor put him on a fairly new anti-inflammatory drug that used a different bio-mechanism. A common adverse effect of this new drug is asthma. The patient almost immediately developed a weird type of orthostatic hypotension and a feeling that he couldn't get enough air. He could no longer walk up a flight of stairs without gasping for breath and having to sit down. He said, "It feels like my life energy is being sucked out of me, and my mind doesn't focus."

Because asthma is a common side effect of the drug, he was diagnosed as having asthma, and was given asthma medications. He was taken off the anti-inflammatory drugs, which hadn't worked anyway. But now, even after two months, since the asthma began, the asthma medications were not helping, and the ankle was still swollen and painful. He tried abruptly stopping the asthma medications, and felt genuinely sick – even though they weren't helping him, he'd become habituated to these powerful drugs. He went back on the medications.

He hadn't golfed in a year when I saw him.

This case puzzled me. His lack of air didn't resemble asthma. Also, the anti-asthma drugs didn't help.

His pulse was weak and tight at the same time. The tightness might have been coming from the medications. His tongue was pale.

I asked questions that related to breathing problems. Emotional upsets at around the time the asthma started? Any sort of flu? Kidney stones? Anything?

I was genuinely stumped. All I could think was that his sympathetic nervous system was not kicking in when it should. When a person changes orthostatic position, or when he climbs a flight of stairs, the heart rate is supposed to increase, the diaphragm is supposed to move more vigorously, and more blood is supposed to go to the head. These things are supposed to happen instantly, activated by adrenaline. But they weren't happening at all. It seemed as if something had gone wrong with his adrenal glands. So the Kidney channel was my first suspect.

I felt the channel Qi in the Kidney channel, but everything was fine, albeit a bit weak. So I checked all the other usual suspect channels that might be related to sympathetic function or breathing: Lung, Ren, Stomach, and Liver. Channel Qi was a bit weak everywhere, but there was no smoking gun, no abrupt break in any of these channels. I had to wonder if this weakness was coming from the drugs. Little did I know.

Next, I felt the Du channel in the areas usually associated with asthma: the cervical vertebrae, the upper thoracic vertebrae. There was almost *no* channel Qi whatsoever in his upper Du channel! Had the drugs somehow damaged his spinal energy?

I ran my hands over the entire length of the Du channel. Strange! Through his clothing, I felt normal channel Qi in the lowest part of the Du channel, but there was no energy past Du-4, at the second lumbar vertabra.

I asked the patient if I might take a look at his low spine, and he lowered his trousers a few inches.

There it was. A fairly fresh scar. The reddish, angry looking scar was over an inch from left-to-right, and almost a quarter of an inch from its superior (towards the head) edge to its inferior edge. It straddled his spine at Du-4.

Of course he couldn't breath! He was practically without life force in the most important channel in his body – the Du channel: the channel that directs all the others. Worse, the location was right over the spot where the adrenal gland-serving spinal nerve emerges from the spine. He basically had no energy flowing to his adrenal gland.

Fig. 10.1 Scarring across the back was completely blocking the Du channel. When I tracked the path of the Du channel, which should flow "upward" (from the anus towards the head), the channel Qi seemed to stop just inferior to the scarring. There was no detectable channel Qi in the rest of his back or head.

The patient had said, "It feels like my life is being sucked out of me."

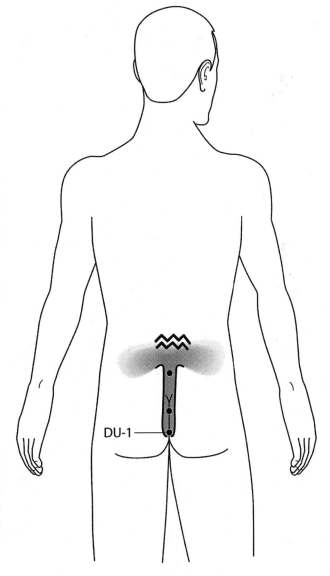

I asked him about the scar: when and why. He'd had a mole removed. It had been a pretty big mole, so the doctor had removed a lot of tissue. It had required five stitches. He didn't remember when. I told him he needed to remember. He mentally walked through events that had occurred just before and after the mole removal, and was able to establish a date. The mole had been removed about ten weeks earlier – *two days before* he'd started the new course of anti-inflammatory drugs.

Scarring from the *back surgery* was the cause of his hypotension and lack of air, not the new anti-inflammatory drugs that he'd started shortly after the surgery.

The drug had not created his weakened lung and cardiac response problems, which had not actually been similar to asthma anyway. (He'd never experienced tightening of the bronchia, and so on.) So now he was habituated to strong anti-asthma drugs for no reason at all!

I inserted needles through the scar. I inserted the needles on the superior side, pushed them through the tough keloid tissue, and into the healthy tissue on the inferior side of the scar. With each needle, he felt as if a stream of cool water was flowing up his back. By the time the fifth needle was in place, he felt better than he'd felt in months.

Over the next two months, he slowly titrated off his asthma medications.

He continued to come in for the ankle problem. I used Yin Tui Na to detect a bone displacement in his ankle. After one session, the ankle bones popped back into place, but the foot still didn't want to bear his full weight. He assumed that he would always have a problem ankle: as a left-handed golfer, he put an enormous amount of weight on his right ankle at the end of his drive.

But a foot *should* be able to take that kind of use. There was some reason his ankle wasn't ready to hold his weight. I felt further down his foot: he had another displacement! It was located at the distal end of the third metatarsal. The following week, I used Yin Tui Na, holding the metatarsal area. After the bones and tissues in that area audibly snapped back into place, he stood up and tested his foot. He was suddenly able to bear full weight on his right foot – for the first time in over a year.

Discussion

This case is a fine example of how scar tissue can create a profound channel Qi blockage. I still have no idea where the excess buildup from the scar was getting shunted. Maybe the blocked Du channel Qi was flowing into some deeper, internal channel, or sideways into the UB channel, and then flowing down his legs. I didn't even take the time to look. In a few similar cases, cases where the Du channel was severely blocked, I've been able to feel Du channel Qi shimmering up, out of the body, into thin air.

So long as that scar tissue was too thick to allow normal flow of channel Qi, the patient was never going to have normal function for any of the organs that are served by the nerves that emerge from the second lumbar. And so long as the scar tissue was so thick that its channel Qi was evidently shunting into another channel, the whole length of the Du channel superior to the blockage was also going to be deficient. This fit the patient's complaint that his "life force was being sucked out."

I perforated the scar in five places – enough to trigger preliminary dissolving of the scar tissue. He immediately felt better. The next week, I needled the area again, just to accelerate the eventual dissolving of the scar.

192

I discovered the scar tissue by feeling channel Qi. I suppose I also could have discovered it by asking the patient to remove all his clothes and giving his body a detailed visual scan. But feeling the channel Qi was far faster and also told me, for a fact, that the channel Qi was not getting past the scar.

If I had fallen back on using acupoints that are indicated for asthma, I would not have cracked this case.

Then again, I might have gotten lucky: if I had remembered that Du-4 was used for "Building Life Fire," and indicated for general fatigue and weakness, I might have been drawn to this point, and then seen the scarring when I tried to insert the needles.

But there are dozens of other points that are also indicated for fatigue and weakness, and it might have taken me a long time to figure out which one was playing the key role in this particular patient.

As an aside, as soon as the scar tissue was perforated, the channel Qi flowed correctly. There was no need to insert any needles to further restore the flow of channel Qi. The same immediacy of effectiveness applied to the foot-bone displacements: Before the Yin Tui Na, the channel Qi was barely detectable in the distal end of the lateral part of his foot. I inserted no acupuncture needles into his foot. After his bones responded to the Yin Tui Na, normal channel Qi flowed perfectly throughout his foot.

Following removal of a blockage, very often the channel Qi will automatically resume flowing correctly. If this occurs, I do not insert a needle to guide the channel Qi into the correct route: *no needle can restore and reposition the channel Qi as perfectly as the body itself.*

4) Channel Qi surging into some wrong neural mode

Case Study #17

High blood pressure while teaching

Male, 61 years old, concerned about his blood pressure. Recently, over the last year, he gets headaches that feel like too much pressure. He'd bought a blood pressure cuff, and had been able to determine that the headaches corresponded to blood pressure soaring regularly to 180/80, and once hitting 220/85. The headaches and surging blood pressure also corresponded to his afternoon students.

He was an internationally acclaimed violinist, and he also taught privately: thirty students per week. The afternoon students tended to be the high school students whose parents wanted them to study with a master, whether or not the students were actually keen on mastering the violin.

Most of the time, his blood pressure was close to 125/80: very good for someone 61 years old. But those students…

As he told me about the onset of the headaches, he was laughing. "There's a student with a concerto in F#. If I ever hear him play it again, I think my head will explode. I'm starting to anticipate with horror that one concerto. I'm truly frightened about my blood pressure when that student walks into my studio. I could have a stroke!"

As an aside, research in 2010 showed that this type of blood pressure irregularity, in which the blood pressure can be perfectly normal and then shoot up dramatically in response to stress, is the type that causes blood vessels to burst from too much pressure: what we used to call "apoplectic stroke," or "stroke from high blood pressure because of strong emotion."

Unmedicated, elderly people whose blood pressure is a steady 170/80 are *not* particularly at risk for blood vessels breaking from the strain of their steady, high blood pressure. If they *do* get bleeding in the brain, it's usually because their blood vessels are leaky. The easily bruised, liver spot-stained hands of an elderly person provide a picture of what is also going on in the blood vessels of the head. The bruises on the hands aren't there because of too much pressure in the hands. The leakiness of these elderly vessels has *little* to do with the amount of pressure in the system. A leaky blood vessel will leak *whether the blood pressure is 120 or 180*. Actually, since higher blood pressure helps most elderly people feel *better*, the improved overall sense of well-being provided by the steady, higher blood pressure may encourage the positive attitudes that contribute to life force in general, and maybe even assist in blood vessel repair and reconstruction.

But all that aside, elderly people usually *need* higher blood pressure to keep oxygen getting to their heads. They need this because of their increasingly *leaky* blood vessel system.

Back in the first half of the twentieth century, when medical models were based on how things actually were, instead on how they "should be," it was recognized that, on average, in our meat-eating, somewhat low-exercise culture, systolic blood pressure tended to go up about 10 points for every decade of life over age twenty. At age 30, systolic pressure, on average, in the US, was creeping up towards 130. By age 70, the average systolic pressure approached 170. This was not considered good or bad, but simply the way things were.

It wasn't until the latter half of the twentieth century that a new theory of health evolved. Helped along by the discovery, earlier in the century, of metabolism-altering substances such as "glands" (as they were then known in the 1920s), then hormones, and then neurotransmitters, plus the parallel development of drugs that could reduce blood pressure, stimulate or suppress hormones, and so on, an entirely new philosophy came into being.

The new philosophy held the following truth to be self-evident: if all the measurable things in a person's body, such as hormones, blood pressure, and so on, were kept, via drugs, at the same levels seen in a twenty-year old, people would be able to maintain the health of a twenty-year old.

This isn't true, of course. We now know that many processes in our body are timed – they are designed to change as we get older. And yet, when it comes to medical philosophy, this foolish model persists even into the twenty-first century.

Today, much of the basis for western medicine's concept of "preventive medicine" consists of just this: measure as many factors as possible in a patient, and then, despite the patient's age or other factors, drug the patient so that the measurements of these factors match those of the average, healthy twenty-year old. This is not preventive medicine; this is insanity. However, that's another book.

Returning to the history, blood pressure was one of the first measurables. Happily, for the doctors of the day, blood pressure could be reduced via diuretics – the first blood pressure drugs. The philosophy was not questioned: since blood pressure *could* be reduced, making it seem closer to that of a young person, it *should* be reduced. It soon became unquestioned medical policy that everyone, despite age or frailty, should try to keep blood pressure at 120/70.

This made no sense then, and it makes no sense now. A delicate 80-year old, who has barely enough pressure in her system to keep her from passing out when she stands up, needs all the blood pressure she can get. She has *deficiency*-type "high" blood pressure: she has low pressure (and oxygen) in the brain, with compensating high pressure in the rest of the body in an attempt to get more air to the brain.

But we never measure the blood pressure in the brain – which is the most important area. We only measure it in the arm, of all places, and then treat accordingly, as if the arm pressure was the same as the pressure in the head – which it is not, especially in older people.

In fact, one of the most common problems with our theory of "ideal, low-end blood pressure" is that elderly people whose blood pressure is as low as the doc can make it tend to get dizzy when they go from sitting to standing – because their blood pressure is *too low* for their age, usually because of their blood pressure drugs. Sometimes, they fall and get head injuries or broken bones. Sometimes they die from the sub-dural hematoma or other sequelae of these falls. And these deaths have been brought about in the name of "better" blood pressure numbers.[1]

Returning to the point, vigorous, excitable people with blood pressure that can blast up into a high range in response to daily stresses (the *excess*-type of high blood pressure) and then swoon back down to normal are the people who tend to form clots in the brain or "burst" a blood vessel. This is the "bad" kind of high blood pressure.

My patient had the bad kind.

---

[1] When I have elderly patients whose doctors have taught them to be terrified of high blood pressure, but who cannot tolerate the effects of their blood pressure medications, I give them cooked, powdered Tian Qi (also known as San Qi). This herb, despite most doctors' misinformation to the contrary, is *not* a blood thinner. (Continued on next page.)

This herb acts as an adaptogen for the blood cells, blood vessels, and clotting function. If a person's blood is clotting poorly, this herb can help increase the clot-ability. If a person's blood is stagnant, forming clots, this herb can help decrease the clotting.

When elderly patients use this herb on a daily basis, it improves the strength and flexibility of the blood vessel walls. Within a week, some patients already notice that they don't bruise so easily, and their existing bruises heal much faster. Soon, as their blood vessels become less leaky, their body automatically reduces the pressure in the blood system. I've had patients' blood pressure drop thirty points and stay there simply by taking Tian Qi for a month or more. In other words, if a person has deficiency-type high blood pressure, he needs *tonics* to decrease the leakiness in his blood system. The blood pressure is high in a deficient person because high pressure is the only way to ensure that enough oxygen gets to the head.

The medications given by the doctors, whether a person is forty with a fiery temper, or eighty-five and frail, are all *drugs*. "Drugs," literally, are system inhibitors – the opposite of tonics. One of the greatest strengths of Asian medicine is that we differentiate between a problem brought about by deficiency, and one brought about by excess. In the case of blood pressure, we treat an *excess* high blood pressure problem (one brought on by, say, emotionalism and/or too much rich food) very differently from how we treat a *deficient* high blood pressure problem (one brought on by leaky vessels and lack of vigor). Both manifest as *high* blood pressure, but one is caused by excessive behavior and the other is caused by deficiency.

Incredibly, despite the absolute illogic, and the devastating side effects, when it comes to blood pressure, western medicine doctors drug our most frail citizens as if they were hot-tempered forty-year olds.

On the afternoons when he had students, he could actually feel his blood pressure mounting, his head starting to throb, an angry temper flickering invisibly around the edges of his thoughts.

As soon as his work afternoons were over, his blood pressure went back to normal.

There was no point in looking for something wrong with his channel Qi. There was no point in treating him with acupuncture. Sitting there in my office, laughing with me, his blood pressure was perfectly normal. There was nothing wrong with his blood pressure system.

The problem was that he tended to shunt into sympathetic mode when he was frustrated. The only problem with that is that he didn't have the liberty of fighting or fleeing his students while he was in sympathetic mode. His body was able to shift beautifully into sympathetic mode, pouring adrenaline into his system and shifting liver channel Qi up into his head, but there was no civilized way for him to use that adrenaline. Instead, he had to stew in his blood-pressure raising adrenaline until the last pupil left.

He did not have a health problem. He had a problem with rampant emotions that came and went. There is no needle treatment for that.

We spoke for a few minutes, and it quickly became apparent that he had never been taught the basic skills for dealing with negative emotions. All his life, he had dealt with negative emotions by pretending they weren't happening, or by suppressing them by "thinking of something else."

I taught him the following exercise.

Exercise for dealing with physical or emotional pain or fear

Location

Physical pain from injury has a fixed location in the body. Pain from emotions also registers in specific locations in the body.

Some people will feel certain emotions as a lump in the throat. Other emotions may cause butterflies (running piggies) in the stomach. Still others will cause pain in the solar plexus. The emotions that strike us most deeply cause pain in the heart. I am not describing a metaphysical pain: I am describing a tangible, physical pain that results from emotions.

In the west, we are often taught to ignore this type of pain, or "rise above it." But, in the words of my most revered teacher, Paramahansa Yogananda, "Truths suppressed lead disconcertingly to a host of errors."

In the east, people are more likely to be taught to notice their pain, and *deal with it* appropriately, so that it doesn't affect their equanimity.

In order to deal correctly with emotional pain, one must first *notice* the part of the body that is tightening up in response to the negative emotion. He must take note of the location, and the sensation, of the physical pain.

196

The something within

Next, he must command himself to feel the expansion in the chest. "Expansion in the chest" refers to the thrilling physical sensation that one experiences when beholding something of great beauty, for example, or when hearing beautiful music.

Most languages have a name for this tangible feeling. This feeling has no name in English. In Latin it is *Spiritus Sanctus*, traditionally translated into English, since the first King James edition of the Bible, as Holy Ghost. I shall refer to this tangible sensation as "heart feeling."

In Chinese, the word for "happy" is made up of two words, Kai and Xin. Kai means expand, in the manner of a flower bud expanding into a magnificent flower – as it gets bigger, its beauty and energy increases. The bud's beauty and energy does *not* become diluted as it expands. Xin means heart. The characters for "happy," Kai Xin, are literally, "expanding (like an opening flower) heart." Nice.

Horribly, in the west, many people are taught that this feeling only occurs when they experience something of great beauty or grace: they are not supposed to induce this sensation without some external trigger. Just the opposite is true. We have the biological ability, the legal right, and the moral responsibility to initiate the feeling of expanded heart as often as possible, *regardless of circumstances.*

If a person has *ever* felt a thrilling expansion in his chest, his brain remembers this event, and is capable of reproducing it on command. With conscious training, the ability to expand the chest on command, even in the face of difficulty, becomes increased. The size of the sensation can also be increased, through practice.

Dealing with pain: two sensations at once

After a person has noticed the place in his body that is feeling pain from physical or emotional cause, 1) he should concentrate on *feeling* the pain, while 2) simultaneously expanding his heart feeling. He must make the heart feeling large enough to encompass the pain.

He must *simultaneously* feel the pain *and* the expanded heart feeling surrounding the pain.

At first, the pain may seem the stronger sensation of the two. Over time, the heart feeling will become stronger. One cannot actually focus continually on a specific physical pain for more than about forty-five minutes. Either the person will pass out from the pain or his mind will start checking out other areas, and flit from thought to thought, coming back to revisit the pain at intervals. The brain is designed to get distracted and look for other things to worry about after enough pain signals have gotten through. However, *with training*, the mature, well-trained *heart feeling* can continue unabated indefinitely.

It takes work to focus simultaneously on both the pain and the heart feeling, but eventually, because the heart feeling can go indefinitely, and the pain cannot, the heart feeling will win out, every time.

How it works

The physical mechanism at work in this heart-feeling exercise is one of resonance. For this to work, the heart feeling, made of wave energy, must cover an area physically larger than the waves generated by the electrical systems involved in the pain feeling. If the area that contains tangible heart-feeling waves is significantly larger than the pain area, the pain-feeling waves very quickly become resonant with the heart-feeling waves. When this resonance occurs, the pain signals cease to be part of a sympathetic-mode story line, and are converted to a parasympathetic story line.[1]

You can think of this exercise as using resonance to shift the pain from the "Oh no!" part of the brain over to the "Huh. That was an interesting experience" part of the brain.

In other words, the person will still have the pain, he won't necessarily forget about the thing that caused the pain, but he will have *processed* the pain – in his brain, he will have moved the pain from the neural panic mode, the fight or flight mode, into the parasympathetic mode: the mode in which healing occurs.

As Paramahansa Yogananda said in a lecture, "In this drama of life, your love must be greater than your pain." He meant it very literally. I have rarely met a westerner that understood this as a literal instruction. It is usually misunderstood; considered to be a metaphor.

Return to the case study

I explained to my patient the above exercise for dealing with pain. Next, I had my patient figure out where, in his body, his students caused him pain. When he imagined the daily blood-pressure raising scenario and allowed himself to actually feel the location of the pain, he was surprised. He felt a ferocious pain clutching at his heart, as if he would die. Then, I asked him to temporarily forget that pain, while he practiced the subtle heart feeling, the "something within."

Then, I had him practice making his heart feeling get large on command. At first, he felt sheepish doing it without some external prompt, but then he announced that he could do it easily by thinking of the previous summer's vacation in Italy. I let him do that for a few seconds. Then I told him that relying on Italy wasn't good enough. He had to learn to produce that expanded-heart feeling on command, for no other reason than that he was commanding himself to re-experience the heart feeling. He was soon able to do this. I told him it still wasn't good enough (and it wasn't).

I pointed out to him that, when his heart feeling got really big, big enough to work for him, it would extend outside the confines of his physical body. When he really got going, the heart feeling should be so big that his wife, sitting next to him on my office couch, would be able to feel it.

He concentrated on making the heart feeling as large as he could, without using memory prompts. His wife and I waited for about fifteen seconds. Then, at the same time, his wife and I both said, "Yes!"

I added, "You did it. Susan and I both felt what you were doing! That's how big it needs to be. Why should it ever be less?"

It was time for him to bring the two sensations together. I had him recreate the pain in his heart, while thinking of his very worst students. Next, I had him make his heart feeling large enough to encompass the entire painful area, and little larger, for good measure.

---

[1] The Heartmath Institute, of Boulder Creek, California, has done beautiful work on the shifts in neural mode function that occur when heartwaves (the electromagnetic waves being given off by the heart) and brainwaves are resonant, as compared with when they are not.

I kept reminding him, "Feel *both* of them. *Feel* the pain. Keep your heart feeling active. Keep feeling the pain *and* feeling the heart at the same time."

In less than a minute, he sighed deeply. "Oh my God, I can feel it coming down out of my head!"

"What's coming down?"

"The pressure, the headache. The pain goes away, I can't feel it even when I try – the heart is stronger than the pain. When I imagined the students, I felt the headache starting. But when I felt at the same time the heart pain *and* my own heart loving my own heart, the sensation of pressure goes down, like a water level is falling in my body. It goes down and down." He gestured with his hand, letting his hand move slowly down from his forehead to the middle of his chest.

"How far down does it go?" I asked.

"It goes to my heart, and it stays there. I feel so much calmer. I feel good! I never knew how to do this. No one ever taught me how to deal with pain! I think I was just expected to ignore pain, or mentally change the subject."

He was so radiantly happy to have learned a new skill, but I made him keep practicing the combined sensations for the rest of our hour-long session.

As they were leaving, his wife said to me, "I can already feel the change in him – he is more like his old self. He has been getting so worried about his blood pressure that he was starting to have high blood pressure all the time – because of fear of blood pressure! Now, I can feel his heart is happier."

My patient was *not* angry about me not doing acupuncture. He understood perfectly well that all the acupuncture in the world would not help him when those students started to play.

He *was* excited at the idea of having a tangible method for dealing with the genuine heart pain brought about by listening to bad music. He hugged me and kissed me on both cheeks, and promised to use his heart feeling, from now on.

As an aside, I'd anticipated that he would be an exceptionally quick student of this technique; professional musicians usually are. Magnificent musicianship is usually contingent upon the musician being able to feel his heart's expressions, so that he can convey, via music, great tides of heart feeling. So when I asked him to make his heart big, he knew very well the sensation that I was trying to describe – he just wasn't used to doing it without music or other external prompts.

Some patients, on the other hand, have no idea what I am talking about when I mention the feeling of expansion in the chest. One patient struggled to understand what I meant for nearly an hour, when he finally exclaimed, "Oh! I know what you mean! I felt it once, when my father unexpectedly showed up after school to bring me home. He was a salesman, on the road a lot, and I almost never saw him. I was six years old, and I remember it like it was yesterday. I felt so happy."

My own heart was physically pained by the thought that this man had only one experience in his entire life when he had felt his heart swell with joy. Still, during the few sessions we had together while he was in California, we were able to work with this single experience and build on it, until he was able to get at least a tiny bit of heart expansion going on command.

Discussion

This case study demonstrates what can happen when a person habitually uses a wrong neural mode. Actually, in this case, the patient's channel Qi wasn't *stuck*, per se, in a wrong mode – he just allowed his moods to drive his channel Qi in and out of sympathetic mode, uncontrollably. I just taught him how to *deal* correctly, maturely, with his pain, so that he could stay in parasympathetic mode despite the genuine discomfort caused by bad music. By learning to deal with his pain, he learned how to reduce his blood pressure.[1]

---

[1] This case study brings to mind one of the most painful experiences I've ever had as an acupuncturist. One of my doctoral program classes was addressing the endocrine system, and included a unit on blood pressure.

The teacher wanted to show how acupuncture works on blood pressure, and asked for a volunteer. My blood pressure is usually fairly low. However, standing in front of a class, I am able to get "public speaking" fear going – one of the most common of all fears – and this would induce a sympathetic mode rise in blood pressure. I had assumed the teacher would understand this, and I looked forward to an intelligent discussion on blood pressure.

Instead, I stood in front of the large class with my heart starting to pound, answering questions about my age and so on, and soon the teacher pumped up the blood pressure cuff. "Very bad!" he announced. My blood pressure had soared to 135/75. Some members of the class gasped in concern.

I was a little surprised. The teacher was wrong. If a person is temporarily in red-alert mode, this is a very reasonable blood pressure.

The teacher inserted a few basic needles: ST-36, Yin Tang, and LI-4. I happened to know that I didn't have any blockages at any of these points, but that was his treatment. Some fellow students pulled a few towels over me, set a heat lamp over my feet, and the classroom lights were dimmed. A few of my fellow students, sympathetic to my "plight," massaged my feet. We laughed and joked for half an hour, then I started to drift off to sleep, when the treatment time ran out. The needles were removed: my blood pressure was back to its usual 120/70.

The teacher announced the results of his treatment, and the class went wild. I'm not kidding. People clapped, and cheered. Several of the people at the front of the class, who I could hear clearly, said, "See, acupuncture *really* works!" "With something like *blood pressure*, that can be measured, you can *prove* that acupuncture really works!" And worst of all, "Acupuncture isn't based on logic: there's no way to *know* how it works…it just *works* … like magic!"

I was outraged. I felt my blood pressure soaring to a level I have rarely experienced.

Were all my dear, loving, fellow students, most of them acupuncturists with more than a decade of experience, truly this incapable of analytical thought? Did it not occur to any of them that my blood pressure would have dropped *without* the needles? I'd had my feet massaged for half an hour, I'd been joking with my friends. When my blood pressure was measured the second time, I hadn't been talking to the class. I was still lying down, still draped with towels, enjoying the still-dimmed lights.

Not one person in the class seemed to understand that the needles might not have had anything to do with my shift back to my normal, relaxed-mode, which is to say, parasympathetic mode-type blood pressure. (Continued on next page.)

Then my glance roved to the back of the room. There, at least, I could see the same disappointment and anger that I was feeling, mirrored on the faces of several of my more thoughtful colleagues. I calmed down and returned to my seat, in the back row. Most of the room was still giddy with this Hard Proof that acupuncture really works!

The genuine pain of this experience was the shameful realization that most of my colleagues, even those in a doctoral program, had little or no understanding of the basic physiological forces that they are working with, or even what constitutes a valid experiment.

200

As an aside, unlike the subject in this case study who was able to shift into low blood pressure when he was content, some patients are stuck in high blood-pressure mode around the clock due to some aberration in their channel Qi that keeps them in sympathetic mode. They may have some bit of channel Qi, or their entire body, permanently stuck in the wrong mode.

If this is occurring because of a physical blockage, illness, or injury, you might be able to fix the problem with acupuncture.

If the blockage is related to some fear, pain, or emotion, the patient might benefit from counseling. The pain, fear, or emotion probably needs to be consciously addressed – it probably won't go away from needles alone. Sometimes the simple act of discussing the source of the blockage can be enough to get rid of it. Other times, a person might need professional help.

At any rate, once the blockage is gone, the patient's channel Qi will, very often, spontaneously revert back to parasympathetic mode. When this happens, the blood pressure will go back to whatever is the best level for this person while in parasympathetic mode.

If you wish to review a case in which a person's channel Qi was somewhat permanently stuck in sympathetic mode, instead of the come-and-go example in this chapter, please review case study #7, in chapter six, p. 126.

A combination of 3) and 4)

The root of the problem, and the treatment, isn't always as cut and dried as these case studies might suggest. The following case study demonstrates how, sometimes, one must look

---

Several months prior to this lecture, my colleagues and I had sat through *painfully* dull, but accurate, beginner-level lectures on concepts such as isolation of variables, and what constitutes a valid experiment. I had just assumed that everyone in the class already understood these basic principles. But evidently, many of my colleagues had not even understood those basic lectures.

Bottom line? Most of my colleagues *wanted* acupuncture to "work." This desire, combined with their lack of understanding and/or analytical thinking allowed them to view this "experiment" as hard proof.

At first, I was angry at their naiveté. Then, I felt shame for my profession, and finally, sadness.

Of course, acupuncturists do not have a monopoly in this arena. I've talked with many scientists and western doctors who are equally naïve about the unproven, often illogical, "facts" abounding in their own professions. I suppose all of us are subject to skewed vision when it comes to our own ugly children.

As Swami Sri Yukteswar said, "Human conduct is ever unreliable until man is anchored in the Divine."

Even so, I had yearned for a *better* degree of understanding than average from my colleagues, my own. My enormous surge of rage and high blood pressure had been caused by temporarily indulging in disappointment and anger: what the ancient sages would have called "attachment to outcome." Evidently, despite the acupuncture treatment that was supposed to have fixed it, my tendency for over-indulgence in the pernicious emotion of anger remained unchanged by mere needles – just as predicted in the *Nei Jing*.

farther afield from the obvious. At the same time, it demonstrates a few methods for tracking down the genuine source of a cryptic problem.

Case study #18

Chronic lung weakness due to faulty electrical circuit at the knee

Male, age 56, history of annual lung infections. The typical pattern was a sinus cold that moved into the lungs and then became pneumonia. This year, he was showing the usual pattern. His MD had given him antibiotics, so the infection had not settled deep in his lungs, but had merely lingered in the bronchia. As a child, he'd had "bronchial asthma." By the time he came to see me, he was nearly better from his most recent bronchial infection. Now, he only had the residual cough, which typically would linger for one or two months. When he came to see me, he wanted help in strengthening his lungs to prevent this pattern in the future.

His pulses were very deficient in the Spleen, possibly because of the antibiotics, but were otherwise harmonized with each other. The tongue had deep teethmarks, also possibly because of the antibiotics. I felt the channel Qi in all the logical places, and found a blockage at UB-13 on the right side. The channel Qi just seemed to disappear at this point.

The problem seemed straightforward: get channel Qi to flow past UB-13, after which, it would flow correctly all by itself – and his lungs would become stronger.

I needled UB-13, and added UB-15 and UB-16. To be on the safe side, I also needled UB-62, to make sure the channel Qi was flowing all the way to his foot, and UB-42, to make sure the "outer row" of points on the right-side UB channel also kept moving nicely.

I asked him to visualize white light in his UB-13 area, which he did. At the end of the treatment, after removing the needles, I massaged LU-1 and LU-2, for good measure.

The next week he returned, very happy. His lungs felt *much* better. He was recovering far faster than usual from the residual cough. However, he still had a cough, with sticky phlegm on his vocal chords.

For starters, I checked to make sure that channel Qi was still flowing past right-side UB-13. To my surprise, it was utterly blocked, the same as it had been last week, prior to treatment.

I inserted a needle at right-side UB-13, and felt for the flow of channel Qi. With the needle in, it was, again, moving correctly. I waited a few minutes – long enough for the initial shock of the needle to wear off. I felt UB-13 again. No channel Qi.

Obviously, something was causing the channel Qi at right-side UB-13 to go somewhere else (to dive interior, to "stop moving" on the surface), even though it *could* go through, *only for a short while*, in immediate response to stimulation.

My treatment, the previous week, hadn't actually attained a lasting result. As far as I was concerned, the treatment hadn't worked. I needed to figure out why.

The patient had easily been able to visualize light and energy in that area, so I could presume that he had no emotional blockage gumming the works.

I wondered if I'd missed a physical blockage just under the skin. I applied Yin Tui Na to the area, but all the tissues felt relaxed and responsive.

I considered a few electrical possibilities. A parallel current can exert an influence over its parallel partner. So I checked the left-side UB channel in the vicinity of UB-13. Channel Qi was flowing just fine on the left side.

The above electrical phenomenon might be referred to as a side-to-side zone of influence. Another electrical phenomenon might be referred to as "length of the current" zone of influence. In this latter type of influence, an electrical glitch located a specific distance from one end of the line can cause a glitch the same distance away from the *other* end of the line.

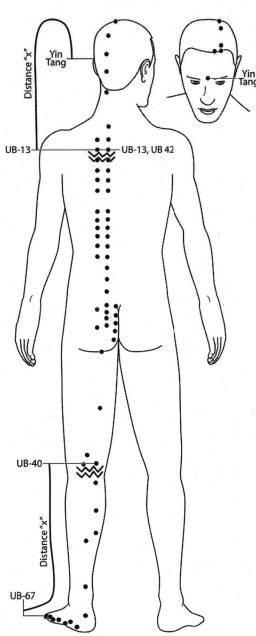

Fig. 10.2 The distance from Yin Tang to UB-13 is nearly the same as the distance from UB-40 to UB-67.

It is not unusual for a glitch some distance from one end of a channel to create a matching glitch equidistant from the opposite end of the channel.

I estimated the distance from UB-1 to UB-13. Then, I tried to picture where that same distance would get me, approximately, if I were to measure backwards, from the end of the UB channel, at UB-67, moving towards to head. My gaze fixed on the most likely spot: UB-40, at the back of the knee.

I gave two seconds of finger massage to right-side UB-40, and checked what the channel Qi was doing up on the back: the channel Qi was now happily flowing through UB-13. Aha.

I had to wonder if this patient's back-of-the-knee stuck place, right at the divergent mode switching spot, was a chronic weak spot for him. What if, after every time he got sick and his body shunted into sympathetic mode to fight the illness, the switch at the right-side back of the knee got stuck in some incorrect setting partway between sympathetic and parasympathetic, and wasn't able to return to full-on parasympathetic?

Evidently, his UB channel had been stuck in some incorrect pattern at UB-40. UB-40 is a key switch-over location during sympathetic mode – the place where, during a fear response, the UB channel Qi is diverted over to the Kidney channel and the adrenals.

Based on what I'd just seen, such a sticking point, or electrical glitch, could cause a corresponding glitch at UB-13 – a point equidistant to UB-40, in terms of their mutual distance to the two ends of the UB channel.

This glitch at UB-40 was causing a corresponding glitch at UB-13, a glitch that shunted UB channel Qi away from UB-13 (the lung point of the UB channel) into some other channel, or even into some other organ. Wherever the glitch was shunting that channel Qi away from UB-13, it was not detectable by hand.

This might explain why he had lingering lung problems after every illness: after his body switched into sympathetic mode at UB-40 at the onset of an illness, maybe it didn't switch back to basic parasympathetic when the illness was ended. Then, the failure of UB-40 to be set straight caused the lung-nourishing point of the UB channel, UB-13, to be deprived of channel Qi.

I inserted a needle at right-side UB-40. The patient screamed and flinched! But in less than a second, he felt very relaxed, and the channel Qi was running correctly the entire length of the channel. Forty minutes later, when I removed the needle, the channel Qi was still running correctly, and he reported that his breathing felt far more relaxed than before.

In terms of resetting his channel Qi at UB-40, I must admit, I had not performed a very subtle treatment – I had caused a localized shock. However, this defibrillation-type treatment had been successful in jolting his UB-40 electrical connections back to parasympathetic mode. I don't know if I actually cured the underlying problem (his body's back-of-the-knee tendency to get stuck in a wrong route after coming out of sympathetic mode). I'll find out if he comes to see me during next year's flu season.

I like this case study. It demonstrates 3) Qi disappearing (at UB-13) *and* 4) channel Qi stuck in a wrong neural mode (at UB-40, stuck in a *post*-sympathetic route, but unable to revert back to full-on parasympathetic).

This case study also allows me to show my thinking in cases where a simple "get the Qi moving past the blockage" doesn't work. When the basic style of treatment didn't give a *lasting* result, I had to keep looking for other likely sources for the channel Qi aberration at UB-13.

First, I assessed his mental willingness to have channel Qi in the area. Next, using Yin Tui Na, I checked to make sure that everything was structurally correct. After that, I went looking for electrical disruptions. I checked the opposite *side* of the body, looking for channel Qi disruption, and I checked the opposite *end* of the body. If those places hadn't panned out, I would have had to keep looking at logical suspects, until I found the underlying problem.

5) Channel Qi attacking another channel

Case study #19

Uterine fibroid caused by Liver channel attacking Spleen channel in the groin and abdomen

Female, 52 years old. Her large, visibly protruding uterine fibroid had been causing severe pain during menses and during bowel movements. Patient was peri-menopausal and preferred to wait out the next few years of menstrual discomfort rather than have a hysterectomy. When she first contacted me, I referred her to a brilliant acupuncturist who specialized in OB-GYN, the late Sharon Feng.

The patient worked for nearly a year with Dr. Feng. She received weekly acupuncture *and* herbal tea made from "loose" Chinese medicinal herbs. While the intense pain during menses had become much less severe, the fibroid had continued to grow in size, and the milder, previously come-and-go, discomfort had become chronic.

After nearly a year, the patient decided to work with me again, despite my confessed relative lack of experience in OB-GYN.

Patient had a history of C-section. A few years earlier, I had needled the patient's C-section scar several times, which had helped her with some other health problems.

This time, when she came in to see me again, I noticed that channel Qi could flow past the C-section scar when needles were in place, but if there were no needles in place, the channel Qi running from SP-10 up to Ren-3 seemed to disappear just past SP-10.

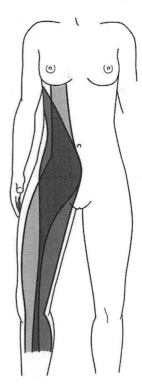

Fig. 10.3 Correct flow of Liver and Spleen channels.
The Liver channel has light shading, the Spleen channel has darker shading, and where the Liver channel overlaps the Spleen, the shading is darkest.

This was not a case of channel Qi being blocked by the scar. Instead, I suspected that the channel Qi of what we traditionally call the Spleen channel (the actual Liver channel) might have been shunting into what we traditionally call the Liver channel. Using my hands, I could not feel this attacking Qi actually flowing into the deeper channel. All I could feel was that, proximal to SP-10, particularly on the right leg (at the spot where she had received a very painful injection during her C-section, and where she had also injured her leg in a car accident at age eighteen), the so-called "Spleen" channel Qi could not be felt – as if it had disappeared. The deeper-running channels can be much harder to feel than the channels that run closer to the surface. A logical conclusion could be that the channel Qi was shunting into the Liver channel.[1]

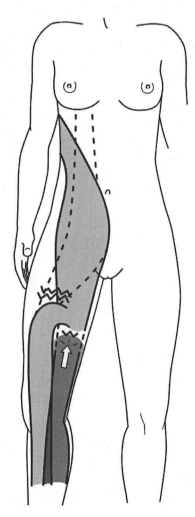

Fig. 10.4

The Liver channel Qi (shown with lighter shading) is attacking the Spleen channel (darker shading). The original blockage (shown with a double zigzag line) is blocking the Liver channel. The Liver channel Qi is flowing into the Spleen channel, causing a secondary blockage that impedes the Spleen channel Qi. The Spleen channel can just barely be seen overflowing its boundaries, seeking a route of decreased resistance. It is also becoming somewhat stagnant, and not flowing very well. Meanwhile, proximal to the blockage, the Liver channel Qi is flowing in the deeper route of the Spleen channel. In the vicinity of the uterus, *no* channel Qi is flowing in the more superficial, Liver channel route. This misdirection causes two problems. 1) The front of the uterus, where the fibroid is growing, is not getting the Liver channel instructions that it needs. 2) The Spleen channel is receiving the wrong kind of channel Qi. Thus the Spleen channel is receiving wrong instructions.

For several weeks, I inserted needles in the upper leg portion of the Spleen channel and Ren-3 and Ren-4. Every time, she felt a surge of "life" flowing up her legs and through the front of her

---

[1] If you consider that the disappearing channel was actually the Liver channel, and not, as taught, the Spleen channel (see chapter five, The Healthy Paths of the Channels), what we had was Liver attacking Spleen, or Wood Attacking Earth: the most common of all attacking scenarios. In general, the Liver channel, because of its powerful connection to self-expression and love for (rather than desire for: Kidney) physical existence, is one of the most powerful channels in the body. It is therefore the one most capable of attacking another channel when it runs up against an obstruction. Therefore, I could conclude that the "disappearing" (actual) Liver channel was attacking the more passive (actual) Spleen channel, at a depth that I could not feel.

uterus, and a sense that the fibroid might be able to shrink a bit if the flow continued. But within a few hours after each treatment, the "surge of life" ceased. The fibroid didn't budge.

On the week that I was writing this chapter, I told her about the relative *depths* of the paths of the actual Liver and Spleen channels. I explained that I thought the channel Qi in the more superficial, more anterior channel of the inner leg was failing to stay in place, and was shunting into the slightly deeper and more posterior channel of the inner leg.

I explained the pathways of these two channels: as these channels approach the groin and the abdomen, the 12th channel, the more anterior medial channel (the actual Liver channel), stays closer to the skin, and the 4th channel, the somewhat posterior medial channel (the actual Spleen channel), flows a bit more deeply, within.

Weeks earlier, I had inserted needles to break up the blockage at the original injury site – the spot where she remembered being violently injected with something during her C-section, the spot where she'd also injured her leg in a car accident. I wanted to assume that the original blockage was gone, and that the real problem, now, was habit – the anterior channel had become so accustomed to flowing into the deeper channel that it just continued to do it, even though the blockage was gone.

I inserted needles just distal to the "disappearing channel Qi," in the actual Liver channel. I asked her to mentally force the channel Qi thus stimulated to stay in the correct channels – meaning, stay close to the surface, at the correct *depth* – as it coursed up to the abdomen. She did so, and the engorged, heavy fibroid started performing muscular contractions! She said it felt very healthy and *dynamic*, and unlike the usual acupuncture stimulation during which she only felt electrical energy moving through the fibroid.

She agreed to practice moving energy in the manner she'd experienced during the treatment – keeping the Liver channel Qi close to the surface of the skin – during the next week. Within a few days she called me to say that the fibroid was regularly pulsing, as if squeezing out fluids, and was getting smaller.

(As a follow-up note to this case study, when I saw her the next week, her fibroid was visibly smaller, and she felt much less pressure from it.)

I continued to work with her, once a week, for several months, and the uterus continued shrinking. Curiously, the previously symmetrical fibroid shrank asymmetrically: the left half of the fibroid is now nearly gone, the portion of the fibroid that used to go right up the midline, along the Ren channel, is now gone, but the right side of the fibroid, after shrinking considerably, has stopped shrinking.

At home, she regularly corrects the flow of channel Qi in the leg and groin. The channel Qi on her right side still reverts back to the attacking mode if she's not thinking about it. Whenever she mentally sends the channel energy into the correct paths, she can feel the energy streaming through her uterus. But shortly afterwards, the channels evidently revert back to their old ways.

The patient is convinced that the right sise is unable to heal because her body was abused by the violence of her C-section, sixteen years earlier. Every week, when I see her, she says that she has "moved on," and is no longer thinking of herself as the victim of the C-section, and wonders why the fibroid is still there.

For my part, the bitter tone in her voice when she brings up the subject of the C-section, and the fact that she still brings it up weekly, suggests to me that she has *not* actually come to peace with her C-section trauma. Certainly, she is not yet able to laugh about it, or talk about it with peace or gratitude. I have to wonder if the remaining chunk of fibroid will remain as-is until such time as her thoughts are at peace with regard to the C-section events.

Still, the fibroid is no longer growing rapidly: it is no longer behaving as if it is a thing apart from the rest of her body.

Discussion

When I was *first* working with her, I chose needles downstream from the points at which the actual-Liver channel Qi seemed to disappear. On her left leg, that was about 4 cun proximal to SP-10. On the right leg, it was about 7 proximal to SP-10. I also inserted needles about an inch proximal to these points, to try to attract channel Qi back into this channel, and keep it there.

Ultimately, however, we were not successful in getting effective amounts of channel Qi moving through until I asked the patient to get *mentally* involved in the process, asking her to keep that Liver channel Qi as close to the surface of the skin as possible. As soon as she became involved in keeping the channel Qi in the right place, she felt the enormous energetic shift in her abdomen. She also felt a bit frightened. The presence of so much channel Qi right out there in the front of her abdomen made her feel "exposed" and a bit vulnerable. However, she was willing to overcome her emotional reluctance and keep the channel Qi where it was supposed to be.

Now, when she forgets to keep the channel Qi at the correct depth, it sometimes returns to its blocked pattern. But she is aware of the ongoing problem, and recognizes it as something that she must conquer. By regularly, if temporarily, returning the channel Qi to the correct area, the fibroid has greatly diminished. She hopes to eliminate the fibroid completely, someday, by retraining her channel Qi and by conquering any residual, surgery-related fear that she may have.

As a curious aside, for years, as long as I'd known her, her heart pulse always felt as if it jutted off, sideways, away from other left side pulses. Because of this, I had treated her for Heart symptoms every once in a while, even though she had no organ, channel, or Heart-system problems.

After the above treatment, during which her Spleen channel was restored to its proper place, her heart pulse became normal. Evidently, at SP-21, where the Spleen channel converts into Heart channel energy, her conversion had been skewed: she had *Liver* channel Qi flowing up to SP-21, and not Spleen channel Qi. Now, whenever she remembers to let the Liver channel flow in its correct path, so that the Spleen channel can flow in its correct path, her heart pulse is in a straight line with the other left-side pulses.

6) Channel Qi running rebelliously

Case study #20

Burning facial pain from Rebellious Stomach channel Qi

Female, age 48, experienced excruciating, "electrical," "burning" sensations on the skin of her chest and on her face, after eating. Her nose and the area from ST-1 to ST-3 would turn bright red, and remain so until several hours after the meal. Also, her legs would become somewhat numb and tingly during this time. Because of the searing pain, she had become afraid to eat most foods, and afraid to eat any food in significant quantity. She was working under the assumption that some particular food was at the root of the problem, and had eliminated nearly all foods from her diet, but still, if she ate more than a few teaspoons of anything, she'd experience the burning. "I burn like a toaster burns! It's electrical heat," she explained repeatedly. Her height was 5' 8". Over two years of this excruciating, "electrical" pain, she'd lost nearly 40 pounds, and was down to 102 pounds.

She'd seen several specialists at a highly respected university medical school, but after dozens of tests showed nothing wrong, all the specialists agreed that they'd never heard of anything like her situation, and therefore, she was psychotically creating the pain and the red face.

When she came to see me, it sounded to me as if stimulation of her Stomach channel, such as from eating, caused her Stomach channel to rebound backwards, electrocuting her face. If this was the case, I had to wonder why her body, at ST-6, wasn't just shunting the backwards-flowing Stomach channel Qi up to ST-8 instead of letting it flow backwards, over her face. I asked her about any medical history relating to her lower jaw. She'd had an extensive amount of dental work on the lower back molars on both sides, including root canals. Very possibly, the tooth surgeries had damaged her body's ability to shunt Rebellious channel Qi of the Stomach channel up to ST-8, hence the horrible burning pain and redness around her mouth and nose whenever that channel surged backwards.

A very quick scan of her Stomach channel Qi showed that no Stomach channel Qi could get past her low abdomen. I asked about C-section. She'd had one.

When I fingered the C-section scar, I was stunned.

The C-section scar was nearly invisible. But beneath the faint line on the skin was a thick wedge of keloid tissue. Immediately under the skin, and extending down deep into the gut, the wedge of scar was an inch and half wide. It felt as if she had a thick, inch and a half wide piece of non-conductive, hard rubber standing between her torso and her pelvic bones. A wall like this could effectively block any Qi flow between her legs and torso. I was amazed that she was a healthy as she was. I asked her for more information about the C-section.

Her C-section doctor had prided himself on making invisible scars. He did not try to connect muscle to muscle, fat to fat, and skin to skin, in any sort of layered effect. Instead, his special technique consisted of turning under, as a massed group, as much skin, muscles, and underlying tissue as possible, so that he could work his stitches on a smooth section of healthy skin, rather than sewing together the raggedy edges of freshly cut skin.

On both sides of the cut line, he'd cut away the "extra" tissue from the pregnancy, then turned as much abdominal tissue as possible to the inside. It had been turned under en masse, or "tucked inside," so that it didn't show, and then he'd stitched up the surface layer. His goal was a simultaneous post-pregnancy tummy tuck *combined* with an almost-invisible scar as evidence of the C-section: two surgeries in one!

The procedure had been performed in Russia. Maybe it was common in Russia, I don't know. But I had never seen this procedure on an American C-section.

And I'd never felt anything as thick and impenetrable as that wedge of scar tissue.

I tried to insert a 1 cun needle into the invisible wedge of scar. The needle bent double. I disposed of it and switched to thicker needles. They bent double. I used my thickest

1/2 cun needles. Of the forty or so 1/2 cun, thick needles I attempted to insert, I was able to get maybe twenty of them inserted a tiny distance into the keloid tissue under the skin, one about every half inch or so, along the length of the scar.

I didn't know what good it would do to have a needle make it such a short distance through the scar, but I didn't know what else to do. I considered using framing nails, but decided to hold off for a few weeks.

Surprisingly, the next week, I was able to get the same number of short, thick needles a little bit deeper into the scar tissue. Again, nearly half of the attempts resulted in a bent and useless needle, but it seemed as if either she was making progress or my needling technique was getting better.

The following week there was a significant difference. The scar tissue was noticeably softer. I was able to insert the needles their full length. I inserted double rows, with the first row of needles aimed at the more superficial level, just under the skin, and a second row, starting a bit further away from the scar, and using longer needles, aimed at the deeper level of the scar.

By the fourth week, the wedge was noticeably softer, and her symptoms ceased. She could once again eat anything without suffering electrical burning in her face and chest or numbness in her legs. She'd been so emotionally traumatized by the excruciating pain, that even with the pain gone, months passed before she dared to eat more than half a cup of food at one sitting.

She continued to come in for treatment to further reduce the rubber wedge.

A few months later, feeling much better and able to eat, once again, she revisited her primary doctor at the university, to pass along the good news. He laughed at her, and assured her that, if acupuncture on her C-section scar had gotten rid of her "electrical burning in her face," a pain that had been triggered by something as innocuous as eating, then she could be *certain* that her problem had been purely psychological.

"The ultimate principle of treatment consists in differentiating the colors and pulses with accuracy." [1]

Chapter eleven

Integrating channel Qi diagnoses with Asian medicine terminology

Translating Channel Qi irregularities into traditional diagnostic patterns

Channel diagnostics is not a separate world of Asian medicine. It is merely an *additional* method for collecting information. Once collected, the channel Qi findings can be translated into familiar terms, also known as "pattern" diagnoses. For example, the terms deficient, stagnation, attacking, and rebellious can be added to channel Qi findings, creating "pattern & channel" diagnoses such as "Stomach channel Qi <u>deficiency</u> starting around ST-16," or "channel Qi <u>stagnation</u> at Du-12," or "Liver channel Qi <u>attacking</u> Spleen channel from LIV-3 to SP-3," or "<u>Rebellious</u> channel Qi in the Stomach channel from ST-42 to ST-40 due to <u>Blood Stagnation</u> at ST-42" – and so on.

By adding the channel Qi findings to the usual pattern diagnoses, one presents an exact *location*, and sometimes even an explanation, to augment the pattern diagnosis. The pattern is no longer just some cryptic generality.

Instead of saying, "It *most likely* is Wood Attacking Earth because we're seeing symptoms that match that pattern, supported by pulse and tongue," you can say, "It *is* Wood Attacking Earth, and here's *where* it's attacking," and maybe even "and here's *why* it's attacking."

It's the same old Asian medicine pattern diagnosis, but with far more information being communicated.

Using the word "channel"

Based on my interactions with students from around the country, and around the world, it seems that many schools of Asian medicine ambiguously refer to channel Qi situations merely as "Qi stagnation" or "Not going through," with no qualifier to indicate whether the stagnant or blocked Qi in question is organ Qi, Zhong Qi, channel Qi, and so on.

---

[1] Su Wen, chapter 13, from *A Complete Translation of Nei-Jing and Nan-Jing* translated by Henry C. Lu, PhD; International College of Traditional Chinese Medicine of Vancouver, 2004; p. 114.

I, too, learned in school to use the word "Qi" in diagnoses without necessarily qualifying, or even knowing, whether or not the problem was originating from channel Qi, organ Qi, nutritive Qi, "upright Qi" and so on.

Looking back, this seems strange. After all, in the very first weeks of school, we had to memorize all the different *types* of Qi. But after that, with the exception of Wei Qi, we only rarely referred to the *types* of Qi in question while working on diagnosis.

During my decades of practicing the medicine, and particularly after meeting practitioners of Asian medicine from various cultures – some of whom *are* careful to specify the type of Qi that's problematic – I've learned that defining the type of Qi I'm working with is extremely helpful in communicating the diagnosis to others and avoiding incorrect conclusions.

For example, some people breezily refer to all stagnant or blocked Liver *channel* Qi problems merely as *liver* problems – leaving off the word "channel." Liver Qi and Liver channel Qi are two very different things:

Technically, the term "Liver Qi blocked (or stagnant)" implies the Qi of the liver *organ* is not moving correctly: which is to say, the liver's organ function (cleaning the blood) is impaired, or the blood's passageways through the liver itself are blocked. Not only does this phrase, "Liver Qi blockage" cause patients to worry about the condition of their liver, causing not a few of them to hie themselves to the doctor for a liver panel, this term is usually incorrect. In most cases of so-called "Liver Stagnation," the liver is perfectly functional – and the practitioner is using the wrong terminology. To be correct, the practitioner should say, the Liver's *channel* Qi is the problem.

In the same vein, some people refer to "Rebellious Stomach Qi" or "Rebellious Lung Qi" without specifying if the rebellion is in the stomach or lung *organs*, or if the rebellion is in the channel Qi of the Stomach or Lung *channels*. It is helpful to be specific: if the backwards movement is in the *channel* Qi, then the diagnosis is Rebellious *channel* Qi. But if an *organ* function is moving backwards, then the diagnosis is Rebellious Organ Qi. For example, coughing and vomiting are backwards motions of the lung and stomach *organs*, respectively.

These examples of terminology are merely presented here to show that, not only can one translate channel Qi findings, when applicable, into the argot of Asian medicine, but by using the adjective "channel," or any of the other qualifiers for Qi, one can make an Asian medicine diagnosis much, much more specific – and more useful.

Of course, a diagnosis may further benefit from even more specifics, such as "Rebellious channel Qi at such and such location, due to Blood Stagnation, which remains unhealed due to Shen disturbance."

But getting back to the main point, we can use the diagnostic lingo and "patterns" that we learn in school, and we can make them communicate far more information by using detail words like "channel Qi" or "organ Qi."

And *if* we know what the problem is with the channels, we can include, in the pattern diagnosis, information as to *where* on the channel the problem seems to be. A diagnosis should bring together as much information as possible.

Combining excess/deficiency and pattern diagnosis

If all channel scenarios are a combination of excess on one place, and deficiency in another, why not include both situations in the diagnosis? For example, instead of merely forming a diagnosis of "deficiency in the Large Intestine channel, warranting stimulation at LI-4," why not add "due to blockage (excess) between LU-7 and LI-4"?[1]

Forming a treatment plan gets easier if one appreciates the channel Qi deficiency problem and location, and the *causative* channel Qi excess problem and location.

The following case is a study in simultaneous excess and deficiency.

Case study #21

Epstein-Barr seen as both excess and deficient

A female, age 18, had been utterly sandbagged by a megalovirus known, in my youth, as mononucleosis, or mono, known as glandular fever in the UK, and more recently (in the 1970s), named Epstein-Barr disease.

By the time I was called over to her house to have a look at her, she'd had almost no energy for more than six months. According to her mother, she'd have spurts of energy every few days, during which she'd be able to sit up and chat, but she would become almost giddy, even giggling hysterically for an hour or two. These good days were followed by days when she could barely eat, speak, or get out of bed. On these days, she stared into space with a blank look on her face. The western medical doctors had said that bed rest was the only treatment – she would get better when she got better, and there was nothing else to be done about it.

I had only been certified for a few weeks when I started seeing her as in my new professional capacity of Licensed Acupuncturist. She had two distinct sets of pulses on each wrist. The superficial pulses were rapid, fluttery and extremely weak. At the same time, on the right side, a very, very deep, very slow, rumbling drum-beat about a finger's breadth directly beneath the superficial pulse seemed to be meting out the core energy that was keeping her alive.

Her tongue was pale and tooth marked.

Of course, with so much deficiency in her symptoms, tongue, and pulse, I started in with vigorous tonifying treatments, both acupuncture and herbs.

---

[1] When we needle LI-4 to get a strong jolt of channel Qi moving, that is exactly what we are treating: a mild blockage – one that arises easily and frequently – between LU-7 and LI-4. By needling LI-4, we drain channel Qi away from the blocked area and, hopefully, break up the blockage.

The purpose of the famous palms-up hand mudra which links the end of the thumb and the tip of the index finger, as when making the "OK" sign, is to implement the flow of Lung channel Qi into the LI channel via the parasympathetic mode, which is to say, through the finger tips. The LU-7 to LI-4 path is a strong way to get Qi moving, but it's also the path used predominantly if a person is *sympathetic* dominant. This path is also one that gets blocked easily if the consciousness is shifting into ego mode. That's why needling LI-4 is so effective for so many problems: when a person gets even a little out of sorts, mentally or physically, but there is no true emergency to deal with and the person tries to suppress (hide) his stress, that path is susceptible to getting a little blocked.

After more than a month of treatments and tonics, she was clearly getting worse. Her family was deeply concerned. I contacted Dr. Tin Lui, one of the most respected acupuncturists in California. He had taught, briefly, at the acupuncture school in Santa Cruz, and was a familiar name in the Santa Cruz acupuncture community. He was over seventy years old.

Dr. Tin Lui was willing to see her, so we made the hour and a half drive to Oakland. I helped carry her up the stairs and into Dr. Tin Lui's office.

Tin Lui spoke little English. I spoke little Chinese. The patient spoke not at all.

Tin Lui felt her pulse for a long time, and then cryptically said, "Emotion."

He put her on the treatment table and gently needled SP-9 on her left leg and LI-11 on her right arm.

I was puzzled. I'd only been out of school a few months, and wasn't thinking in terms of channel Qi. The two points he'd needled are famous for draining excess. At the time, with my limited understanding, I assumed that these points drained energy out of the body, making a person have less energy overall.

I now know that, technically, these points are effective when energy isn't flowing well in the lower leg or arm (moving slowly because of fluid or channel Qi phlegm residue from the pathogen, or even psychologically blocked: in either case, it's an excess condition in the lower half of the limbs). This stagnation can be incited to flow more easily (often described as "stagnation breaking up") when these knee and elbow points are needled. In other words, needles inserted into these two joint-located acupoints will *pull* on the sluggish, stagnant channel Qi (excess) in the upstream (closer to the hand or foot) part of the arm or leg. As some of that stagnant channel Qi in the lower arm or leg gets moving into the upper arm or leg, the congestion (excess) in the lower arm or leg is diminished. The electric attraction of the needle in the joint, just beyond the excess area, pulls some of that excess into the joint. Once the channel Qi has got into the joint, it can flow easily past the joint, and into the upper arm or leg.

The channel Qi sluggishness in the lower arm and leg, in her case, came from too much post-illness debris building up in these areas, causing electrical resistance in the sections of the channels that had to flow through the lower arms and legs: excess.

Thus, although needling these points encouraged a speeded up flow of energy in her upper arms and legs ("tonifying" the channel Qi flow in her upper arms and legs), the flow generated by these needles is *traditionally* thought of as "sedating" the excess in her lower leg and forearm. Again, these points are usually thought of as "sedating" an excess situation. But the excess is only in the lower limbs. The upper limbs have a deficiency. The so-called "sedation of excess" in the lower limbs could *just as easily* be referred to as tonification of the upper limbs.

Again: what we call sedation in one area could just as logically be referred to as tonification in another area: the area into which the channel Qi gets drained off.

But I didn't know that. I only knew that these points "sedated" a person.

And my patient didn't seem excessive to me. She was barely able to move. She couldn't speak louder than a muffled whisper, and yet, to me, it looked as if the doctor was trying to sedate her – which I still thought of as "make weaker." Was this doctor crazy? Why was he "sedating" my patient?

He only used these two needles, and he only left them in for five minutes. I was glad when he took the needles out. With my complete lack of understanding as to what "sedation" meant, I was afraid that if he sedated her much longer, there would be nothing left of her.

But the treatment wasn't finished.

He gently turned her onto her stomach, and massaged a warm (red flower) oil of his own recipe onto her back at UB-23 and vicinity. He then placed a thin piece of cloth over the oil and ignited a moxa burner (a 2-inch by 1-inch brass box with a wooden handle, with lots of air holes for the smoke to pour out after he lit the mugwort leaves he'd stuffed into the box). He rubbed the smouldering moxa burner back and forth over UB-23 area and environs for nearly ten minutes – she never exclaimed against what I thought must be excruciating heat. (Later, she told me that it hadn't even felt warm until the very end. Her back had been cold and numb.)

I was staring at him rubbing vigorously back and forth on her back with the moxa burner when it hit me: he wasn't just tonifying. Prior to this bit of tonification, he'd taken care to "sedate" an excess: which is to say, get Qi *moving* past a blockage.

Had it been due to my failure to "sedate" the excess that she'd had her bouts of hysterical giddiness? I'd been doing her harm by tonifying an excess condition!

Admittedly, she was very weak, so he'd only sedated the excess (drained the sluggish channel Qi) for a few minutes. He'd only used two of the many possible elbow and knee points, and he'd needled one of the two points on the right side only, and the other point on the left side only. He'd only left the needles in for a few minutes. This was extremely *minimal* "sedation," to be sure, but it was sedation, just the same. He had started by reducing an excess, not by tonifying. It took me a few minutes to wrap my head around this.

Though she appeared to me to be deficient, Dr. Tin Lui *began* her treatment by draining the hidden (hidden from *me*) excess.

Then, *after* the sedation, he began to tonify: he introduced powerful heat and channel Qi-moving moxa smoke and applied it for nearly ten minutes.

It was safe to tonify in this manner because he'd started the treatment by first draining the stagnation in her limbs. If he had only used moxa, without first sedating the excess, he would have been tonifying an excess condition – causing excess Qi to build up even more in her arms and legs, thus preventing channel Qi from getting to the head and torso. *That* type of build up was exactly what I'd been doing.

I hadn't realized that she'd had both an excess and a deficiency. What I know now is, there's almost always an excess and a deficiency. Except in conditions such as old-age weakness, physical exhaustion, severe blood loss or malnutrition – the types of conditions that we call *true* deficiency, excess and deficiency go together.

Although her utter lack of energy had been screaming "Weakness," to me, Dr. Tin Lui also heard a voice crying "Excess!" (Maybe when he'd said, "Emotion," he was pointing out to me the excess nature of her condition. Mental and emotional strains are always a form of excess. I will never know for certain why he said "Emotion." However, I have since observed that people under a high level of emotional stress sometimes have a far worse time of mono than people who, as soon as they get sick, are able to relax, go to bed, and stay there, while being waited on hand and foot.)

He started her treatment by draining the excess – making the channel Qi able to move past the blockages.

Watching him apply smoking moxa to her back, I was stunned as I realized all the implications of this treatment in which he treated first the excess and then the deficiency. I exclaimed with joy, "Brilliant!"

Dr. Tin Lui had been treating this case with great seriousness. But when I blurted out my stunned appreciation for his mixed treatment, in which he was treating both the channel Qi stagnation in Spleen and Large Intestine channels, and the subsequent Kidney channel Qi deficiency and related kidney organ weakness, he turned and smiled at me. I felt a wave of blessing pass from him to me.

After ten minutes with the moxa, the small room was filled with choking smoke. The patient turned her head to look at me, and she look slightly stronger.

I asked Dr. Tin Lui, "Gui Pi Tang?"

By this, I was asking if I should give her an extremely gentle herb formula named Gui Pi Tang, a formula that strengthens digestion, making it easier for a weak, malnourished person to absorb their nutrients. He shook his head as if I should have known better. So much for the blessings. My stupidity had clearly flung me into disfavor.

He said sternly, "Too strong!"

Now I didn't know *what* to think. If Gui Pi Tang, one of the mildest possible tonic formulas, was too strong, what could she possibly ingest?

As if in answer to my question, he said "Oatmeal. Only oatmeal. Honey OK. Small amount of oatmeal every time. All day."

I replied, without thinking of his language limits, "No one could possibly induce a teenager to eat nothing but oatmeal!"

The patient then spoke for the first time since I'd lugged her into the office. Softly, she murmured, "That sounds *good*."

That evening, I spoke with a fellow acupuncturist and told her about the oatmeal diet. She replied, "Brilliant! He's using the goopy, easy-to-digest muck from the oatmeal as a tonic, and the roughage from the oats will keep her bowels moving, keeping them as cool as possible. He's tonifying her with food while he's sedating her large intestine with roughage at the same time! "

"Oooh," I thought to myself. "Why didn't I think of that!"

Within a week the patient was sitting up, and when we went to see Dr. Tin Lui again, she was able to navigate his office stairs under her own steam. She added raisins to her oatmeal. Over the next few weeks she made daily, visible progress, and returned to school the next semester.

This case study shows that, even in a case of such glaring behavioral deficiency, in terms of channel Qi both excess and deficiency were in place. The real deficiency was in her

216

adrenal glands. Her Bladder and Kidney channel had become profoundly deficient during her illness, but they could not get back up to speed because of the build up of debris in her arms and legs. I noticed that, even though Dr. Tin Lui had tonified the Du, UB, and Kidney channels, by using moxa at UB-23 and environs, he had chosen sedation for the arm and legs points that did *not* directly increase flow into either the UB or KI channels: he hadn't used Small Intestine elbow points (which flow, after Yin Tang, into the UB channel), or Kidney knee points. In other words, he kept the sedation work far away from the tonification work.

And yet, overall, her system benefited from having some small amount of drainage, and some small amount of tonification.

Putting all the above into a "pattern" diagnosis, we might say the patient had stagnation (excess) in the lower parts of the arms and legs, especially in the lower limb parts of the Large Intestine and Spleen channels, creating a deficiency throughout the rest of those two channels, and the channels that derive from them: the Stomach and Heart. The deficiency in these two channels was depleting both appetite for life (Stomach) and joy of living (Heart). As the *consciousness* related to these two factors was diminished, the Ren (physical strength, guided primarily by consciousness) and Du (strength of pure consciousness) channels were inhibited.

To reactivate the will to live, tonifying the Will to Live (Gate of Fire) at UB-23 would be the most direct approach, once the blockages had been loosened up. Also, the UB channel is the farthest removed, in terms of sequence, from the two channels that were most blocked.

Or, to shorten it, the diagnosis was Stagnation in channel Qi just prior to SP-9 and LI-11, and channel Qi deficiency everywhere else, including at the Gate of Fire.

As an aside, Dr. Tin Lui must have been very concerned about her. Four days after her first treatment, a few bags containing two *very* mild, Qi-moving herbs (*not* tonics) showed up in my mailbox with a note. A woman from Santa Cruz had been in Oakland to see Tin Lui, and he'd asked her to deliver these herbs to me, for "the girl."

I sent word back to Tin Lui, through this woman, that the girl was improving, and I would always be deeply grateful for the huge lesson he had taught me. I am grateful that writing this book gives me the opportunity to pay homage to this brilliant, warm-hearted doctor.

The importance of feeling pulses

Veering sharply off the subject of excess and deficiency, this case also gives me a chance to discuss the extreme importance of learning to feel pulses.

When I first started studying Chinese medicine, I made an utter pest of myself by constantly feeling the pulses of family members, friends, neighbors, members of the PTA: anyone I could get my hands on. By the time I was licensed, I don't think there was anyone in the immediate neighborhood who had escaped my grip.

The patient in the above case study was a neighbor. I dropped in on her nearly every day during her illness, and felt her pulses every time.

Her right-hand pulse was peculiar. I might best describe it as two pulses. At the more superficial level, the pulse was extremely rapid, thin, and floating. But just below this flashy pulse, a very weak, slow, steady, drumbeat. The lower beat was a completely different tempo from the upper one. It was extremely slow, and seemed utterly unrelated to heart rate. It seemed to be coming from somewhere deep beneath the earth, something primitive, ancient, and not related to her conscious self. I'd never felt anything like it.

I must have felt her "mono pulse" many dozens of times.

Just a few months after my experiences with her at Tin Lui's office, I got the benefit of all that pulse taking. My home phone rang at ten o'clock on a bleak November night. The nice young man who worked at the local auto shop, who did the tune-ups on my car, was on the line. The last time I'd been to the shop, I'd chatted with him for quite a while about the relative strengths of both Asian and western medicines.

He blurted out, "My mother is dying. The regular doctors can't help her anymore. You're a different kind of doctor. Can you please help her?"

What could I say? I hadn't been practicing very long, really, but I felt I had to attend. I drove to the other side of town...

Case study #22

"Can you save my mother's life?"

The atmosphere in the apartment was hushed. My patient was lying on the living room sofa. She looked to be about 40 years old and looked as if she'd been athletic prior to her recent decline. Now, she was pale, very thin, with shallow breathing, not moving, not talking. Her relatives, gathered in the room, had flown in from out of state because she was dying. They spoke Russian, not English. Her husband spoke broken English, but the son's English was excellent. Supposedly, the mother spoke very good English, but she was not speaking at all. I had no idea what to do. I stood there, stupidly looking around, when the son spoke up: "Can you save my mother's life?"

My heart was breaking for him, but my inclination was to say, "I don't know what to do here, take this woman to the hospital," so that I could get out of there as quickly as possible. Instead, in an attempt to show respect to the son and to the situation, I decided to behave like a doctor for a few minutes, prior to sending her to the emergency room. I pulled a chair over to the sofa, and started feeling her pulses.

I asked the son for her recent medical history, and kept my hand on her right-hand pulse, though I wasn't paying much attention to the pulse. I was more focused on the history that he told me.

Four months earlier, back in August, she'd been feeling depressed. This was unlike her, so she'd seen a doctor. Because she claimed to have no emotional issues, the doctor diagnosed her as having "chemical depression," and prescribed Zoloft. After two weeks of taking the Zoloft, she started feeling light headed and dizzy. The doctor decided that she probably had some heart problems, so he prescribed her a beta-blocker. Within a month, she was extremely weak, wobbly and couldn't stand up. The doctor prescribed an additional antidepressant.

After that, she'd quickly gone downhill. For the last few weeks, she'd been lying on the sofa, unable to move, with no interest in food or talking. It had been three months since she'd begun her decline.

218

The family was not going to take her to the doctor again, because the doctor clearly had not helped. It was obvious that there was nothing left for the doctor to do.

They were all watching me, expectant. I had no idea what to do. I was terrified. I wanted to flee. But I was bent on going through the motions of being a medical professional, to show I was giving the case my best shot. I nodded in what I hoped was an intelligent manner, and continued to feel the pulse. By now, I'd already been pretending to feel that right-side pulse for nearly ten minutes. After he'd told me everything he knew, no one spoke. I needed to keep my mind busy while making a show of feeling the pulse. So my thoughts started to ramble. My late-night thoughts scooted around in a dozen directions having nothing to do with the dying patient.

Just about the same time that my mind was saying, "It's late, but Safeway's still open. I can pick up stuff for the kid's sandwiches on the way home..." I suddenly heard my own brain interrupt my thoughts: "You've felt this pulse before!" I silently said to my brain, "Huh?" The memory sector of my brain repeated its message: "You've felt this pulse before!" I started paying some attention to the pulse.

By letting my mind wander, I'd been able to let my deeper level of consciousness kick in. I've since used this wandering-mind technique of pulse diagnosis now and again, sometimes with good results. But when I brought my mind back to bear on the pulse, I realized I *could* feel something that I hadn't noticed before. She had two pulses. One was floating and very weak and thin and rapid, and the other was deep, somber, slow, like a death-knell drum. My subconscious mind made the connection.

I exclaimed to the assembled crowd, "She's not dying! She has mono!!" They looked at each other. The son looked at me, baffled. "Huh?"

I told him that she had been misdiagnosed, and she had a treatable illness. I asked him to translate for me, and I started to grill the whole family using the son as translator. Did anyone remember how she'd been doing in *August*, when she'd first felt so tired? Had she had a *cough* in August? I imitated the peculiar mono cough. Her mother spoke up, "*Da!*" The mother recalled that she'd had that cough while talking on the telephone. I asked of the husband, "Had her skin been slightly yellow? Had her throat glands been sore in August?"

With every question, I got a "Yes" reply. As I continued asking questions about symptoms of mono, and getting "yes" each time, it was clear that I had picked up on something. I could feel the family's hope rising.

I explained, through the son, this woman had a bad infectious illness in August. She had been *sick*, not depressed. The antidepressant had forced her into parasympathetic mode, when she had needed to be 1) in bed, and 2) in sympathetic mode, to fight the illness. By taking the drive-inhibiting drugs, she'd allowed the infection to get deeper into her system. She'd felt weaker because of the Zoloft. Next, when the doctor gave her the beta-blocker, inhibiting her *heart*'s ability to support sympathetic mode, she was even more susceptible to the profound weakness that this pathogen can induce, if bed rest is not immediately applied. Finally, the second layer of antidepressants had pushed her over the edge: she could no longer move.

I instructed the family, she must stop taking those drugs. They were killing her. At this point, she spoke weakly, for the first time, saying, "The drugs are the only thing keeping me alive." I told her she could keep taking one drug, any drug, but that the other two would have to go. She chose the Zoloft. (I no longer advise anyone as to prescription medications.

Legally, as an acupuncturist, I am breaking the law if I even make prescriptive *suggestions or comments* about pharmaceuticals to a patient or *to an MD*.)

Next, I tried to explain a little about this very common illness to the family. It turns out, mono is *uncommon* in Russia. Oppositely, in the USA, testing of military recruits suggests that 95% of the population has been exposed to mono by age 18. Maybe the bug doesn't survive well in Russian winters. At any rate, no one in the well-educated Russian family was familiar with this illness – but the America-raised son thought he might have heard of it.

I knew what to do. I gave her the same needle treatment I'd learned from Dr. Tin Lui, but I didn't have any moxa with me. Instead, I rubbed her back at UB-23 with as much warmth as I could muster. I told them to put her on the oatmeal diet. They were extremely dubious. I could tell that their faith in my idea was waning.

I was desperate to make them believe me. I exclaimed, "You must feed her a small amount of kasha every hour, and I will treat her every day, with needles and moxa. *In one week*, she will be walking!"

My confidence level encouraged them. A week later, family members burst into tears as she very slowly got up from the bed and, for the first time, walked the length of the hall, to greet them.

After that, my patient continued to see me once a week, for two months. I asked her to get blood work done, to check for a recent mono infection. I was stunned when she reported back, "My doctor refuses to test me for that." I told her to demand a test. Again, the doctor refused. I instructed her to say, "I will sue you if you don't test me." So he tested her. After a month, he still hadn't called her with the results, and the nurses would not tell her the results. I asked her to, once again, threaten a lawsuit. After making this threat, she was finally given the results: the tests showed that she'd had mono, and *recently*.

The doctor had clearly been afraid of a lawsuit from his glaring misdiagnosis of her original problem. But he should not have been. In this country, mono at age 40 is very rare. It is a teenager's disease, in this country, and so it was understandable that the MD had missed the diagnosis.

And now for the point of all this: if I had not felt pulses every chance I got, I too would have missed the diagnosis. What with the obscuring effects of the medications, I could not easily make sense of her tongue and symptoms. Her pulse, and pulse alone, had told me exactly what she had. We were lucky, in that regard. She was too exhausted to have any ability to mentally "disguise" her pulse. And I was lucky when I stopped paying attention to her pulse and, instead, pondered on whether Safeway was open 24 hours.

There is no way that I would have guessed "mono!" based on words like "wiry, slippery, deep," and so on. Only because I had already felt that particular pulse dozens of times, and knew exactly what that pulse signified, was I able to use that particular bit of pulse knowledge.

So, even though I've stated that pulse is usually, for most practitioners of Asian medicine, a highly inexact, overly generalized, and often misleading, method of diagnosis, you *must* still practice feeling pulses. Don't try too hard to assess them. Don't think about whether they are wiry, or what slippery feels like. Just *feel* them. Thousands of them.

Even if you "only" save one life by virtue of recognizing a peculiar pulse, you've done something brilliant. *Do* keep feeling pulses. *Do* learn to read tongues. Don't worry if you don't know what you're feeling or seeing. Just keep feeling pulses and looking at tongues, accumulating subconscious memories.

Summary

When channel Qi runs awry, both excess and deficient areas of channel Qi are present. In nearly all cases, the overall amount of channel Qi in the system holds steady. There is no absolute excess or deficiency. The channel Qi is always being replenished, via wave energy entering the body, and is always being converted into matter, as needed. Any excess is always being released out of the body in the form of static, via the fingers and toes and to a lesser extent, through the rest of the skin.

In terms of basic, pure channel energy, there is always conservation of energy. Unless a person is suffering from a *true* deficiency, an actual absence of some crucial life-providing substance, he will have *both* excess and deficiency of channel Qi flow.

His problems come about if the *distribution* of channel Qi has become stuck or otherwise aberrant: not going through. The stuck, or slow, place is the site where channel Qi is building up or even getting tangled, congealing: conditions we call excess. The resultant failure to go through *correctly* creates the subsequent deficiency somewhere else.

"Perseverance is more prevailing than violence; and many things which cannot be overcome when they are together, yield themselves up when taken little by little"

Plutarch's Lives ; Sertorius

Chapter twelve

Treating scar tissue with acupuncture

Introduction

The non-conductivity of scar tissue renders it a significant impediment to the flow of channel Qi. In many cases, scar tissue can prevent the flow of Qi and may contribute to health problems. Needling scar tissue correctly may reduce the density of the keloid tissue and may reduce related health problems.

While other impediments to the flow of channel Qi are usually discussed in schools of Asian medicine, scar tissue is often not mentioned. Therefore, this chapter and the next will discuss scar tissue in depth.

Be aware that the acupuncture academic community is divided on the subject of whether or not scar tissue should be needled. Due to fluctuating historical and political trends in Asian medicine, various schools of thinking now co-exist. Some practitioners of Asian medicine say that scar tissue must be needled. Others say that scars should never be needled. Some say that scar tissue poses no energetic problem, and doesn't *need* to be needled, but, if the scarring is at an acupoint location, that acupoint can be needled, if needed; the scar tissue in this case should be treated as if it were normal skin.

The academic differences on the scar tissue question are inherently related to the ongoing academic debate regarding the existence of channels. After all, if channel Qi really doesn't exist, then scar tissue can't be blocking the flow of channel Qi.

Apropos this issue, I enjoyed hearing, twice in one year, revealing statements by famous Chinese acupuncturists who were visiting the American acupuncture school where I teach. Both doctors said, at some point in their lectures (I paraphrase), "For this health condition, you should consider needling either of these two adjacent points, both of which are on the same channel. It doesn't really matter which of the two points you use, or if you locate the point exactly according to the book. The most important thing is that you get the needle somewhere on the *channel*."

At each of the two lectures, in immediate response to the professor's clear statement about needle contact with the *channel* being more crucial than the exact location of the acupoint, I raised my hand and asked, "Do channels exist?"

The response, in both instances, was a quick and adamant. "No! There is no such thing as a channel!"

I had to wonder if, even from their safe podium in the US, these doctors were worried about the political fallout and damage to their careers should the Chinese authorities somehow discover that these doctors were referring to the officially disproved concept of channels.

Getting back to the point, the measurable physiological events that can occur in the vicinity of unhealed scar tissue or in the aftermath of scar tissue treatment, in many cases, seem to validate (politically incorrect) channel theory. Therefore, these events are necessarily controversial from the academic-political perspective.

Let the academic and historical arguments continue, by all means. As the Chinese once took pride in saying, "Let a hundred flowers blossom, let a hundred schools contend." Of course, this was in the Hundred Schools period, the period of five hundred years prior to the snuffing of all political dissent during the self-named "Great Unification" of approximately 221 BC. After the "Great Unification," the glorious age of great philosophical inquiry and debate, the "Hundred Schools," was renamed the "Warring States" period, as a means of justifying the carnage wrought during the "unification."

I like to think that, at least in the USA, we are once again able to debate openly as to the value or need of needling scar tissue. And while we do so, I vote that people who have health problems that stem from or are augmented by the blockage of Channel Qi due to scar tissue can and should be treated.

This chapter includes case studies from my own practice that suggest some of the objective, measurable benefits and risks of needling scar tissue.

My introduction to needling scar tissue

The first time I needled into a patient's scar tissue, I had a hard time inserting the tine into her dense, rubbery scar. I bent and ruined several slender needles trying to get them into the keloidal tissue, the residue from a childhood surgery. Finally, using my thickest and shortest needle with a lot of wristy follow-through, I got a needle through the wall of scar tissue. My patient, felt a terrifying, *slicing* pain *cutting* through her skin, a pain *not* consistent with the pricking insertion of my needle. She broke into a cold sweat and her eyes rolled up into her head.

I assumed that she was experiencing needle shock, a phenomenon that occurs on rare occasions. I repositioned the heat lamp closer to her feet, laid a towel over her to keep her warm, and did not insert any more needles.

She quickly came back to full alertness, but was slightly shaky for the rest of the one-hour session. The next day, completely restored to calmness, she dropped in to my office with a story to share.

A few hours after her acupuncture treatment, she had uncontrollably re-experienced her childhood surgery. The memory was so realistic that she felt she was in two places at once: she was simultaneously sitting in her apartment and she was on a gurney in the hospital. She was not *remembering* being on the gurney: she was *on* the gurney. She could feel the

224

cold hard pressure of the gurney on her back, she could feel the thin sheet over her bare skin. Her nostrils filled with the smells of the surgery room, and then with the smell of the anesthesia. Her eyes were simultaneously seeing the walls of her living room and the corridors of the hospital as she was wheeled on the gurney. Her ears were hearing her home radio and the conversations of the hospital staff. Her heart was pounding with terror.

She momentarily feared that she was going crazy, but the two-places-at-once experience ended after about ten minutes. She was so shaken by the seeming hospital visit that she called her mother even though it was mid-afternoon on a weekday. She asked her mom to confirm details about the surgery, the appearance of the doctor, and all of the surgery-related events that she had just experienced in what had seemed like "real time." Some of the events of her recall were not in her *conscious* memory – including sensations and conversations that had occurred while she was presumably unconscious from anesthesia.

This had been my first experience with needling scar tissue. I had been hoping to stimulate the Qi flow through an acupuncture point, a point that just happened to be located on her old surgery scar.

I had been as supremely confident in my ability to "first, do no harm" as only a newly licensed acupuncturist can be. So when, following her acupuncture treatment, she momentarily thought she was going crazy and experienced fear, pain, and other unexpected sensory effects, I wondered what I had done wrong. I did not, at that time, suspect that *my* needling of her scar tissue had anything to do with her hospital memories. I reviewed her case notes:

Case study #23

Kidney troubles following childhood ureter surgery

The patient was a twenty-seven year old female with frequent kidney and bladder infections. She had been born with a bifurcated ureter: the tube coming off her right kidney broke into two branches, both of which connected to the bladder. One of the bifurcating branches was extremely narrow. When she was young, the narrower ureter was a frequent site of infection: therefore it was surgically removed when she was seven years old.

When she came to see me for help with her recurring kidney infections, the surgical scar was still visible: a nasty, reddish, tough gash of scar tissue several inches long and about half an inch wide running across her lower abdomen. The scar started at a point several inches below the belly button and extended laterally for several inches, heading over towards the right hip.

I wished to needle the Bladder-regulating acupoint on the Ren channel (the channel that runs up the front of the torso, neck and face, from the pubic bone up to the lower lip). The Bladder-regulating acupoint on the Ren channel is located on a spot that, in her case, was traversed by her surgical scar. I decided to insert a needle into the acupoint despite the scar tissue.

Being only recently graduated from a Master's program in basic Asian medicine, I was only mildly aware of the somewhat obscure controversy around whether or not scar tissue should ever be needled. Carefree and confident, I attempted to pop the needle into her "Front Mu of the Bladder" acupoint. I planned to slide the needle right through the scar tissue and into the tissue beneath. I assumed that she would have the usual fleeting and minimal sensation of needle penetration, and then she would relax and take a nap with the needle in place.

She had not had the "usual" sensations, nor had she experienced the normal, relaxing sequelae of needling.

Then again, after the treatment, her kidney pain had ceased. The presumed infection cleared up overnight.

Hypothesis

Since this first event, I've seen many similar instances where needling scar tissue caused the patient to experience a pain consistent with the sensation of the original injury. I've also seen instances in which the patient had been numb in the area of the scar, and regained feeling after the scar was treated.

Most doctors assume that the numbness in the vicinity of a scar is caused by nerve damage. The nerve was cut at the time of injury. However, this idea does not hold up. If this were the case, a person should have numbness in the area of the scar, and in all areas inferior or distal to the scar.

Instead, based on what I've seen, I propose that scar tissue occurs when a person has an injury that must be healed quickly. The body throws down a mat of crisscrossed, strong fibers, because it can't take the time to do the job right. *At the same time*, the trauma that caused the scar tissue also causes a matching black-out in that portion of the mind that registers sensation for that exact area.

In other words, when channel Qi ceases to be able to flow in a specific, injured spot, the parallel channel Qi system in the brain that pays attention to that spot is also denied flow of energy.

If, subsequent to healing, a person revisits the scar and the scar-producing event via massage, acupuncture, cupping (in some cases), meditation, and so on, channel Qi will be restored to both the memory and the injured tissues.

Scar tissue is non-conductive. Channel Qi cannot flow through scar tissue. It makes sense that the associated *mental* bit of energy becomes blocked when the channel Qi in the injury area becomes blocked. In fact, we have to wonder which blockage comes first.

If the pain of an event causes the mind to temporarily block out its awareness of its associated body part, it may be that the subsequent lack of channel Qi guidance in the area causes the body to form random tissue (scarring). We can hypothesize that a person of great spiritual calm, who is able to experience a traumatic injury without "shutting down" the part of the brain that registers the experience, will also be able to consciously direct healing in such a way that no scar tissue forms.

Certainly, we see that, by processing (treating) the scar tissue, some patients are then also able to process pain that was hidden, that was not yet experienced, that was hiding in their minds.

Then again, many scar tissue patients do *not* experience flashbacks or memories of trauma.

The reason for the warnings?

I have to wonder if the ancient injunctions against needling scar tissue are related to the "crazy" mental recall of injury such as that experienced by this patient. During her recall phase, she had thought she was going crazy. The Chinese were very wary of anything that looked like "Shen disturbance" (craziness). Historically, it is very possible that some Chinese doctor decided that scar tissue should not be needled, following some patient's "crazy" recall of trauma.

Also, the sensations experienced when scar tissue is needled don't always "make sense." If a person, while having scar tissue needled, feels the slice of a surgeon's knife, or feels a burn, when he *should* be feeling only a mild needling sensation, this too suggests Shen disturbance.

Case study #24

"Incurable Crohn's disease" and a history of appendectomy

In my second year of practice, I saw a thirty-one year old woman who had recently been diagnosed with Crohn's disease (inflammation in the large bowel – an incurable condition). She was changing jobs and feared that her new work-based insurance company would consider her Crohn's to be a "pre-existing condition," so that her Crohn's-related problems would not be covered by insurance.

She asked me if acupuncture might be helpful in easing the symptoms of Crohn's, even though the condition was incurable. I didn't know for certain that I could help, but offered to give it a try. This was several years before I'd learned to feel channel Qi.

As part of the diagnostic process, I palpated her abdomen through her shirt and noticed a deep indentation on the right side. I asked if I might look at her belly. She warned me that it wasn't pretty, but I was welcome to look.

She had a huge scar on the right side of her abdomen. I asked her if I was looking at an appendectomy scar. She replied that, at age six, she'd been diagnosed with appendicitis. The doctors had opened up the abdomen and found nothing wrong. However, a few days after the surgery, she had another bout of severe abdominal pain. The doctor reopened the abdomen near the original incision site and found a raging infection. The infection was cleaned out and the incision site re-sewn. Several weeks later, she was hospitalized with very high fever. The abdomen was opened again at yet another location. The appendix was inflamed and the infection had spread to the sides of her uterus and one ovary. The appendix and ovary were removed, the uterus was scraped clean and scrubbed with antibiotics, the abdominal cavity was cleansed, and she was sewn back up again.

The infection never returned, but the incision sites had not healed neatly. Instead, the taut and abruptly indented scar tissue on her abdomen suggested that adhesions had formed between the skin layer and some reproductive and/or abdominal organs.

I inquired about her other health conditions. She told me that her periods had been excruciatingly painful all her life. She was very healthy, in general: she was a brilliant skier, competed at a semi-professional level in Tennis, and had a college degree in Physical Education. Even so, she often fainted during her periods and had regularly missed school or work because of severe menstrual pain.

Because of the menstrual pain, she had been put on birth control pills during her early-teen years. She stopped taking birth control pills in her mid-twenties because of her concern about continual hormone therapies.

When she was a teen she had been told that, due to her menstrual and uterine problems, she could never have children. So when she stopped taking birth control pills, she and her husband did not feel the need to use another system of birth control. They had no children.

She also had a "delicate stomach." She ate tiny meals, and only ate very mild food. She could be incapacitated from intestinal pain if she ate a bit too quickly or a bit too much. Recently, her "delicate stomach" had become "delicate intestines." Just before coming to see me, she'd seen an MD about her increasingly poorly controlled, painful, bloody stools. He had diagnosed her with Incurable Crohn's.

Crohn's is sometimes attributed to emotional fragility. I had known this patient for years before she came to me with her intestinal trouble, and she was *not* emotionally fragile. Her robust energy was combined with a glorious sense of humor.

I had treated several problematic scars since my early days with that first scar-tissue patient, so I assumed I was ready for anything. But when I first beheld her abdominal scars, I tried to hide my shock and my concern at the extent of the scarring.

I had not yet seen any scar tissue with this degree of adhesions. (I have since seen far worse scars in terms of diameter and general ghastliness, but none in which the skin of the abdomen was pulled so tightly down to the internal organs, making one side of the abdomen look caved in.)

Whether or not the scarring was the cause of the Crohn's or even a contributing factor, I could not begin to guess. I had not yet learned how to detect the flow (or non-flow) of channel Qi with my hands, so I did not determine if the channel Qi of the abdomen was impeded. But I was pretty sure that scar wasn't helping matters. Due to her extremely delicate stomach, she did not think she could handle the Damp-Heat herbs that are sometimes used to treat intestinal problems such as Crohn's.

I decided to needle the scar.

Her scar was not a neat, straight line. The center of the scarred area was over an inch in diameter, and rays of scar tissue stretched out from the center in several directions. There was no one "line" to bisect.

I decided to start by traversing the diameter of the scar at its widest part. A half-inch needle could not traverse the diameter of the scar, so I used a "threading technique" in which a series of needles is inserted in a linear pattern.

Threading technique

In threading technique, a series of needles can be inserted in such a way as to behave like a much longer needle, of small-angle insertion. For example, several half-cun needles ("cun," pronounced "soon" or "tsoon," means "inch") or several one-cun needles can be threaded in such a way as to traverse three or four inches of skin – giving the same effect as if one had used a four-cun needle. A four-cun needle is unwieldy. A half-cun needle allows for excellent control. The first needle is inserted almost to the hilt using a small angle insertion

(in which the under-the-skin needle shaft is as close as possible to parallel to the surface of the skin.)

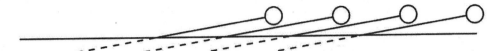

Fig. 12.1 "Threaded" needles

The length of the needle does not go deep down into the underlying tissue, but travels just below the skin. The second needle is inserted directly over the place where the tip of the first needle has come to rest under the skin, again using a small angle. The second needle is also inserted almost to the hilt, bringing the effective "tip" of the combined needles farther along than might have been reached with only one needle.

The third needle is inserted over the resting point of the tip of the second needle, and so on. By "threading" the needles, a line of needles can traverse an area several inches wide even if short, half-inch or one-inch needles are used.

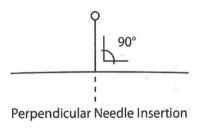

Perpendicular Needle Insertion

Fig. 12.2 "Small-angle" insertion, and comparisons with other insertion angles.

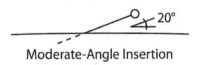

Moderate-Angle Insertion

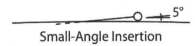

Small-Angle Insertion

Getting back to the patient with Chrohn's

In treating this case study's patient, eight half-inch needles were needed to traverse the widest part of the scar. I also traversed the scar at many other, narrower locations. I used the needles to recreate what should have been lines of channel Qi flowing over her abdomen.

I treated her once a week for four weeks. I repeated the original needling each time. The deep indentation of the abdomen became steadily less severe. When I saw her the fourth time, the taut, stretched scar tissue had definitely begun to soften. It had lost some of its red, shiny and fibrous appearance. Her digestive problems had begun to ease after the first week. Her next menstrual period was much less painful. A few weeks after the four treatments, I saw her again, socially, but did not treat her again. She assured me that her health was steadily improving.

A month after our first session, she asked me if she should get regular colonoscopies so that she could follow any changes occurring in her large intestine. Concerned about the insurance implications that might occur if her scans showed even a receding level of inflammation, I suggested that she not have any scans for at least six months, so that the gut had time to finish the healing that apparently was now under way.

I also suggested that she find a new gastroenterologist to work with; her previous GI (gastrointestinal) specialist might have a hard time admitting that he'd made a "mistake" when he'd diagnosed her with an incurable illness. Of course, he had not made a mistake of diagnosis. His mistake was in thinking that Crohn's is incurable. However, I have seen repeatedly the following cultural phenomenon: if an "incurable" disease is successfully treated and goes away, the MD can then be blamed for having misdiagnosed the illness – even if the actual diagnosis *had* been correct. And some MDs, possibly because of our lawsuit-happy population, are hesitant to admit to diagnostic error. And so I suggested that she go to a new doctor for her follow-up colonoscopy.

Six months after her first treatment, six months after her diagnosis with "incurable Crohn's disease," she had her first intestinal scan under the auspices of a new GI doc. There was no sign of any inflammation or disease process. She informed the doctor prior to the scan that, although a previous doctor had suggested a diagnosis of Crohn's disease to explain a bout of intestinal trouble, her intestinal pain and bleeding had long since stopped, and that her bowel movements were once again regular and healthy.

The doctor wrote on her chart that any previous diagnosis of Crohn's was obviously incorrect: clearly, she had only had a passing intestinal infection; she had never had Crohn's disease. Her insurance worries were over.

I want to emphasize that Crohn's disease is *not* always caused by childhood surgery, nor am I suggesting that needling scar tissue is the way to treat all cases of Crohn's. In *this* case, the Qi blockage from scar tissue may have contributed to her body's steadily decreasing ability to maintain healthy physiology in her abdomen. But, as always in Asian medicine, the doctor needs to figure out what is causing the decline in health in the individual, the root cause of the disease pattern. The original underlying *causes* of even very common disease patterns such as irritable bowel or Crohn's disease may be somewhat unique to each individual.

Getting back to this case study, it may be that, in this patient's case, the severe blockages of Qi flow in her abdominal region evidently played a part in her increasingly weak digestion, her painful periods, and her intestinal degeneration. The scar, or to be more specific, the channel Qi disruption resulting from her mass of nonconductive scar tissue, may have contributed to that blockage.

Several years after I first treated this patient, she gave birth to a beautiful baby boy.

The value of treating scar tissue

These two case studies demonstrate how helpful the treatment of scar tissue can be. I have met acupuncturists who insist that channel Qi – if there is such a thing – is not impeded by scar tissue. This is correct inasmuch as the causal and astral currents *can* penetrate scar tissue. However, the other three types of current, which use electrons as the basis for their currents, can only flow through this non-conductive area with difficulty. Possibly more significant, so long as the parallel obstruction in the mind is still in place, the causal and astral currents will not flow correctly past the area occluded by the scar tissue.

But despite the differing opinions on the subject, I have seen lasting improvements in the flow of channel Qi, and the diminishing of troublesome symptoms, in response to direct treatment of scar tissue. Even more compelling, it's easy to *feel* the channel Qi blockages that are created by scar tissue. It's also easy to *feel* that the blockages cease following direct treatment of a scar.

"One should observe minute and trifling things as if they were of normal size; and when they are thus treated they cannot become dangerous"[1]

Chapter thirteen

Scar tissue needling techniques

Needle size

When you first start needling scar tissue, you will find that most of your needles bend and kink when they hit the "wall" of rubbery, tough scar tissue. These needles must be discarded. To combat this textural resistance, use the thickest, and the shortest needles that you have on hand. If you only have 36 gauge needles, consider buying one or two boxes of the thicker 32 gauge, just to use on scar tissue.

Even when using thicker, shorter needles, penetrating scar tissue requires a very steady hand and strong control of the needle. If one's concentration wavers and the scar is really tough, even the short, thicker needle will bend and kink up, becoming unusable, when it hits the subdermal wall of keloid tissue. The bent needle must be discarded. One has to start over. If you simply cannot penetrate through the scar, but you can get needles a small distance into the keloidal tissue, just leave the needles there, as far in as you can get. Even this tiny amount of penetration may provide some benefit. A week later, during the next session, you may find the scar has softened up just a bit, so that subsequent needling is easier.

Insertion depth

Insert the needle into healthy skin about a quarter of an inch away from the scar, to a depth of an eighth to a quarter of an inch or so. Then, keeping the tip of the needle under the skin and after lowering the needle handle to a position almost touching the skin surface (so that the needle is nearly parallel to the skin, or at a "small angle"), slowly advance the subcutaneous needle tip into the scar tissue, approaching the scar tissue from the side instead of trying to perforate it from the top. The needle depth does not necessarily ever go deeper than the original eighth or quarter of an inch or so: the needle shaft, underneath the skin, stays more or less parallel to the surface of the skin plane.

You do not need to go *beneath* the scar tissue – go *through* the scar tissue.

---

[1] Su Wen, book 2, from *The Yellow Emperor's Classic of Internal Medicine*, translated by Ilza Veith, 2002, University of California Press, Berkeley, p. 124

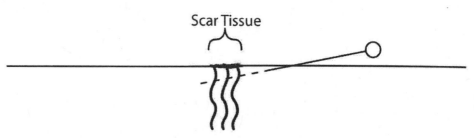

Fig. 13.1 The needle enters into healthy tissue, perforates the scar tissue, then rests in the healthy tissue on the other side of the scarring. This creates a hole through the scar tissue, along the sides of which the channel Qi will be able to flow.

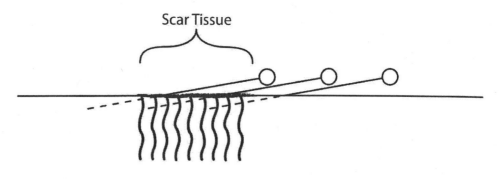

Fig. 13.2   If the scar is too wide to be straddled with a single needle, threaded needles can be applied. So long as the first needle is inserted into healthy tissue and the last needle perforates through to healthy tissue, the channel Qi will be able to get through. The channel Qi will make the very tiny jumps from one needle to the next, thus traveling the full width of the scar.

Scar tissue can be very difficult to needle into; it is usually easier to use several very short, easily controlled needles, instead of trying to get a long (several inches) needle through the keloid tissue.

Choosing sides
    If the needle is inserted on the downstream side of the scar, the patient will usually experience no sensation, or only a mild sensation. This makes sense: downstream from the scar the patient usually has a small, channel Qi-free zone – and the resulting numbness.

234

Oppositely, if the needle is inserted on the upstream side of the scar tissue, the patient will usually experience a momentary, unpleasant shock of electrical pain. This results from needling into an area that is blocked and excessive: using the needle to attract, or "call" channel Qi into an area that's already congested (excess).

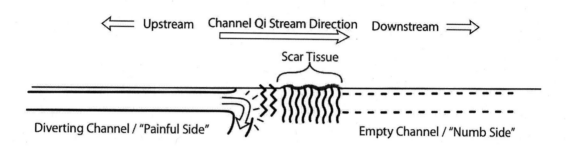

Fig. 13.3   The upstream side of the scar tissue is the painful side. The downstream side of the scar tissue is the numb side.

When needling scar tissue, the needle (or the collection of threaded needles) must form a bridge from healthy skin on one side of the scar into healthy skin on the other side of the scar. Channel Qi will be able to stream along the metal needle, opening a route through which blocked channel Qi can flow.

Do not cause the patient any unnecessary pain: insert the needle into the side of the scar that is deficient. Push the needle through the tough, rubbery, keloid scar tissue, and keep pushing until the needle penetrates the healthy skin on the other side of the scar.

After the needle contacts the healthy skin on the upstream side of the scar and the channel Qi immediately starts to flow, the patient often feels a rush of coolness, or "running water," or something best expressed in terms of "flowing," into the area that had been numb, on the downstream side of the scar.

Example: C-section scars
A C-section scar often bisects many channels: Ren, Kidney, Stomach, and sometimes Spleen, Liver, and even Gallbladder.

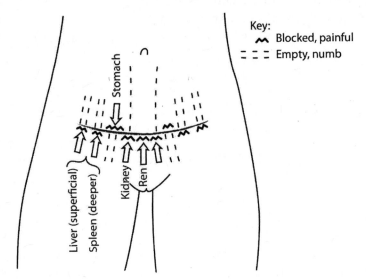

Fig. 13.4 Showing the directions of the channels that bisect a "bikini cut" C-section scar. The wide band of numbness, and possibly diminished channel Qi flow, located superior to the scar, spanning the the frontal midline includes the Ren channel *and* the left- and right-side Kidney channels.

The Ren channel runs from the crotch to the head. Therefore, the scar will have an area of excess on the inferior (farther from the head) side of the scar, and an area of deficiency on the superior (closer to the head) side of the scar.

This excess and deficiency can usually be felt by hand.

I usually start needling a C-section scar at the center, along the Ren channel, and work my way laterally.

The needle bridging the scar tissue along the Ren channel should be inserted on the deficient side: the superior side of the scar. The needle should then be worked through the scar, emerging into the healthy, but excessively charged, tissue on the inferior side of the scar.

The Kidney channels run in the same direction as the Ren. Therefore, the needles bridging the blocked Kidney channels should also be inserted on the superior (deficient) side of the scar.

However, the next needles to be inserted will bridge the blocked Stomach channels. The Stomach channels run from head to foot – the opposite direction of the Ren and Kidney channels. Therefore, the channel-Qi deficient area of the Stomach channels will be on the *inferior* side of the scar. The superior side of the scar, in the Stomach channel areas, will be excessive. Insert the needle into the deficient area, on the *inferior* side, and work it through to the superior side.

By always inserting the needles into the deficient side, you avoid 1) tonifying an excess condition, 2) causing unnecessary pain to the patient.

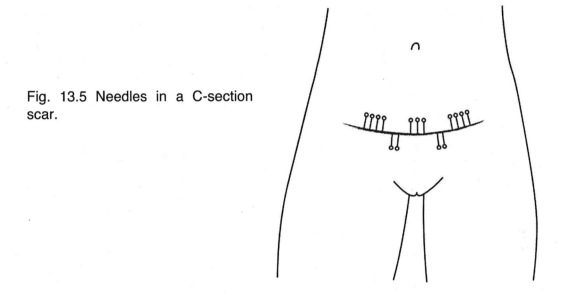

Fig. 13.5 Needles in a C-section scar.

In rare situations, because of the location of a scar, the deficient area is not physically accessible. If you can't needle into the deficient area, you must needle into the excess area.

Fine. Do it, if you must. The channel Qi will quickly become harmonized on both sides of the scar tissue.

But be prepared for the patient to experience some pain: warn the patient that there may be an electrical shock at the moment of insertion, in addition to the weird, "recall" pain that *might or might not* be experienced as the needle passes through the scar tissue itself.

Choosing distances

How closely together should the needles be placed? It depends.

An obstruction of a quarter inch can be significant on the fingers or in areas where channel Qi runs in a narrow path. Then again, where channel Qi is running widely, channel Qi might be able to get through fairly unimpeded even if the scar tissue is a quarter of an inch across.

The number of needles also depends on how much the patient is willing or able to tolerate the experience. With large scars, such as those left by C-sections, needling every quarter inch would require twenty to thirty needles! Therefore, for the first scar tissue treatment, you might choose to only insert one pair of needles for each of the pairs of channels, even if this leaves gaps that are nearly an inch across. You can needle other parts of the channel during subsequent treatments.

How do you know if you've opened up enough of the scar tissue? At a following session, feel what the channel Qi is doing. If the channel Qi seems to divert around the scar or slow down in the vicinity of the scar, the scar needs more work. On the other hand, if channel

Qi is roaring happily through the scarred area, your work is done – even if there is still visible scar tissue.

Choosing the angle of approach

Most scars are somewhat linear – long and thin. Strangely enough, many scars also seem to bisect a channel at 90 degrees. (Maybe skin tears that are *parallel* to the channel are able to heal without scarring?) With linear scars that are bisecting a channel, the goal is to bisect the scar – breaking the line in half. Very often, I insert the needle at 90 degrees to the scar: perpendicular.

However, this is not always the case. The needle must run along, or parallel to, the path of the nearest *channel*. Therefore, depending on location and accessibility, the needle may or may not run at right angles to the scar tissue.

If the scar tissue is blocking the path of a major channel, causing a gap in the flow of the channel, locate the needle approximately along the path of the channel, thus bridging the channel's gap with the needle.

Staying parallel to the line of the channel is *more* important than staying perpendicular to the line of the scar. For example, if the scar is running at an oblique angle to the channel, the needle will need to intersect the scar at an oblique angle.

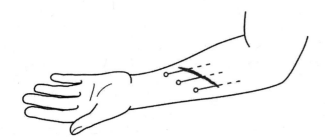

Fig. 13.6 Oblique scar, with needles parallel to the lines of the channels

Also, I always insert needles perpendicular to the scar in the healthy tissue at both end edges of a linear scar. Even though channel Qi can flow past the end edges of a scar, the channel Qi often flows in a whorled pattern in this area – just as water flows in a whorled pattern at the very edges of a spill. By inserting needles here, the small amount of channel Qi that is still diverting around the edges of the scar, if any, is encouraged to stop running in whorl, and helped to resume its flow in the straightest, most efficient manner possible.

If a scar is not linear, but covers a large area, thread needles along the paths of any and all primary and/or extraordinary channels that traverse the scar area. Make sure that the line of threaded needles starts and ends in healthy tissue: the first needle in the thread series goes into healthy tissue on the deficient side tissue and the last needle of the thread series ends in healthy tissue where the channel Qi had become blocked (excessive).

If the scar is very large, you may need to traverse the scar in several lines, reconstructing several channels.

238

First treatment

Needling scar tissue can be highly traumatic, and extremely painful, especially if the scar is the result of surgery, a terrifying accident, or abuse. Therefore, I will usually not needle scar tissue on a patient's first visit.

When I do decide the patient is ready for scar tissue work, I share all of the following information with the patient:

1) At the moment the *scar* tissue is perforated, some patients experience *not* the normal sensation associated with skin perforation by an acupuncture needle, but sensations of pain appropriate for the pain experienced during the *initial injury*. For example, if the source of the scar was an incision, a slicing-type pain might briefly be felt. If the scar was the result of a burn, a burning sensation might briefly occur.

2) The progression of the scar tissue needling experience can be as follows: after insertion, there may be almost no needle sensation, because of channel Qi deficiency in the insertion zone. As the needle is pushed, with firmness and good control, into the keloid tissue, a sensation of original injury may occur.

3) The patient can cry out when he feels this pain – he shouldn't hold back.

4) As the needle continues to be pushed and moves into the healthy tissue on the other side of the scar, a very quick flash of electrical "contact" *might* be felt by the patient, followed by the sensation of something cool or warm flowing over the needle and into the tissue on the deficient side.

In summary, there can be up to four distinct sensations: insertion sensation, penetration of the scar tissue pain, the electrical contact as the needle penetrates into the excess area, and finally, the flow of something "good."

Because of the complexity of the sensations, and the very real likelihood of a flash of pain while perforating the scar tissue itself, I usually will not needle a patient's scar tissue in his first meeting with me. Unless the scar is clearly the main cause of the person's problems, I will do some other, gentler treatment, and save the scar work for next time.

I usually tell the patient that I intend to work on the scar in the next visit, but that the experience will be too raw for a first-timer. I want the patient to feel safe, and not frightened.

Of course, sometimes, patients will insist on having a strong treatment even if they are new to acupuncture. In this case, I will comply. But at least the patient is aware that he is experiencing something outside the usual realm of acupuncture experience.

In all cases when I am about to needle scar tissue, I do warn the patient of the rare possibility of re-experiencing the pain of the initial injury or surgery. I also warn about the very *rare* possibility of a short-term, experiential, "you are there" flashback.

Most patients, when warned, still give permission for you to needle their scars. In fact, many patients, when they *don't* experience anything remarkable or weird, aren't grateful: they're disappointed!

On the lookout for scar tissue

Although I do not needle scar tissue on a first visit unless the scar tissue treatment is crucial to the patient's health complaint, I *do* needle scar tissue in patients who come on a regular basis, whether or not the scar tissue has anything to do with the patient's original complaint.

For example, if I'm working with a patient for several weeks for her shoulder injury, and I happen to notice that she has a C-section or appendectomy scar, I will suggest that we work on that scar tissue after the more pressing shoulder problem is resolved.

As an aside, I *strongly* encourage all women with C-section scars to have the scars broken up with acupuncture.

The women who get these scars treated are often astonished at the emotional and physiological changes that they experience following, or even during, the treatment.

For example, one woman told me during her C-section scar treatment, "I just felt a rush of energy going up to my heart, and I can feel my heart opening up again! My heart has felt closed off for five years, since my daughter was born. I can feel emotion! After my daughter was born, it seemed strange to me, but even if a friend was having a hard time, I didn't feel any compassion in my heart. I just assumed my new lack of compassion was because I'd become a mother, so I had become more detached from other people's feeling. And now, with those needles in the scar, I can feel something relaxing and opening up: feeling is coming back into my heart."

Stories like this one, and dozens of variations, on surgeries ranging from knee surgeries to heart surgeries to seemingly "unimportant" mole removals, have convinced me that everyone should have acupuncture to break up scar tissue, following *any* surgical procedure.

As an aside, a scar that runs *parallel* to the flow of channel Qi might not cause much of a blockage. I usually don't bother needling scars that run parallel to the channel Qi unless there seems to be channel Qi deficiency in the nearby area, or unless there are cosmetic reasons for reducing the size of the scar tissue.

Healing of scar tissue: growth of new skin

Very often, after having been needled, scar tissue will begin to replace itself with healthy skin.

Sometimes, the skin heals only in exactly those locations that had received needles. For example, if three needles had been inserted, traversing a linear scar in three places then, a few months later, the scar may have three small zones of perfectly healthy skin in the locations that had been needled. This causes the scar to look like a line of small dashes made of scar tissue, instead of one, solid line.

Sometimes, this zone of healthy skin continues to spread, healing the scar tissue on either side of the healthy zone, until the scar becomes almost invisible.

Even though channel Qi can get through the breaks in the line-of-dashes, you may want to decrease the line-of-dashes effect. In any subsequent needlings of that scar, choose insertion sites slightly to the side of the previous insertions. These needles will encourage new zones of healthy skin, so that the remaining "dashes," if any, will be even smaller, and the healthy spans will be wider.

Results are worth the time it takes to learn

Needling scar tissue can be challenging. My own technique has improved slowly over the years, but I still kink a fair percentage of needles if I'm working on a particularly beastly scar. But although it took years for me to develop my manual skill at getting needles smoothly through keloid tissue, the patients' health benefits, in response to needling scar tissue, were glaringly obvious from the beginning.

Back in my pre-med, undergraduate days at the university, and in my private study of western medicine theory, I had learned that keloidal (tough, rubbery) scar tissue could never transform into healthy tissue. I was astonished, therefore, to see the speed with which healthy skin could replace scar tissue when properly stimulated by needles.

I certainly hadn't learned that Qi, palpably blocked by the presence of non-conductive, rubbery scar tissue could once again flow easily as soon as the scar tissue was opened up via needling. But I learned through observation that not only could the scar tissue soften or heal and the Qi flow be restored through correct needling, but that this corrected flow of Qi often had powerful consequences in terms of reversing pathologies that had been set in motion or had been negatively effected by the scar-induced Qi blockage.

Since that time, since observing the many benefits of needling scar tissue, I have spoken with many acupuncturists on the subject. Some are afraid to needle scar tissue. Others insist that no benefit derives from its treatment. Some insist that, since channel Qi can get through at the end of a channel, despite a scar somewhere along the length of the channel, there is no harm done by having a small distance of channel Qi being temporarily diverted out of the way.

This last bit of specious thinking is incorrect. Any diversion of channel Qi has the potential to contribute to other patterns of disarray. For example, if a scar is causing a diversion of channel Qi five inches from the beginning of the channel, a matching aberration in channel Qi flow is likely to occur at approximately five inches from the end of the channel. And/or a channel Qi aberration may show up on the opposite (left/right) side of the body. For example, an aberration at SP-6 on the right leg can create an "echo" on the left leg at SP-6.

Our job is to clear up irregularities in channel Qi, so that the patient's channel Qi can "go through" to the greatest extent possible. Treating small situations that have not yet created obvious problems is a powerful form of preventive medicine. Patients are often amazed at the subtle change in the overall feeling of their bodies when small corrections are made in their channel Qi flow, especially if the channel Qi has been blocked or flowing incorrectly for many years.

Practice feeling scar tissue impediments

Do not take my word for anything in this book. Feel for yourself whether or not scar tissue creates impediments in the flow of channel Qi.

Scar lines are actually an excellent place to practice feeling the flow of channel Qi. When feeling channel Qi in scarred areas, see if you can detect the chaotic channel Qi on the upstream side that is being dammed up by the scar, and the whorls of Qi that spin off laterally at the edges of the scar tissue, where the channel Qi is streaming around the sides of the obstruction.

"Those who are wise inquire and search together, while those who are ignorant and stupid inquire and search apart from each other. Those who are stupid and ignorant do not exert themselves enough in the search for the Right Way, while those who are wise search beyond the natural limits."[1]

Chapter fourteen

Wrapping things up

When you think of acupoints, don't think of them only in terms of the point indications. Think of a given point in terms of where its channel Qi comes from and where it goes. Think of the role the point plays in all the various neural modes, and mode transitions.

For example, don't just remember "LI-4 is good for headache."

Also think "LI-4 is on a channel that supplies the head. It receives Qi predominantly from LU-7 or from LI-3, depending on whether or not a person is relaxed. Therefore, stimulation of this point can attract Qi from LU-7 or from LI-3. If no channel Qi is moving into this point, there will be pain in the channel, at some point somewhere between the hand and the side of the opposite nostril, or maybe even *everywhere* along the length of the channel. If Qi is blocked and stagnant at this point, or running backwards into this point from LI-5, something must be wrong farther up the channel.

Think to yourself, "This point can pull channel Qi out of a stagnant Lung channel, and can therefore treat those symptoms, including headaches, caused by Exterior Wind attacking the Lung channel and making it stagnant while simultaneously making the LI channel deficient."

Remind yourself, "This is a strong point: stimulating this point can send a shock wave of channel Qi all the way down to ST-45, on the other side of the body, *if* there is no blockage between this LI-4 and opposite side ST-45. I can see if those two channels are flowing correctly by inserting a needle at LI-4 and counting the number of seconds before one of the three medial toes on the opposite foot moves the tiniest bit in response to the surge of channel Qi."

(The normal time span for channel Qi to flow from LI-4, on one side of the body, down ST-44, on the other side of the body, can range from two to twenty seconds.)

We can think of acupoints in the context of their roles in the highly flexible electric schema of the body. We can understand *why* certain points have certain traditional indications

---

[1] Su Wen, book 2, from *The Yellow Emperor's Classic of Internal Medicine*, translated by Ilza Veith, 2002, University of California Press, Berkeley, p. 121.

– and whether or not those indications are likely to be incorrect. We can understand why certain point prescriptions work…but only work sometimes. [1]

Why point prescriptions work sometimes, or not

You have enough information now to start figuring out why some treatments work and some don't, depending upon circumstances. Acupuncture will not necessarily be helpful if the problem is 1) structural (displaced bones or twisted fascia), 2) nutritional (malnutrition or toxins), or 3) psychological (whether from determination to avoid some body part, or thinking based on indulgence in negative emotions.)

In other baffling cases, the problem may seem to be structural – an ankle injury that won't heal. Or the problem may seem food-related – as in a case of "oversensitive gut." But it's perfectly possible, in both of these cases, that the underlying problem has a psychological origin. *If* so, acupuncture will probably *not* be able to do anything about the ankle's inability to heal, or the gut's oversensitivity – until the psychological choices have been addressed.

For difficult cases, the most important diagnostic work will always be tracking down the actual *origin* of the problem. A seeming structural problem may have a nutritional origin. A seeming organ problem may have a channel Qi origin. Never make assumptions. You must track down the original cause of the problem, or you will not be able to crack the case.

This book is directed primarily at problems that have, at their origin, an aberration in channel Qi.

In these types of cases, treatments that actually remove the channel Qi problem, in a lasting manner, will work.

In these types of cases, treatments that do *not* realign the channel Qi and take steps to ensure that the realignment is lasting (get rid of any blockages) will *not* have lasting benefits.

Carefully observe the traditional treatments your teachers perform in clinic. Try to guess whether these treatments might or might not be helpful. See if your hunches were correct when the patient comes the next week for follow up.

Given that most practitioners don't bother to feel channel Qi, and often have no idea where a patient's blockages are, why do so many practitioners get results? In my many years of experience, I've seen that most acupuncturists have very uneven results, being successful with fewer than half of their patients, or being successful after a very long period of time (when time, the great healer, may be accorded some of the credit). However, they do have some happy successes. It's important to understand why, using nothing but guesswork and local points, an acupuncturist may be successful. The following section will show why, from the perspective of various schools of theory, the acupuncturist may often "get lucky."

TCM

We've already discussed one of the favorite TCM point combos, LI-4 and LIV-3, and how it actually works: it's a defibrillating shock treatment.

---

[1] For the state board exams, do memorize all the point indications even if you know they don't actually work! Do not use any information from this book when taking the state boards.

Many of the TCM treatments are either defibrillating, by using strong acupoints (points in a vicinity of significantly lowered electrical resistance), or they are local points.

In either case, the shock of needling these points is sometimes able to correct the aberrant flow of channel Qi, and the problem is solved.

Five Elements

Now let's consider why some Five Element treatments are effective, even though many of them are merely pat formulas revolving around the five transport points, or formulaic treatments such as a Shen circle (Aggressive Energy) treatment.

Five Element acupoints formulas very often include transport points near the fingers and toes, or else the knees and elbows. We know that stimulation of the fingers and toes temporarily pulls a person back into parasympathetic mode. In sympathetic and dissociated modes, channel Qi is diverted away from the extremities. Stimulation of the extremities can force a person *back* into parasympathetic. By forcing a person into parasympathetic mode, very often, his body will begin, or accelerate, healing.

Oppositely, the Source points and the points around the knees and elbows have greatly lowered resistance. When needled, they yield a good jolt: they are good defibrillators.

Thus, *if* there are no significant structural or dissociation blockages to deal with, and *if* a person's channel Qi is just mildly stuck somewhere, either in a wrong mode, or from sequelae of some external Evil (pathogen, rough weather, injury, and so on) or *remembered* emotion, most Five Element point combinations of transport points, whether they are referred to as Mother and Child combos, Husband-Wife combos, Over-acting combos, and so on, are bound to hit at least one point that can either pull a person back into parasympathetic mode (toe or finger points) *or* defibrillate him out of a stuck channel Qi situation (source points and Sea points) – and one lucky point might be all you need. [1]

More importantly, Five Element practitioners are trained to indulge in a little bit of emotional probing and counseling. In cases of mild emotional blockage, this can sometimes

---

[1] My first acupuncture treatment was Five Element style. The doctor was an MD, as well as a Five Elements practitioner. He was extremely kind and thoughtful, a very good questioner and listener. I'd been dealing with chronic fatigue for nearly two years. We didn't discuss much of anything, as I was too tired to care.

Based on Five Element pulse theory and moxa heat-testing, he treated SP-1, LIV-8, and several UB points (probably UB-13, 15, and 17). In terms of channels, his treatment was remotely similar to the treatment Dr. Tin Lui gave my patient: Spleen and UB channels featured in both of their treatments. In my case, the treatment worked – within a few days, energy started moving in my spine and my brain clicked back on. Energy returned almost immediately after the spinal currents resumed. This treatment started me on my quest to learn about Asian medicine.

Subsequent treatments by him, for back muscle spasm due to displaced vertabrae, were always pleasant, but never helpful. I also saw a TCM practitioner for back spasms, to no avail. My intermittent back problems were finally resolved working with a very gentle, activator-method chiropractor who also studied craniosacral therapy and reflexology. He found the chronic tendency toward spasm in my psoas muscle and taught me a simple, quick method to release and retrain it.

I have since attended doctoral level Five Element seminars and observed hundreds of Five Element treatments, performed by Five Element faculty, while getting my doctoral degree.

My master's degree in acupuncture and herbology was based primarily on TCM texts, but I also sought out other schools of thinking.

be very helpful. (In this context, "mild" emotional blockage refers to those that are related to habit or memories that can be accessed. "Severe" emotional blockages are those that cannot be accessed due to dissociation or unconsciousness at the time of trauma.)

If you combine the counseling with the needle-directed shift back into parasympathetic mode, you have a combination that might well help restore a person's channel Qi to healthy, parasympathetic flow – if the blockage was merely electromagnetic, or was emotional and resolvable by talking, and/or did not have a significant physical component.

As an aside, some students and some patients are fascinated with the relationships between the elements. However, the element selection so critical to Five Element "theory" is not actually significant in terms of acupuncture: to bring someone back to parasympathetic mode, it doesn't really matter *which* transport points are used, so long as they are on the three medial toes (the two lateral toes are also helpful, but weaker), or *any* of the fingers, *or* at the elbows and knees. They all "transport" a person back to parasympathetic. So long as points on or in the vicinity of the three medial toes or any of the fingers, or at the elbows or knees, are selected, the results will be the same no matter what elements are considered – so long as the problem was a basic situation in which a person was wedged into a non-parasympathetic mode due to *mild* channel Qi blockage and/or *mild* emotional stress.

Also, artificially attributing self-induced emotional problems to an imbalance of elements can be *very* helpful for establishing a context for a blame-free and guilt-free discussion of emotional issues. If the patient can think of his emotional issues in terms of Fire or Water, instead of blaming himself, or Aunt Evelyn or "the jerk who did this to me," he can often get to the bigger picture, and clear it up, much faster – no matter *which* elements are attributed to the problem.

Magic points and combinations

Various schools of "magic" abound. A quick examination of these "new, magic acupoints" or magic combos will show why they offer up good odds of bringing about an effective treatment.

Sometimes, to make an acupoint "magical," or "more effective," the acupuncturist is advised to insert the needle a quarter inch away from the nearby traditional point, or an inch or two upstream from a traditional point. First, from a point location standpoint, it often doesn't really matter whether or not a needle is inserted into the traditional point, or alongside it, or downstream or upstream from the point location. The channels are wide enough that they can be affected even if the needles are outside the traditional location. And the whole point is getting the channel Qi moving – so it doesn't really matter, from a basic, defibrillating standpoint, exactly *where* in the channel the needle is inserted.

Still, I've met acupuncturists who were powerfully swayed by the idea that someone had "invented" new, "magic" acupuncture points that worked as well as the old ones.

As for the magical combos, these combos usually include points from opposite sides of the body, or opposite extremities. For example, a left hand point must be combined with a right leg point. In other words, they are variations of the Four Gates type of combos – such as LI-4 with LIV-3.

Next, from a basic, defibrillating standpoint, by needling both sides of the body, and both the upper and lower body, the odds are very good that something, somewhere, in the body will be shaken up a bit. If the patient was going to respond to a defibrillating treatment, these combos are usually well-designed enough to ensure that a large area of the body will be shaken up, with a minimum of needles.

The magic combo adherents sometimes suggest that, if the first treatment didn't work, switch over to the next group of channels. In other words, if you didn't get lucky with the first pair, or group, of wide-ranging generalized mini-shock treatments, try a different pair, or group. For these "schools" of medical theory, precise diagnostics have been thrown out the window.

And if a person's channel Qi does happen to get shocked back into health by these strong, though random, treatments, it does indeed seem magical! But when these treatments don't work, as they often don't, there is no way of knowing why not.

The magical treatment may also benefit from another highly important factor: practitioner focus. This factor may also play a huge part in holographic acupuncture.

Holographic acupuncture

Based on the idea that every cell in the body contains a potential electrical map of the entire body, many schools of holographic (everywhere the same, or from the same origin) acupuncture have arisen. The most widely studied holographic system studied is ear acupuncture, in which the ear is understood to represent the entire body. By needling the "ankle" point on the ear, pain in the ankle can be suppressed.

Other holographic systems use the hand, or the foot, or the area around the belly button, or the abdomen, the buttocks – or any part of the body, so long as the practitioner is holding in mind an image of the whole body at that smaller part, and needling into the portion of that area that represents the problem. Holographic acupuncture does work. It can be particularly effective in treating pain.

One of the most fascinating studies of holographic acupuncture came to an utterly unsuspected conclusion: the more holographic points that were needled, the more effective the treatment was. In other words, if a person had ankle pain, and was needled at the ear point for ankle, and the holographic hand point for ankle, and the abdominal point for ankle, and the foot point for ankle, he would have a much better result than if he was only needled in one, or maybe two, holographic points. It turned out that it didn't matter which holographic points were used – the number of holographic points was the greatest determinant of whether or not the patient's pain would go away.

This raises a very interesting question. Is it possible, that the practitioner's focus is playing a crucial part?

When needling a holographic point for, say, ankle, the practitioner is thinking, "I am imagining this to be the spot for ankle." The practitioner is busy imagining the ankle, its relative location on the body, and its role as ankle. He is thinking of an idealized ankle.

By comparison, if the practitioner is needling locally, putting needles into and around the injured ankle, he is thinking, "Ooh, this ankle is swollen; I'm going to try to avoid hurting the patient; this ankle is such a mess."

It is perfectly possible that the thoughts of the holographic practitioner, focusing on the idealized body part, may be responsible for helping the patient re-tune his own thoughts.

The proximity of the practitioner's thought waves may help the patient return his own thought waves back to "idealized ankle," thus getting away from "injured ankle."

We know that, ultimately, all existence is a delusion, created from the particular perspective that allows us to perceive waves as matter.

If, as practitioners, we keep our own minds always focused on the idealized form of the body, we are offering that ideal to the patients. The patients have a choice as to whether or not to accept the ideal, but it is good for us to make the offer.

In the end, this rather suggests that every acupuncturist, not just the holographic practitioners, should, while working on a patient, be mentally beholding the patient in an ideal state of health, rather than in an injured state.

In addition to the idealized thinking, the holographic practitioner's treatments may also benefit from the defibrillating effects of the needles.

A TCM – Five Element comparison

A very common back-treatment for calming mental stress often works very well. In TCM (Traditional Chinese Medicine, which is the name for the modern, People's Republic of China version of Asian medicine), this treatment is called a Shen circle treatment. In Five Element lingo, with a few modifications and with observations of the amount of pinkness brought to the surface of the skin, it's called the "Aggressive Energy" treatment. This acupoints combination could also be called the "stuck in fight-or-flight" treatment, or "sympathetic mode" treatment.[1]

This treatment for getting a person back into parasympathetic mode approaches the underlying problem (mental or emotional stress, or poor organ function or sleep or whatever, because of too much mental or emotional stress) by shaking up the sympathetic mode "alarm" points in the Bladder channel.

Instead of trying to pull a person into parasympathetic via the transport points, the Shen circle treatment serves to powerfully defibrillate the blockages that may arise in the UB channel during sympathetic mode: blockages that can keep a person stuck in some aspect of sympathetic mode.

If there is no physical blockage (displaced bones or soft tissue, or scar tissue) and no unresolved emotional blockage, shaking up the "stuck" sympathetic mode points by using the Shen circle can often help a person *quickly* settle back down into parasympathetic.

It doesn't matter what you call the treatment – if you stimulate the points along the bladder channel that are particularly affected by the surge of Bladder channel Qi that occurs during sympathetic mode, you can help any glitches at those locations become unstuck by defibrillating them with a needle. Then, the patient will shift into parasympathetic mode – no matter what school or theory you attribute to the treatment.

---

[1] One of the basic Shen Circle "needle formulas" is made up of inner *and* outer UB channel points, both left and right side, across from vertebrae T-3, T-5, T-9, T-11, and L-2, plus one to four other points, often various combinations along the Du or Kidney channels. Variations abound. Various schools of thought each have their own rules regarding the sequence and timing of needle insertion and removal. Regardless of which school's schema is followed, the treatment is usually very effective at temporarily helping a person get out of sympathetic mode.

Finally, I want to include the following case study just because it may remind students that a cursory, quick scan of the largest segments of a channel may not yield enough information.

I had a patient, female, age 14, with a recent onset of violent panic attacks. The attacks had become so severe that she could no longer be alone in her room, at home, or even stay in the classroom if the room was darkened for watching a video. Over several weeks, I asked hundreds of what I thought were clever and insightful intake questions, and gave her several ineffective acupuncture treatments and herbal teas.

I was certain that some psychological problem or internal stagnation causing "Heart Qi Deficiency, or Heart Qi Excess, or even Heart Yin Xu Heat" was the root cause of her sudden onset of Shen Disturbance. But she had no history of anything that could remotely be related to my understanding of Shen disturbance. She was perfectly self-controlled, mentally, but her physical body responded with terror to nearly everything.

In addition to working with me, she was having appointments with a psychiatrist, who wanted her to start antidepressant medications.

Finally, after several fruitless weeks, I asked her to remember what she'd been doing every moment of the day, two months ago, on the day the panic attacks first began.

She laughed cheerfully and said, "That will be easy. The panic attacks started on the first day of school, so I remember everything I did that day. I know exactly what I wore to school – it was the first day. I even remember, I had a bagel for breakfast. I was holding the bagel in my hand, and sliced it with a knife. I accidentally sliced my hand, too!"

I nearly jumped out of my chair. You sliced your hand? Where? Show me!"

She pointed to a short but knotted scar running across P-8 on her left hand.

I had previously checked the channel Qi in her arms, but hadn't bothered to check it all the way out to her fingertips. Her Pericardium channel, the "Protector of the Heart," was utterly blocked at one of its most perceptive points. No wonder she was panicked: her heart constantly was feeling under attack.

I treated the scar in her hand. Needling this area caused her extreme, but fleeting, pain. I told her to massage this area and fill it with loving light as often as she felt like. Her panic attacks ceased.

The above case study appeared, at first glance, to have a psychological origin. But it did not. Technically, it was a Blood Stagnation (physical injury) problem.

If I had continued treating her based on point prescriptions for Shen disturbance, she might never have gotten better.

I will add, I have *never* seen a point prescription for panic disorder that said, "needle P-8, if injured, and if there's a scar there, bisect it." On the other hand, I'm also certain that other acupuncturists, over the centuries, have treated Shen disturbances that arose from injury to the Pericardium channel. But many of the old anecdotal case studies have not have made it into the modern lore. Especially because channel theory has become increasingly ignored, there is no current method for understanding why a scar at P-8 would cause Shen disturbance-type behavior.

Back to root causes

Channel theory is the basis for effective acupuncture.

But channel theory and acupuncture alone, whether based on TCM, holographic points, muscle channel theory, Five Element acupuncture or you name it, don't work very well for problems of a more structural or nutritional origin.

For example, if a person's foot problem is being caused by a displaced anklebone or scar tissue blocking the channel, the generic point prescription treatments of *any* school tend *not* to work. In the same way, if a person has rickets from a vitamin deficiency, acupuncture isn't going to help, no matter which school is adhered to, and no matter how "magical" the points are.

But sometimes – often – channel theory can get to the root cause faster than any diagnostic method short of intuition.

For example, consider a case of Blood Stagnation causing back pain – a common diagnosis. Even though some students think that the "fixed, stabbing pain" of Blood stagnation can *only* be the result of externally-caused injury, channel Qi blockage, ultimately, is at the root of any fixed stabbing pain. A fixed, stabbing pain can develop even where there is no actual injury or technical condition of Blood Stagnation.

Consider: if UB channel Qi is physically or mentally blocked, for whatever reason, for a long time on only one side of the spine, the channel Qi on that one side of the Bladder channel can be said to be "not going through." In consequence, the muscles on that side become weaker from lack of invigoration via channel Qi.

Eventually, the muscles on the *opposite side*, being relatively stronger, pull the vertebrae toward the stronger side. If these bones are pulled too far out of alignment, nerves emerging from the base of the vertebrae can become pinched. A fixed, stabbing pain ensues: by definition, this is Blood Stagnation pain.

The *root* cause of this Blood Stagnation pain is *not* the pinched nerve, or the misalignment of the bones. The *almost-root* cause is deficient channel Qi in the section of the UB channel that allowed the muscles along the spine to become weak. The *root* cause is the blockage, either physical or emotional, that is *causing* the UB channel Qi to be deficient.

To treat this person *correctly*, whether we apply acupuncture, herbs, Tui Na, magnets, lasers, or teach the patient appropriate Qi Gong exercises, we must address that which is causing the UB-channel Qi blockage. When the cause of the blockage is gone and channel Qi flow has been restored to its correct flow, all the side effects of the deficient channel Qi will be very easy to treat – and will not return.

That blockage in the UB channel on the side of the head might have started with driving with the window open on a frosty cold night. It might have started with a seemingly insignificant bump on the head from a cabinet door (I've seen this in my practice). It might have started with an infection on the head from a tree limb scratch. It doesn't really matter what started it – the important thing is to get as close to the root cause as possible. Hopefully, when you get really close to the root, the problem will become obvious, and the roots of the illness can then be torn out. In this example, by discovering the deficient flow of Bladder channel Qi, the root cause of the back pain can be discovered.

In many cases, knowing what the channel Qi is doing is one of the best ways to track the root of an illness to its origin.

For another example, Stomach Yin deficiency or even Stomach Qi, Blood, or Yang deficiency can all arise from deficient channel Qi in the stomach due to constant emotional stress or fear (which diverts Stomach channel Qi to the heart, a sympathetic mode divergence).

All the possible conditions of wrong health have at their root, an incorrect distribution of channel Qi.

When channel Qi is flowing in some unique pattern due to external or internal "Evils," or when channel Qi has become stuck, inappropriately, in what is normally a "healthy" divergence pattern, then poor health, or "pain" ensues. Go through, no pain; No go through, Pain.

In other words, channel Qi, which "goes through (parasympathetic mode)," or which *fails* to go through (anything other than parasympathetic mode), lies at the root, or very close to the root, of all physiological conditions: both health and "pain."

Assignment

When you are observing a teacher, either in clinic or the teacher's private practice, try to figure out the teacher's TCM point prescriptions, or Mother/Son combos, or "classical treatment" formulas work, *or not*, in a given patient.

By "work" I mean "yields a favorable response" as opposed to, say, causing a traveling electrical pain response. Very often, if the underlying channel blockage has been successfully broached, the patient will notice an immediate change, the pulse will improve and, best of all, you will be able to feel the channel Qi suddenly flowing correctly. Notice, in particular, responses to local points or Four Gates combinations. See if they happen to inadvertently rectify an aberrant channel Qi situation, or not. If *not*, try to figure out why not. Have fun!

After all my hours of observation of practitioners of Five Element and TCM theory, muscle channel theory, local point theory, magic point theory, O-ring theory, muscle testing theory, and on and on, I've seen that, when treatments are based on generic point indications, pre-packaged formulas and/or theories, *without actual knowledge of exactly what is going on with the patient's channel Qi*, they are essentially guesswork treatments.

One guesswork system is pretty much as good as another: sometimes you get lucky.

Emotional support

I've also noticed, in terms of style and success rate, *if* a patient's problems are coming from the types of emotional issues that can be solved via talking, *any* practitioner who includes a lot of listening and a bit of counseling with his treatment might be better than a practitioner who doesn't want to "waste time" listening to the patient, regardless of what theory group the practitioner belongs to.

A TCM practitioner who is able to make the patient feel heard, and who offers concrete, practical suggestions for dealing with emotional problems, may have much better results with a patient's emotion-based problems than a Five Element practitioner who is brusque. A Magic Point practitioner who teaches an emotional patient how to retrain his emotions will have better results than a Classical Acupuncturist who hammers his patient with haughty instructions about emotional control.

In other words, if the problem is a simple question of emotional education, the practitioner's individual style will have a far greater influence on the patient than the practitioner's school of theory.

No matter what school of medicine we adhere to, our patients deserve both technical competence in acupuncture, and offerings of the wisdom that can lead to emotional retraining.

In gratitude

I can't possibly thank enough people in this short book. But the following two examples, drawn from two of my own teachers, help demonstrate further the significance of working with channels *and* emotional support. The third example demonstrates something else again.

Dr. Jeffery Pang, internal medicine

When Five Branches College of Traditional Asian medicine, where I got my Master's degree, was just getting off the ground, Dr. Jeffery Pang, LAc was the *brilliant* teacher who developed the theory, herb, and herb formula classes.

Dr. Pang is a master of theory and of acupuncture, but in practice, he is primarily an herbalist. He knows the classic herbal lore inside and out. Dr. Pang's success rate, even with very difficult cases, is very high. He is a deeply intuitive doctor, very loving, and dedicated to helping students master Asian medicine.

I have been practicing Asian medicine for nearly twenty years and if, after I've had two or three visits with a patient, I am uncertain of my diagnosis *and/or* not getting good results, I refer them out to Dr. Pang – so I can find out what I've missed or done wrong.

Knowing of my interest in channel theory, one of the senior-year students at my school mentioned to me, "I'm just starting to recognize that Dr. Pang's *extremely* effective herb formulas are based on what *channels* the herbs go to. When I learned the herbs, I always thought that the channel information was an afterthought, and not too important. Since I've been thinking in terms of channel theory, I've realized that Dr. Pang's herb formula selections and modifications are all about the *channels*, and not necessarily the herb indications."

Dr. Lucy Hu, pediatrics

Dr. Lucy Hu, like Dr. Pang, was both western-medicine trained, in China, *and* TCM-trained. Her utter humility as she listens keenly and patiently to the mothers of her young patients, never rushing, never interrupting, and her simple, opening pronouncement when the patient is done speaking: "I'm not sure… but *maybe* we can help," nearly always elicits a deep sigh of relief from the patient's mother, along with the light of hope in the eyes.

Dr. Lucy Hu is legendary for her ability to reduce a screaming frightened child or baby, in theater classes, no less, into a lump of shy giggles, even while quickly poking the infant with needles. She is able to calm even the worried mothers. For the most part, her treatments are mundane. Yet her results are as good as those of the other teachers. Her patients, both mother and child, are certainly among the most contented and grateful, by the time the treatment was over. Contentment and gratitude are conditions in which healing can most rapidly occur.

She never comes across as a strict adherent of any particular school of thinking. Increasingly over the years, I've noticed that her treatments are very simple treatments – just a few of what she called the "most popular" acupoints, and plenty of gentle, pediatric style (skin rolling) Tui Na alongside the spine, over and over. Much of the treatment time is devoted to giving helpful dietary and behavioral advice to the concerned mothers of her little patients.

Her patience, kindness, and loving humility are as much a part of every treatment as the medicine.

Several years ago, one of my students confessed the following anecdote: "The other day, I was wondering when we were going to start learning about the spiritual part of this medicine. I mean, I was getting frustrated after three years of study, but no classes on learning the spiritual stuff. I happened to be in the herb room with Dr. Lucy Hu – *Lucy Hu*, of all people. I demanded to know when we were going to learn the spiritual stuff. Why weren't they telling us about the spiritual stuff? Was it going to stay some kind of darned secret?"

"And then I stopped. She was looking up at me with those gentle eyes, with so much compassion for my frustration. She said, "I don't know.""

"I was instantly *so* ashamed of myself. Duh! She'd been modeling the "spiritual stuff" for me for three years. I'd never realized that she was teaching by example.""

Paramahansa Yogananda

An unfinished case study featuring Wind-Heat and subsequent sepsis was presented in a footnote in chapter three, page 56. We had left that patient with racing heart, irregularly irregular heartbeat, palpitations, severe low blood pressure, insomnia, and the need for steadily increasing doses of Tian Wang Bu Xin Dan. These herbs are supposed to tonify Heart Yin, but evidently, the tonification was not leading to a calming of his symptoms. His symptoms would stop for a few hours after taking each dose, and then return, exactly as before, when the herbs wore off.

His channel Qi was blocked or missing in nearly every channel, rendering hopeless an accurate channel Qi diagnosis. Previous attempts to straighten out the many, various kinks in his channel Qi had obtained only temporary, fleeting results. He was still hoping that I had some sort of trick of Asian medicine up my sleeve, but I felt I had nothing more to offer.

Of course, I did still have one more source for help. I could ask my spiritual teacher for advice. I had already asked him, politely, for help on this case, but had received no reply. I decided, finally, to demand some answers. I spent four hours arguing, pleading, and trying to negotiate with my teacher. Maybe I wore him down because, during a pause in my petitioning, I was told, "Think about what is happening to him. When he takes the pills, his symptoms wane. When they wear off, his symptoms return. What, in his case, are the pills doing? What does that tell you?"

As usual, his long-awaited answer to my pleadings had been cryptic, but it assured me 1) there is a logical solution to this problem and 2) I *could* figure it out.

Within a few minutes, a new idea seemed to manifest in my mind. Maybe the pills worked, temporarily, because they temporarily moved his channel Qi more towards parasympathetic mode, with a leaning towards sleep mode. In other words, keeping him out of sympathetic mode. When the pills went into effect, within a few minutes of each dose, his heart worked perfectly well. This told me there was nothing really wrong with the heart. Realizing this was huge. If there was nothing really wrong with his heart, then some electrical snafu somewhere *outside* the heart was causing the problem.

When the pills began to wear off, his symptoms returned. When the pills wore off, he had crazy irregularities in an otherwise perfectly healthy heart. His heart was receiving a wrong signal from somewhere, a signal that was overriding his healthy heart rate. Also, he'd noticed that, every time the heart symptoms returned, he would feel, physiologically, as if he were mildly panicked, even though he was emotionally calm.

It was as if, when the pills wore off, and his body reverted back to a capability for sympathetic mode, all his symptoms returned. If this was the case, the underlying electrical glitch that was throwing the heart off was most likely somewhere in the channel system that regulates sympathetic mode.

My thoughts sped up. My teacher had planted enough thoughts in my mind to get me going, and from here, I could apply my training and logic.

Possibly, my patient, in response to the toxic sepsis, had developed a glitch in the nerves that go to the heart from the spine: the nerves that emerge from the 4th and 5th thoracic vertebrae. If this were the case, pills that kept him in parasympathetic mode would enable him to avoid hitting this glitch. Then, when the pills wore off and and channel Qi resumed flowing more vigorously in the spine, the glitch would trigger, again, all the violent heart symptoms.

I called the patient. I asked him if he could imagine sparkling white light traveling down his back, a few inches lateral to the spine, particularly in the area of the lower part of the shoulder blades.

He replied that he could not – he even felt uneasy when he tried to do so. Both sides of the Bladder channel were affected, with the right side being even worse than the left.

I suggested that he really needed to get energy flowing all the way down his back, and in this area, in particular.

He came over to my house, and I did acupressure on this area, while he worked to mentally restore wholesome movement of light past this blocked area. It was highly unpleasant – his mind was resistant to entertaining notions about this part of his body. His years of yogic practice stood him in good stead, however, and he was able to override his mental fear.

After nearly ten minutes of intense mental focus on his part, he announced that he was suddenly feeling the mental light and energy flowing all the way down to the back of his knee. He said it felt wonderful. At the same time, he felt his heart rate normalize, and his palpitations ceased. His pills had just begun to wear off when we'd started this treatment, so the improvement was clearly coming from his own work on his channels.

As quickly as that, the heart symptoms were healed. They did reappear, faintly, a few hours later, and again the next day, but a quick mental restoration of energy flow past UB-4 and -5 set things right again, in both episodes. Within a week, his blood pressure was normal, he was exercising, even running, again, and his weight had stabilized. Channel Qi flow resumed in his arms, and flowed correctly in all the channels that had seemed blocked or had reduced flow.

There had been nothing wrong with his heart – the problem had been coming from an aberrant signal that was going to his heart from his spinal nerve. All the subsequent channel Qi irregularities had been derived from the constant heart irregularities.

That's all great. But the greater point is, as doctors, we always have recourse to a higher power.

It is said that every illness already has a cure: the cure is floating in the ether, in the form of vibrations. These specific vibrations make up the antidotes to each illness.

Call it what you will: God, or Universal Love, or the Om, or the Tao. This wisdom knows what the causes and cures are for every illness. If you only read your books, and never open your heart to a higher source for information, you are ignoring the greatest teacher of all.

I recommend that any student of medicine learn to meditate and pray. The universe holds many answers that, as yet, can only be obtained through the wordless language of the heart.

You may think that prayer is not scientific, or not "real." But the underlying Love that sustains this universe has created this universe in a very scientific manner. If we want answers about the deepest sciences of the universe, why not go right to the source?

And in all my years of practice, when I've asked patients with difficult problems if I might pray for their health during my evening prayers, I have never once been told no.

This gratitude section of this chapter, in which I get to name just a few of those generous souls who have taught me, is also the place where I now declare my deepest homage, love, and devotion to my spiritual teacher, Paramahansa Yogananda. Without his guidance, I could not have written this book. Without his prodding, I would not have become a practitioner and teacher of medicine. Without his love and teachings, my life would be a wandering in darkness.

In closing

Do not take *anything* in this book on blind trust. Experiment on your own. Learn to feel channel Qi. Prove to yourself whether or not the ideas in this book are correct or not, or if they are helpful.

Practice Asian medicine as if it is a science, not a collection of random tricks and magic formulas. Prove to yourself that it is a science that honors the universal laws of cause and effect, including the causative power of thought waves; a science that acknowledges both the Spiritual Pivot, which is to say, the influence of consciousness on the constant transformation from wave energy into matter, and back *and* the Dragon, the actual currents created by those transformations. *Feel* those currents: know what they are doing.

With difficult cases, be a detective who never gives up: make sure you know *when* the symptoms started, and what the patient thinks might be at the root of it. The patient might be wrong, at first, but the process might start you both thinking in terms of *logical* sequences and consequences. Keep thinking, but also keep listening to your wisdom-driven intuition. And based on the information you gather, choose where to start *feeling* the flow of the currents.

When you treat patients based on their channel Qi aberrations, always confirm, right then and there, if the treatment is working, by checking on the local flow of channel Qi after you've put the needles in, and yet again, after you've removed the needles, to see if the channel Qi aberration has corrected itself in a lasting manner.

Combine the practical and the spiritual. Use knowledge of physiology, physics, modern medicine, Asian theory, pulse, tongue and channel Qi, while treating the patient as honored guest.

Behold within every patient, no matter how troubled, the immortal, ever-healthy radiance of Divine Love, also known as Wei Qi, protecting and blessing the patient, and blessing you. That Love is holding you in the palm of its Divine Hand.

As you continue to practice medicine and, hopefully, grow in humility, you will increase your ability to feel that Love. If you learn to focus on that feeling, or, as it says in the *Nei Jing*, "exert yourself enough in the search for the Right Way," your own channel Qi increasingly will flow correctly. Your own Dragon will dance with the joy of your unique soul's self-expression.

Blessings.

Appendix

with

Maps of the channels

The channel maps in this appendix are provided to give a general idea of point locations and the *main* paths of the channels. For *very* exact, anatomical descriptions of the acupoint locations, please use the internet or *A Manual of Acupuncture*, by Peter Deadman and Mazin Al-Khafaji, 1998.

Bilateral symmetry

Each of the twelve primary channels has a left side channel and a right side channel. However, for an uncluttered look, the maps show each channel on only one side of the body.

Yin and Yang

For purposes of artistic variation, the Yang channels are shown on male models; the Yin channels are shown on female models. But all humans, male and female, have all twelve channels.

Acupoint nomenclature

In modern times, for English speakers, the acupoints have been assigned names based on the channel they sit in, and their sequence on that channel.

The spelling of the acupoint name uses an abbreviation of the channel name, and the number is represented in numeral form. However, the point names are always *pronounced* by saying the whole name of the channel, followed by the number. For example, the first point on the lung channel is written as "LU-1," but pronounced "Lung one," not "L"-"U"-"one."

Chinese acupuncture students tend to learn the old, classical names for the points. These names describe the points' uses or locations – these names have nothing whatever to do with the English nomenclature. For example, the point on the inner canthus of the eyes is named, in Chinese, Jing Ming, or "bright eyes." In the English system, it is named UB-1, suggesting that this is the first point of the Urinary Bladder channel.

In point of fact, this point is actually on the Stomach channel, not the Urinary Bladder channel. However, in the modern "traditional" books, in accordance with the modern numbering system, the Bladder channel is drawn as if it starts out with a downward dive for a few inches, going down to the inner canthus of the eye at Jing Ming, before it turns on its heel and climbs up to the forehead to UB-2.

This is not actually how the Bladder channel behaves, but this is how the Bladder channel is currently drawn in the books that claim to be based on tradition.

The actual paths of the channels can be easily perceived. As it turns out, the actual paths of the channels make more sense – they are flowing lines with gentle curves, not harsh zigzags that jerk back and forth.

This appendix has maps of "traditional" channels, as they are taught in acupuncture schools, side by side with maps of the actual paths of channel Qi flow.

Channel nomenclature

The twelve primary channels, their abbreviations, and their Chinese names (which are significant) are, in order:

Channel name	abbreviation	Chinese name
1. Lung	LU	arm Tai Yin
2. Large Intestine	LI	arm Yang Ming
3. Stomach	ST	leg Yang Ming
4. Spleen	SP	leg Tai Yin
5. Heart	HT	arm Shao Yin
6. Small Intestine	SI	arm Tai Yang
7. Urinary Bladder	UB	leg Tai Yang
8. Kidney	KI	leg Shao Yin
9. Pericardium	P	arm Jue Yin
10. Triple Burner	TB	arm Shao Yang
11. Gallbladder	GB	leg Shao Yang
12. Liver	LIV	leg Jue Yin
Ren	Ren	extraordinary Yin
Du	Du	extraordinary Yang

The Traditional channel maps

In this book, the Traditional Channel maps of the twelve Primary channels and the Du and Ren channel include all the acupoints that are traditionally (in modern times) considered to be located on the skin-portion of these channels. On these maps, lines linking the points are shown in their traditional presentation, showing the presumed routes of the channels.

As an aside, the traditional descriptions of each of the primary channels often include routes of channel Qi that travel deeply interior and routes of channel Qi that vary depending on a person's activity level or state of mind, such as the Luo channels and the channels that travel back and forth between Du-14 and the Yang channels. However, for purposes of this book, which instructs in feeling just-under-the-skin routes of the channel Qi, the traditional maps in this section only include the main portions of these "surface" routes.

The traditional channels, as described in most of the current literature, tend to be portrayed as point-to-point connections from a channel's first point to its last point. For example, the Lung channel runs from LU-1 to LU-11 (LU-11 being the last point on the Lung channel). The Large Intestine channel runs from LI-1 to LI-20 (LI-20 being the last point on the Large Intestine channel). And so on.

All of the locations of the acupoints mentioned in this text can be found on the "traditional channel" maps.

Actual channel maps

Maps of the actual channel pathways show the paths of channel Qi that can easily be felt, by hand, when a person is predominantly in parasympathetic mode.

Several of these paths are very different from the traditional channels. What we now refer to as the "traditional" paths of the channels have been codified relatively recently, after having been passed down for thousands of years, incorporating inadvertent errors, guesswork, political preferences and, very possibly. faulty original scholarship.

In addition to the probable compilation of errors regarding the traditional ideas about the channel locations, the relatively recent designations of western-language names for the acupoints has created many new, implied, errors. Examples abound in which acupoints that have an modern, western-language-style name, a name that suggests residency on a specific channel, are actually located on a different channel.

Remember, the original names of the points did not specify which channel, if any, the point was located on, or even near. I have no idea what criteria were used when the modern, or "channel name + numbered sequence" nomenclature was put in place, but matching up the new names with the obvious, feel-able paths of the channels was clearly *not* a consideration.

For example, the channel Qi flowing over points SP-17, -18, and –19 is moving downward, towards the toes. These points are obviously a part of the downward-flowing Stomach channel. These points are *not* on the Spleen channel, which flows upwards from the feet.

Do not take my word for it: anyone who can feel channel Qi can quickly prove to himself the actual locations of the channels, and which points are most logically associated with which channels.

The boundaries of the channels

The maps of the Actual channels in this text are necessarily abstractions and approximations. The maps, if taken literally, would seem to suggest that the channels have hard edges: specific, unchanging boundaries. In fact, the channels abut, and even bleed into, each other. There is no inch of skin that is not traversed by channel Qi from the Primary, Ren, and Du, and Dai (belt) channels.

For example, in the Actual channel maps, a moderate degree of separation between the torso portions of the Stomach channel and the Gallbladder channel is suggested. In fact, the lateral edges of the Stomach channels actually meet and mingle with the anterior edges of the Gallbladder channels.

In these boundary areas, the channel Qi can be more difficult to feel. The flow of channel Qi is usually easiest to feel in the areas directly over the acupoints.

To be completely accurate – and to follow boldly when we track aberrant channel Qi, which is to say, channel Qi that is not "staying in the right place" – we need to know that there are no hard and fast boundaries to the energy that flows just under the skin.

Depths of the channels

Not only do the channels of the same type (either Yin or Yang) meet at the lateral boundaries of the channels (Yang channels can all meet and slightly mingle with other Yang channels, at their borders, and the Yin channels can all meet and slightly mingle with other Yin channels, along their borders), the various channels flow at various *depths*, in various areas.

For example, we read in the classics that, in the vicinity of the pectoral (chest) muscles, the Liver channel flows "deep." The Liver channel flows *under* the pectoral muscles. The Stomach channel flows *over* the pectoral muscles, just under the surface of the skin.

In *general*, if there's a question of overlapping channels, those channels with the word "Yang" in their title flow closer to the surface, while those channels with the word "Yin" flow deeper inside.

In the pectoral muscle example, where both the Liver channel and Stomach channel flow in the same general area, the Chinese channel names tell us which channel is closer to the skin, and which channel flows deeper inside the body: the Stomach channel, as seen in the above channel chart, is named leg Yang Ming. The Liver is leg Jue Yin. Yang channels nearly always flow closer to the surface, relative to any nearby Yin channels. By looking at the names, leg *Yang* Ming (Stomach) and leg Jue *Yin* (Liver), we know that, wherever the Liver channel and Stomach channel traverse the same area of the body, the Liver channel will be the one to flow deeper inside, flowing "under" the Stomach channel.

Traditional Lung Channel

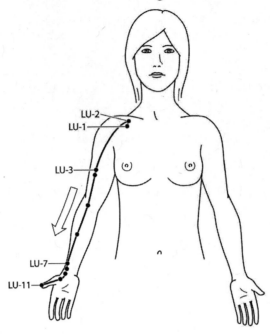

Actual Lung Channel

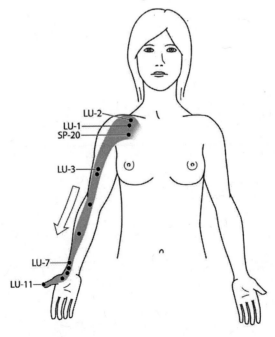

Traditional Large Intestine Channel

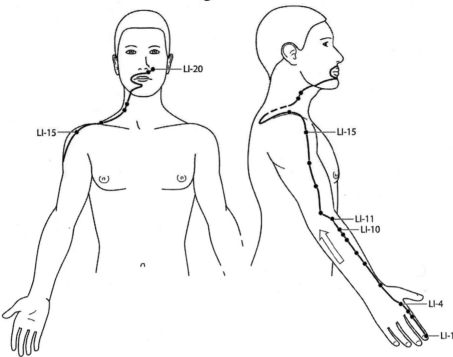

LI-20

LI-15

LI-15

LI-11
LI-10

LI-4

LI-1

Actual Large Intestine Channel

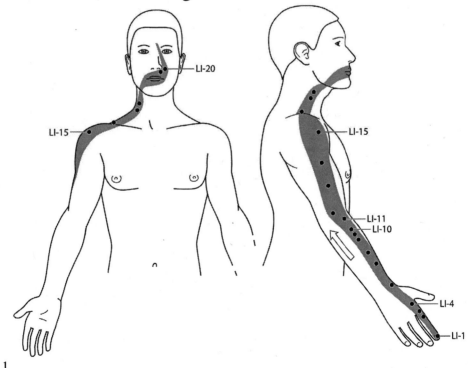

LI-20

LI-15

LI-15

LI-11
LI-10

LI-4

LI-1

1

Traditional Stomach Channel

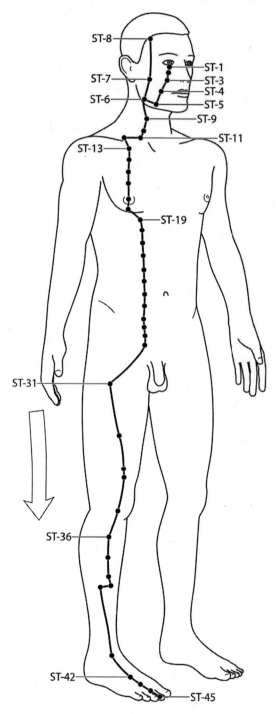

Actual Stomach Channel

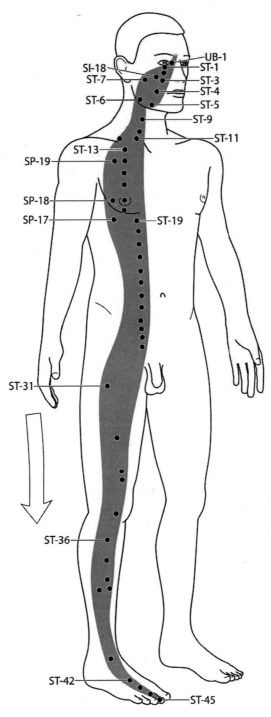

Traditional Spleen Channel

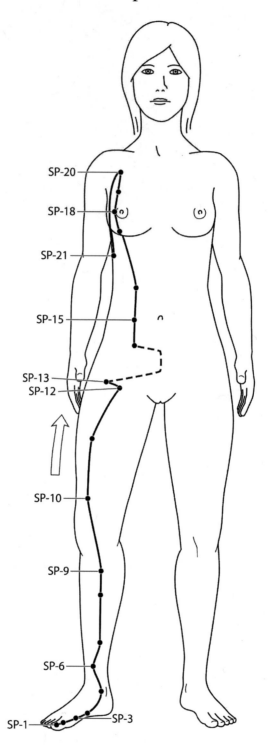

SP-20

SP-18

SP-21

SP-15

SP-13
SP-12

SP-10

SP-9

SP-6

SP-1 — SP-3

Actual Spleen Channel

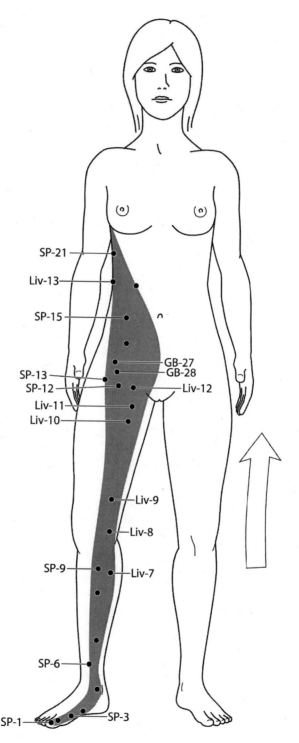

SP-21
Liv-13
SP-15
GB-27
GB-28
SP-13
SP-12
Liv-12
Liv-11
Liv-10
Liv-9
Liv-8
SP-9
Liv-7
SP-6
SP-1
SP-3

Traditional Heart Channel

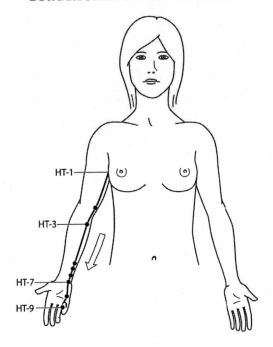

Actual Heart Channel

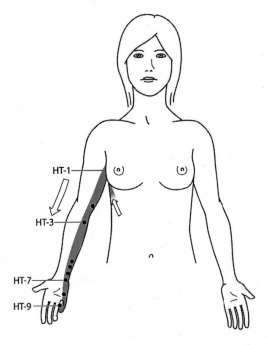

Traditional Small Intestine Channel

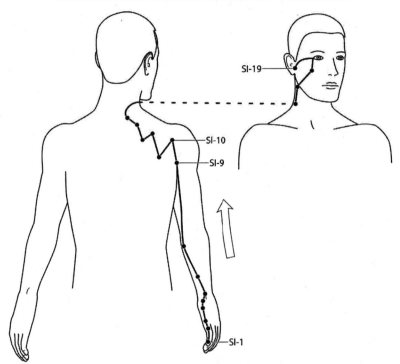

Actual Small Intestine Channel

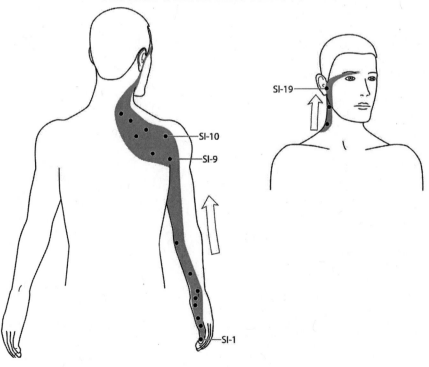

Traditional Urinary Bladder Channel

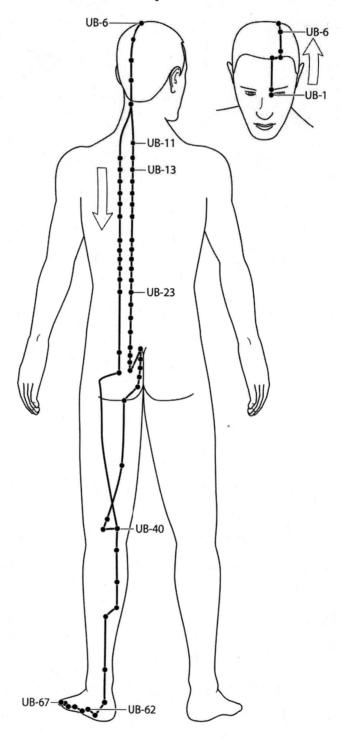

Actual Urinary Bladder Channel

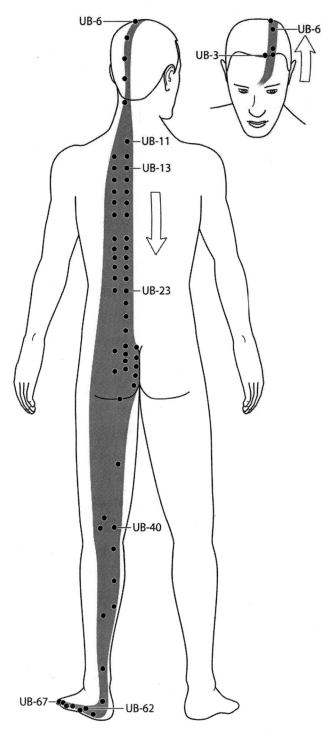

Traditional Kidney Channel

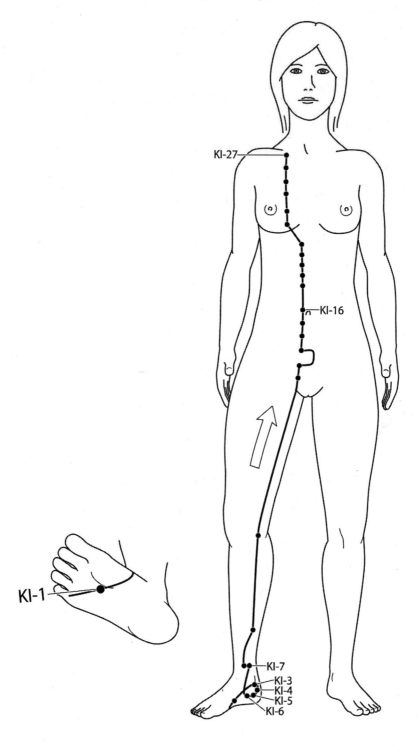

KI-27

KI-16

KI-1

KI-7
KI-3
KI-4
KI-5
KI-6

Actual Kidney Channel

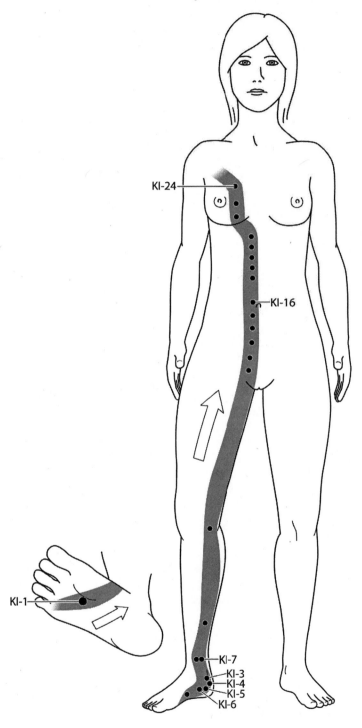

KI-24

KI-16

KI-1

KI-7
KI-3
KI-4
KI-5
KI-6

Traditional Pericardium Channel

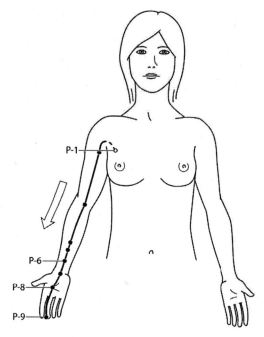

Actual Pericardium Channel

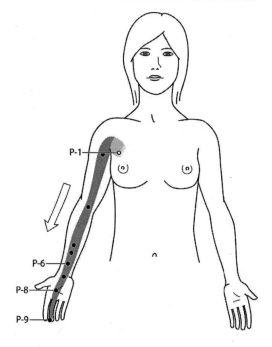

274

Traditional Triple Burner Channel

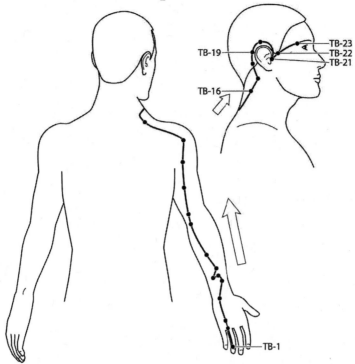

Actual Triple Burner Channel

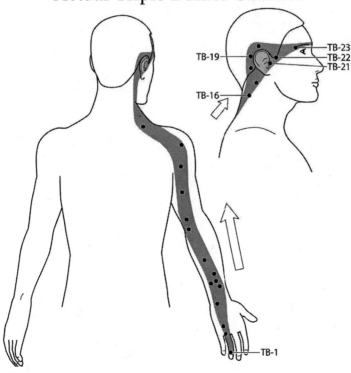

Traditional Gallbladder Channel

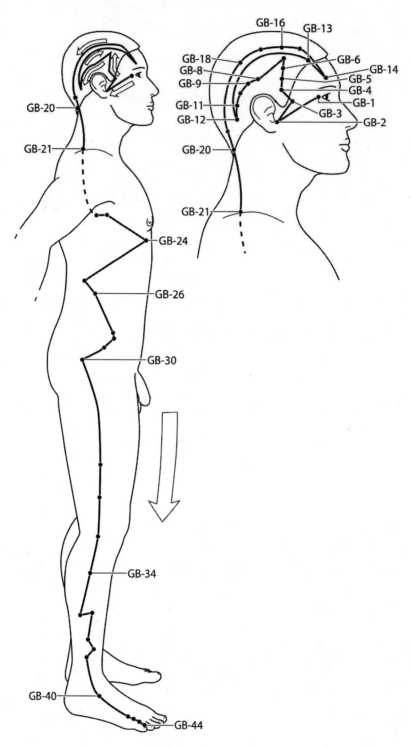

Actual Gallbladder Channel

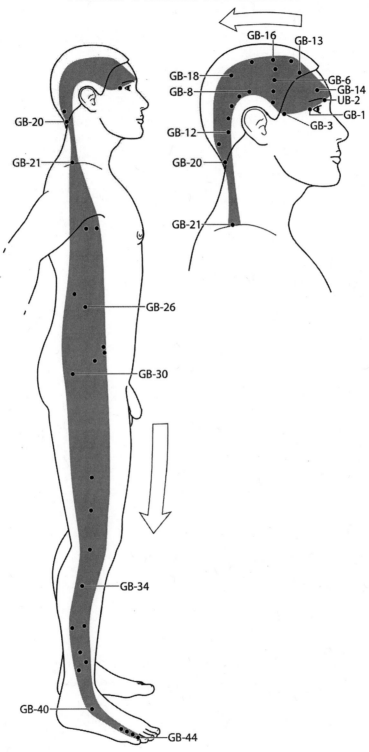

Traditional Liver Channel

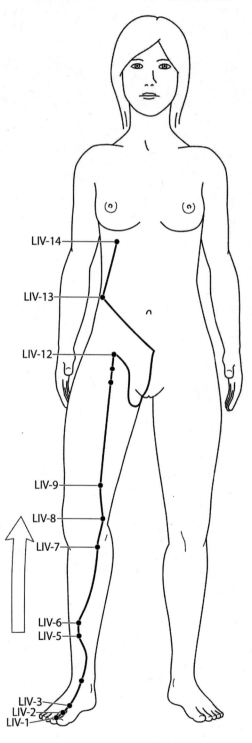

LIV-14
LIV-13
LIV-12
LIV-9
LIV-8
LIV-7
LIV-6
LIV-5
LIV-3
LIV-2
LIV-1

Actual Liver Channel

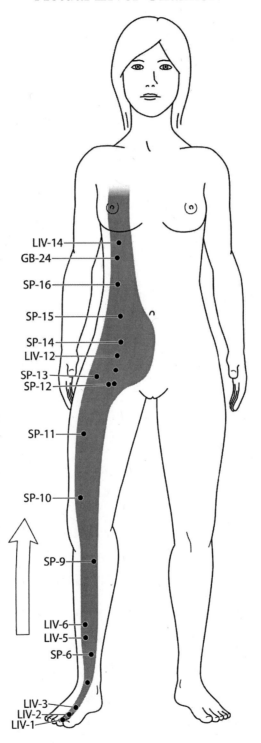

LIV-14
GB-24
SP-16
SP-15
SP-14
LIV-12
SP-13
SP-12
SP-11
SP-10
SP-9
LIV-6
LIV-5
SP-6
LIV-3
LIV-2
LIV-1

Traditional Ren Channel

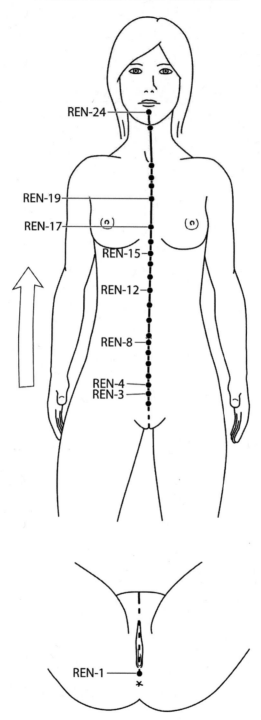

REN-24

REN-19

REN-17

REN-15

REN-12

REN-8

REN-4
REN-3

REN-1

Actual Ren Channel

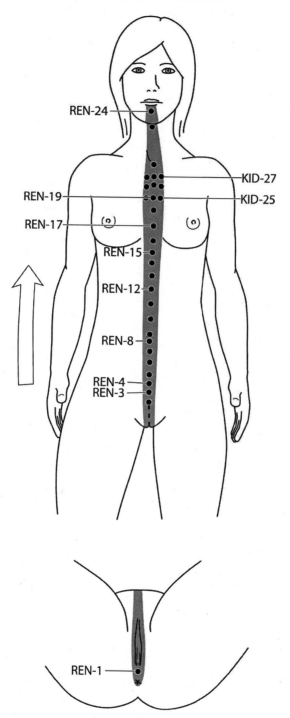

REN-24

KID-27

REN-19

KID-25

REN-17

REN-15

REN-12

REN-8

REN-4
REN-3

REN-1

Traditional Du Channel

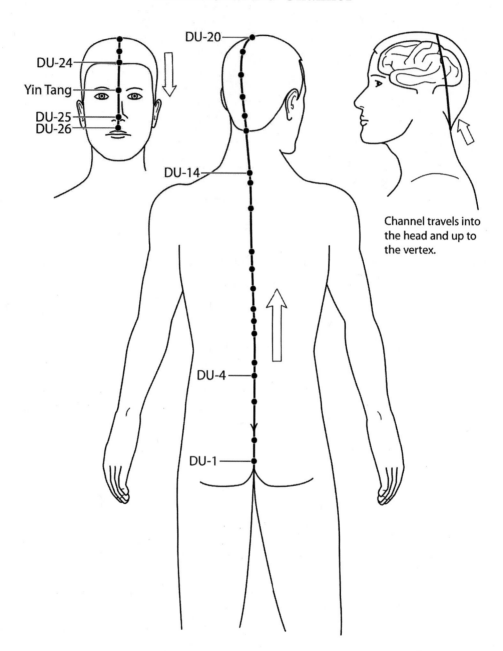

Channel travels into the head and up to the vertex.

After the main branch goes to the vertex, it "winds its way to the forehead." The assumption is often made that this translates to "The channel then flows over the top of the head (the vertex), from Du-20 to Du-21, to Du-22, and so on, to the end of the Du channel. See the written material on page 98.

Actual Du Channel

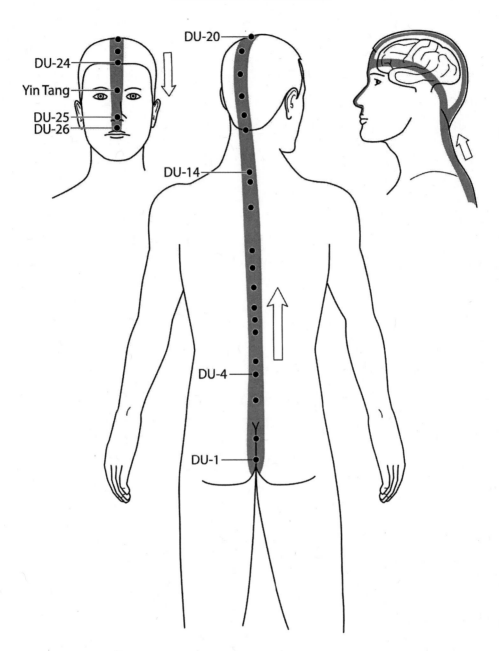

For more information about the variations in parasympathetic paths of the Du channel, please read the material on page 98.

Index

About the author –

Dr. Janice Walton-Hadlock, DAOM, earned a BA in Biology at University of California, Santa Cruz, in 1974. While there, she also studied History of Science – ancient and modern. She obtained a Master's degree in Traditional Chinese Medicine at Five Branches Institute in Santa Cruz, CA, and a DAOM degree (Doctor of Acupuncture and Oriental Medicine) at Five Branches University in San Jose, CA.

She has been teaching at Five Branches, an acupuncture college in Santa Cruz, California, since 1998.

Her research articles have been published in the peer-reviewed *American Journal of Acupuncture*, *The Journal of Chinese Medicine*, and other journals in the field. A "commentary" on a piece of published research was published in the *New England Journal of Medicine*: she was the first non-MD acupuncturist to be accepted for publication in that journal.

She has lectured extensively, at home and abroad. In China, she learned an expanded way of using pattern diagnostics, an expansion that revolutionized the way she understood Chinese medicine.

She brings to her study of Chinese medicine a passion for modern physics and for ancient languages and scriptures.

Other books by Dr. Janice Walton-Hadlock, DAOM

Trouble Afoot: finding the cause and an effective treatment for Parkinson's disease

Medications of Parkinson's Disease or Once Upon a Pill: patient experiences with dopamine-enhancing drugs and supplements.

These books are both available for free download at www.pdrecovery.org., the website for the non-profit PD Recovery Project, founded by Janice Walton-Hadlock in 1998.

Published by FastPencil
http://www.fastpencil.com